# Your Midlife Anti-Aging Plan

Natural Ways to Slow the Aging Process

Linda Posnansky, B.S., NC.

*To my loving and patient son Forest,*

*You inspire me everyday to be the best person I can be. I love you.*

**Disclaimer:**

The information provided in this book is intended for informational purposes for those wishing to know more about health issues, and is not meant to substitute or conflict with the advice from your health care providers. You should not use the information in this book for diagnosis or treatment of any health problems. Please consult with your health care provider before attempting any practices in this book. We strongly recommend that you follow your physician's advice in all health matters. This book is not meant for pregnant or nursing women. Information in this book is general and to the best of our knowledge is true and complete, and is offered with no guarantees on the part of the author. The author disclaims all liability in connection with the use of this book.

Copyright © 2015 by Linda Posnansky. All rights reserved. No part of this publication may be reproduced or distributed in any form or by any means without the prior written permission of the publisher.

ISBN: 978-1-68111-019-6
Library of Congress Control Number: 2015932532

www.VibrantHealthConsulting.com

# Table of Contents

Introduction ............................................................................................................... 4

Chapter 1   Vibrant Aging and Wellness ..................................................................... 7

Chapter 2   Aging & the Mind/Body/Spirit Connection ............................................. 13

Chapter 3   What is a Healthy Diet? Nutrient Density and Healthy Aging ................ 22

Chapter 4   Macronutrients: Our Primary Food Constituents (Proteins/Digestion) ... 38

Chapter 5   Fats and Healthy Aging ........................................................................... 63

Chapter 6   Carbohydrates and Healthy Aging .......................................................... 76

Chapter 7   Carbs, Middle-Age Weight Gain and a Dysfunctional Metabolism ....... 100

Chapter 8   Our Modern Diet vs. the Health-Giving Properties of Traditional Diets .... 124

Chapter 9   Common Nutritional Insufficiencies in Midlife ..................................... 135

Chapter 10  Free-Radicals, Antioxidants and Aging ................................................. 145

Chapter 11  Cellular Aging and Our Body's Internal Antioxidants .......................... 159

Chapter 12  Mitochondria: Our "Cellular Batteries" ................................................ 165

Chapter 13  Telomeres and Our Anti-Aging Enzyme ............................................... 168

Chapter 14  Alkalinity, Mineral Reserves and pH .................................................... 172

Chapter 15  Hidden Inflammation and Immune Balance .................................................... 176

Chapter 16  Nitric Oxide and Optimal Circulation ............................................................. 182

Chapter 17  Exercise, and the Anti-Aging "Human Growth Hormone" ............................... 185

Chapter 18  Chronic Stress, the Adrenals, and Sleep........................................................ 190

Chapter 19  Reducing "Total Load," Liver Cleansing and Detoxification............................ 201

Chapter 20  The Digital Age: EMF's, Electro Pollution and Electro Sensitivity .................. 218

Chapter 21  "Earthing:" the Ultimate Anti-Aging Agent ..................................................... 225

Chapter 22  Female Health: Menopause and Hormone Balance ...................................... 229

Chapter 23  Male Health: Andropause, Hormone Balance and Prostate Health ............... 238

Chapter 24  Graceful Aging; Delaying the Visible Signs of Advancing Years .................... 243

Chapter 25  Putting It All Together: Key Vibrant Aging Takeaways ................................... 251

Resources ........................................................................................................................ 279

Vibrant Aging Functional Self-Assessments ..................................................................... 284

Vibrant Aging and Wellness Health Goals Worksheet ...................................................... 304

Vibrant Aging and Wellness Plan (template) .................................................................... 306

References ....................................................................................................................... 320

About the Author .............................................................................................................. 332

# Introduction

Many of us have been conditioned to believe that we are "over the hill" when we turn 40, and that we might as well learn to "live with" low energy, poor mood, aches and pains, weight gain and declining health as a usual part of growing older.

But this scenario doesn't have to be an inevitable consequence of midlife aging. There is solid scientific evidence that proves that how we live greatly controls the speed at which we age. Prevention is the key word here, and the most important piece to healthy aging. If we take preventative measures now in midlife, such as eating well, keeping active, managing our stress levels, getting proper sleep, and living in balance; deteriorating health and accelerated aging can be minimized and even reversed.

*Prevention is always easier and frequently cheaper than treatment.*

The first step toward vibrant aging and wellness is awareness. Brain authority Dr. Daniel Amen believes that consciousness is the number one predictor of longevity; therefore the aim of this book is to help you take charge of your health by increasing your awareness about the contributing factors that can speed up your aging, and the parts that they play in your current state of health. By bringing light to these issues, your awareness and understanding will grow; and as your awareness grows, your motivation and well-being will increase also. To that end, this book is written as an easy-to-follow plan that will give you the information and the tools you need to protect your health now and in the future.

The reality is as we get older we frequently start to experience more symptoms of poor health, and often want quick symptom relief; but most conventional medical protocols are solely symptom-driven, (pharmaceuticals) and only offer a band-aid solution. They don't address the underlying problems that trigger symptoms; and often, unfortunately cause even more adverse conditions and symptomology.

This book, on the other hand, offers a natural, whole-person oriented comprehensive approach that addresses the root causes of illness and aging; characteristic of integrative, holistic, and functional health modalities. A time-honored natural approach offers health benefits that balance our whole system, and work <u>with our body</u> as opposed to against it, unlike pharmaceuticals. Whole life-giving foods are the major players in this plan; coupled with regular exercise, relaxation, good sleep, stress-reduction strategies, toxin elimination, and the judicious use of dietary supplements and botanicals. Interestingly, there is an overwhelming amount of up-to-date scientific research that finds this natural approach far more effective than medications or surgery in many circumstances.

Declining health and accelerated aging in midlife often is not triggered by one organ or factor, but numerous influences owing to the fact that every part of our body is connected and functions together. Integrative/holistic/functional medicine believes that illness is a dysfunction and imbalance of the whole person, (body, mind and spirit) and that ill health manifests when there is an imbalance in a few key elements; usually caused by too much of something, (poor diet, stress, toxins, alcohol, over-work, over-eating, destructive habits, negative thought patterns, dysfunctional belief systems etc.) or not enough of something. (whole foods, nutrients, water, exercise, relaxation, sleep, optimism, positive social connections etc.)

This book is centered on helping you to discover the root imbalances and weak links of your own system; and providing you with as many resources and solutions possible to help your body to come into balance; enabling it to thrive, not just to survive or avoid disease. When we are truly healthy and thriving we experience vibrant energy; a calm, sharp mind; ease of movement; restful sleep; freedom from pain; glowing skin and healthy hair. All products of healthy living habits.

The present health and diet industry tends to follow a cookie-cutter health model using a "one-size-fits-all" approach; but this method is generally not effective for most people because it doesn't recognize the scientific concept of "biochemical individuality." We all have a unique bio-chemical make-up as a result of our genetics, metabolism, diverse lifestyle habits and environmental conditions. This difference means that every person has distinctive nutritional and lifestyle needs that must be met in order to achieve optimal health. The info in this book is designed to help you discover your own "biochemical individuality;" and to help you to shape an individualized health plan that will aid you in making suitable nutritional and lifestyle choices for yourself.

The book is divided into several segments. The back of the book contains **functional assessments (quizzes)** that will help you identify lifestyle and health areas that may need more focused attention and balance. These assessments will also foster your interest in each health topic. You can do these quizzes all at once (right away) or do them sequentially as you progress through the related chapters. A chart is also provided to record your progress. Reviewing these results with your health practitioner may also be of benefit.

**Lab testing information** is also supplied in this book, as lab analysis can give you a more precise picture of what is occuring in your body, and any underlying issues that may be accelerating your aging and poor health. Lab results will then enable you and your medical practitioner to tailor specific targeted whole-foods, dietary supplements, herbs, and personalized lifestyle modifications to enhance your health. Later on, you can retest again to monitor whether the methods are working.

There is a large amount of detailed information in this book; thus to facilitate reading I have included many charts that summarize the info in an easy-to-read format. If you don't want to read all the medical details-you can go right to the charts to easily understand the information. Additionally, I recommend reading only a few pages at a time to absorb the abundant information.

There are also many health recommendations presented in this book; however they are meant to be used as a framework only, and are not all intended to be followed by the letter. Often, your intuition will guide you on what is best for you. The aim is to be mindful, but not overly worried or obsessed about your health. If you set an intention to lovingly and joyfully care for yourself, your body will be happy with any new self-care routines that you put in place.

This book also provides numerous **exercises** to help you create your **personalized wellness plan**, and includes a **health plan template** at the back of the book to go along with it. You will be signaled by this icon: to fill in targeted personalized nutrition and lifestyle info into the template. The plan is very lengthy, and doesn't have to be filled out completely to be of benefit. It is suggested that beginning health-seekers only read up to page 158, to avoid overwhelm. Reading the fitness/exercise chapter and chapter 25 is also advised. After your health plan is finished, you can start making appropriate lifestyle choices and begin feeling better right away.

Your body wants to be whole and healthy, and if you give it the opportunity- it can start to come into balance within a few months of whole-foods, rest, and healthy living habits. You will then be able to see dramatic improvements in your energy levels, body composition, mood, memory and well-being. However, it is advised to be patient with yourself. Reversing negative habits and societal conditioning about eating can take some time.

It is my hope that this book goes a long way towards giving you the tools that you need to have a long, healthy, well-lived life. We are all masters of our own body and lives, and we have the power to make major changes in our health. I encourage you to give yourself and your loved ones the gift of vibrant health.

I look forward to helping you reach your health goals. So turn to the functional self-assessments page, (284) and take the first step toward vibrant aging and wellness.

Note: Consult with a physician if taking medications before using any supplements/herbs.

*Chapter One*

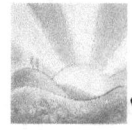
## Vibrant Aging and Wellness

There is nothing more universal than the desire to live a long and healthy life. It's just part of human nature to want to feel and look our best for as long as we can. The good news is that with a little consistent effort it is totally feasible to enjoy long-lasting wellness, vitality and longevity. It is not too late to make major shifts in our health, or to reverse premature age-related declines. Fortunately, there are many natural strategies that can help us to maintain and even regain our health.

However, in order to be successful, we <u>will</u> need to make "<u>taking care of our health</u>," our top priority. Taking our health for granted isn't an option for us in middle-age. We just can't do the same health-depleting things we did when we were younger, and expect to remain well. We have to put our wellbeing on the top of our daily "to-do list" if we want to forestall the ill effects of aging, and be alive and well for our loved ones into our elder years.

Cultivating good health as we age also has an additional benefit, as it affords us the <u>energy</u> to function at our peak creative, intellectual and spiritual levels. When we are healthy and strong, we are more apt to live out our lives to our fullest potential; thereby increasing our life-satisfaction and fulfillment.

The stage known as midlife, encompassing the ages from forty to sixty-five is typically the time when signs of physical degeneration begin to appear. Particularly around the late forties or early fifties many people start to experience an unexpected and often abrupt worsening in their health. This is because when we were younger our body was tougher, and was able to roll-with-the-punches more. It wasn't impacted as much by the stressors that we put on it; it was able to recover more easily. But, aging speeds up as we get older, and by middle age we start to see and feel the results of prolonged poor lifestyle habits, stress, insufficient exercise, nutrient deficiencies, or inadequate digestion.

However, middle age is not a stage to be feared or dreaded. Declining health and energy levels can be a "wake-up-call," motivating us to take charge of our health and well-being. Studies show that most debilitating chronic diseases and premature deaths are caused by poor lifestyle choices that could have been prevented if individuals had practiced healthy-living habits. Hence, the earlier we take the time to reassess our lifestyle and make significant changes, the better our midlife, and senior years will be.

Midlife can also be a time of great fulfillment and pleasure. Successfully navigating through all of life's challenges has the potential to enrich us and allow us to acquire wisdom, patience and depth. Hopefully, as a result of overcoming our numerous challenges; aging has humbled and mellowed us too.

Middle-age can also be a wonderful chance for us to grow as persons, and an opportune time to investigate our inner-dimensions and life purpose; maybe even to become who we truly want to be. Many of us have worked hard in our lives to get to where we are today; low energy and waning health don't have to get in the way of enjoying the growth, wisdom, and success that we have gained.

This book is not advocating self-deprivation however. The key to healthy aging is balance, not self-denial. Taking pleasure from our eating and leisure activities is what makes life worth living at every age. Nevertheless, optimal aging depends on moderation and making good decisions about our lives. By focusing on preventative measures such as eating well, getting regular exercise, controlling our weight and living sensibly; we will be able to tap into our body's own natural ability to repair and revitalize its self. As a result, we will be strengthened to have many more years spent in our prime; living our fullest life.

Change isn't always easy however, but we have the capacity to modify our eating habits and behaviors with minimal effort. Research finds that we can "rewire" our thoughts, and behaviors to a more health enhancing state, just by making small incremental changes, and by doing health promoting activities on a regular basis. Some experts assert that we can form new healthful habits in a few weeks of consistent effort.

It's helpful to think of our self-care endeavors as putting money away in a bank. The small health supportive efforts that we make every day, we will be able to draw upon in our later years; and reap substantial rewards for our efforts. Remember, our best investment is in our own health!

## What Is Aging?

Aging, the degeneration of our cells and body systems is happening all the time. Aging can't be put off forever; **BUT** aging can be slowed down or accelerated by the supportive or harmful things that we do, and by our feelings about the aging process itself. Aging or more importantly *"staying young,"* in many ways is a state of mind; as our true age (our functional age) really doesn't have to correspond with our chronological age. Our true age is more about our attitude, our vitality, our physical capabilities, and how we go about living. Conversely, not being in good health can be a major downside as we get older.

Studies reveal that people who had a positive attitude about aging, and who took a preventative approach to their health were inclined to be healthier and lived longer. They also were able to postpone end-of-life debilitating diseases to a far later date. Research completed on aging, and longevity by the McArthur Foundation, and the Institute of Gerontology, respectively, concluded that lifestyle factors were more significant than genetics in determining our longevity and health as we age.

The new science of epigenetics, which literally means "control above genetics," proposes that environmental factors greatly influence the expression of our genes and our health. The environment in which we expose ourselves to such as: our dietary choices, toxins, and activity levels, and even our stress levels and emotions effect the expression of our genes, and direct which genes get turned on or off. This means that we can turn on the genes that stimulate vitality and a long life, and turn off the genes that cause damage. In essence, our genetic makeup may **predispose** us to certain conditions, but it doesn't have to **predetermine** declining health and disease as we get older.

For that reason, we don't have to accept the common heritable diseases of aging, such as heart disease, cancer, diabetes, stroke, or osteoporosis, as inevitable. We also don't have to believe that a premature death is inevitable, due to our parents' untimely demise. We have the power to turn off our disease triggering genes, and extend our lives by making positive lifestyle choices.

What **does** determine our health as we get older is the degree of restoration and renewal vs. the degree of abuse, damage and deterioration our body experiences. Essentially, we begin to age when our body ceases to repair itself. So, the ideal goal is to have our deterioration, or breakdown proportionate to our restoration; or even more favorable, more repair than deterioration. If we actively center our energies on our body's repair and regeneration; degeneration and premature aging will be diminished.

### *Factors that Determine Rejuvenation and Health*
**Bestowing youthful looks and vibrant energy**

| Eating nutrient dense whole foods and drinking ample purified water | Living in balance and keeping active | Maintaining an optimistic attitude and staying young minded |
|---|---|---|
| Stress management and relaxation | Sleeping 7 to 9 hours nightly | Evading and neutralizing toxic compounds |

### Factors that Determine Degeneration, Premature Aging and Disease:
Causing us to feel and look older than our age

| Poor nutrition and hydration | Nutrient mal-absorption (poor digestion) | Trauma (emotional and physical) | Stress |
|---|---|---|---|
| Addictive behaviors | Toxicity | Poor sleep/lack of down-time | Inactivity |

### Major Causes of Aging

There are simple measures we can do to protect and enhance our health. In this book I will be addressing the major scientifically-researched theories and causes of pre-mature aging. I will also be sharing optimal aging principles, tips, and plans on how to achieve a long "**health span**," as opposed to simply achieving a **long lifespan**. Enjoying a long vital "health span," also known as "compression of morbidity" is the result of delaying degeneration and chronic illness until as late in life as possible, due to a healthy lifestyle.

When we gain an awareness and understanding of the reasons why we age, we are more likely to be motivated to take better care of our health.

### Causes of Premature Aging

| Poor nutrition/nutrient insufficiencies | Glycation/insulin resistance |
|---|---|
| Poor digestion/absorption | Imbalanced gut flora populations |
| Acid/alkaline imbalances | Inflammation |
| Free radicals and oxidative stress | Decreased mitochondrial functioning |
| Telomere shortening | Inactivity/lack of exercise |
| Stress/negative thought patterns | Poor circulation/low nitric oxide levels |
| Hormone imbalances | Obesity/dysfunctional metabolism |
| High toxic load/poor liver functioning | Disconnection from nature, sunlight, the earth, and social support |
| Poor sleep/lack of relaxation | Poor immune functioning |

However, there are **five key areas** that need to be optimized in order to slow the aging process and prevent age-related diseases. They are:

1. Optimize positive thoughts and keep stress levels down
2. Ensure optimal digestion and gut functioning
3. Ensure optimal nutrition
4. Keep physically active
5. Avoid free-radicals and toxin exposures/Detoxify daily

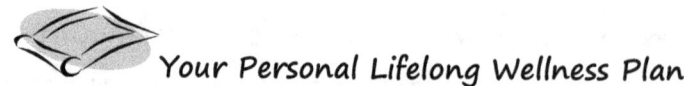 Your Personal Lifelong Wellness Plan

Preparation and planning are an essential component of accomplishing any goal, and so I have provided you with a health plan template to help you design and implement your own wellness program. Having a health plan is a practical way to give you the structure that you need to guide your personal wellness journey. Throughout this book, I have provided you with self-care exercises to help you gain awareness and record information to facilitate your health maintenance or transformation process. Your health plan template is provided at the back of the book, and you will be writing in information sequentially as you progress through the book.

There is quite a lot of information in this book to take in. It may take you some time to integrate this knowledge into your understanding. Don't be concerned about this. Rereading this information over time will help the comprehension process. Therefore, if you don't want to read through all the nutritional details in this book right away; you can go right to the charts and writing activities so that you can design your own wellness plan immediately. When you have finished this book, you will have designed a workable plan that will optimize your body's innate healing ability; thus making lifelong wellness and longevity a likely reality for you.

All practice activities contain this exercise icon: ☺ Go right to these icons if you choose to skip ahead..

## Motivation and Commitment

Motivation and commitment are crucial to the success of any wellness program. A useful exercise to help encourage you to make healthy lifestyle choices is to write down your <u>motivation for wanting to experience vibrant health and longevity</u>. It will be sort of like your "bucket list." This list should state very specific goals and outcomes that you would like to achieve in your life. One may be: "I want to be healthy enough to travel throughout Africa after I retire," or "I want to be able to have the energy to play with my new grandchild" etc. This list will become your inspiration to help you make important changes in your life. Consider reading these 5 reasons in the morning, and at night before bed. Refer to them when you need encouragement. By reading this list daily; your mind will accept the suggestions for change.

I want to stress however that health is a process, not a one-time event; and we all make changes at our own pace, and when we are ready. There are three distinct stages we go through before a positive change fully takes hold in our lives. They are:

1. <u>Awareness</u>: Being conscious that a change is necessary.
2. <u>Commitment</u>: Committing to making the change happen.
3. <u>Adopting the change as habit</u>: Making change take hold in our lives.

There may be times in the future, especially during times of stress or change that you may break your healthy habits and fall back into your old bad habits and dysfunctional behaviors. This is human nature. But don't lose heart or punish yourself; just cut your losses and start over. The above stages may be cycled through repeatedly, but all the while a gradual shift will be taking place in your consciousness. If you maintain the resolve to start over and over, you will eventually accomplish your health goals.

*Exercise 1: Complete: "My personal motivators"* –Why I want to experience vibrant health and longevity. Go to your health plan template (page 306) now and complete this exercise.

---

*"Things that matter most must never be at the mercy of things that matter least."*   Goethe

Chapter Two

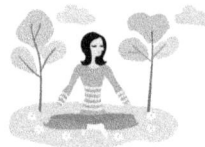

# Aging and the Mind/Body/Spirit Connection

The impact of our attitude, thoughts and feelings on our health has been well recognized for centuries in many cultures, and Western science is now acknowledging this link. The new field of psychoneuroimmunology studies the interconnectedness of the mind and body to the health of our immune system. Psychoneuroimmunology proposes that our body responds to our thoughts, just as it responds to nutrition, light and temperature; and recent research is now revealing how the power of our beliefs can affect our biology and immunity either towards health or disease. The science finds that there are certain people who exhibit a "self-healing" or "disease-resistant personality." These individuals benefit from better health than the general population due to their upbeat attitude. Some of the traits that these people exhibit are:

## Traits and Attributes of Healthy People

| Enthusiasm | Alertness | Responsiveness | Curiosity |
|---|---|---|---|
| Security | Self-esteem | Contentment | The ability to express anger assertively (not hold it in) |
| The ability to resolve fears | The ability to manage loss | The ability to forgive self and others | The ability to see the world with hope |

Unfortunately much of our thinking today is negative, fraught with worry, resentment, hopelessness, and anxiety. In fact, studies show that a typical woman has 60,000 thoughts a day, and 80% of them are negative! Having self-defeating and unconstructive thoughts can sap our energy levels and make us feel stressed. Not good for our wellbeing!

Biologist Bruce Lipton, author of the book: *Biology of Belief- Unleashing the Power of Consciousness, Matter & Miracles,* believes that it is not our genes, but our beliefs that control our lives. He contends that our nervous system, cells and biological behavior are profoundly influenced and controlled by our thought patterns and perceptions about our environment. He has observed that our cell receptors are like antennas that can read invisible vibrational energy fields from our thoughts- just as they can from other physical molecules, like pharmaceuticals. Dr. Lipton has found that our body's cells are either in a growth response or in a protection response; and he has discovered through his study that constant worrying and anxious thinking about our lives carry a frequency that activates our self-protection response.

When our cells pick up fearful signals due to some perceived threat, they automatically shut down for self-protection. Unfortunately, this inhibits our cell's growth and life-giving healing energy; which makes our body more vulnerable to disease. Dr. Lipton believes that reducing our negative thought patterns and stress levels, and actively seeking loving, joyful, fulfilling lives will stimulate our cells "growth response;" helping our body's cells to grow healthy.

Stress and chronic worry have also been shown to impair our brain cells; however, studies have found that our brain health can be restored when we try to limit worry and emotional upset. Additionally, our nervous system is influenced by our moods and thoughts. Excessive stress, worry, anger, and anxiety can trigger the release of adrenalin; also called the fight-or-flight system. This emergency state tears down our body, and diverts our energy and nourishment away from our vital organs, thus reducing our self-healing capacity. However rest, relaxation, and peaceful and joyful thoughts move our nervous system into a relaxed state (also known as the parasympathetic state.) This calm state can facilitate our healing and help us side-step our health hurdles.

Psychologists have also long supported the belief that we attract to us what we think; also known as the "self-fulfilling prophesy," or the "law of attraction." Many of us as we get older habitually think fearful and glum thoughts about the health of our body; but according to this law, these thoughts may be unwittingly attracting increasingly poor health. Not what we want!

Fortunately, we have the power to change our negative thought patterns. Our body has a remarkable capability for self-healing if we shift our mindset and refocus on positive, optimistic thoughts. As a bonus, cheerful thoughts produce feel-good endorphins and neurotransmitters; the same chemicals produced during exercise, meditation and love making. However, it is important to be mindful of our thoughts. So many of us go throughout our day without ever noticing our self-defeating and unconstructive thoughts. There is a wonderful book by Michael Singer called *The Untethered Soul: The Journey Beyond Yourself,* which can help us to learn how to observe and free ourselves from self-limiting thoughts.

Another way to consciously challenge limited thinking and negative thought patterns about our life or health is by immediately replacing or "reframing" negative thoughts with upbeat helpful ones. Instead of obsessing about aging and possible illnesses, or an earlier diagnosed illness- don't identify with them or give them any focused attention. Instead focus on your assets; acknowledge your health strengths, and the aspects of your body that are functioning well. For instance, as soon as you start having negative thoughts about your physical condition, immediately reframe the thoughts and state your health strengths such as: "I am doing everything necessary to support my health and healing;" or "My body is strong; I have great eyesight; I sleep really well; I heal fast or I have great digestion" etc. It is always important to focus on what you do <u>want</u> in your life, not what you <u>don't want</u>; as whatever you focus your attention on grows. By doing this, you tell your body that it is possible to heal; and you affirm that you are <u>more</u> than any health challenge that you experience.

*Exercise 2a: List 5 of your current "Health Assets/Strengths"* gleaned from the "Longevity self-Assessment" and from your own appraisal about your health. You will be reciting these health assets daily as positive affirmations to encourage an upbeat attitude about your wellbeing.

---

### Having a Health Vision

Numerous studies demonstrate the health benefits of guided imagery, and many hospitals are now incorporating imagery as a treatment tool. We can actually use our senses through imagery, affirmations, and meditation to create a different reality for ourselves. Studies show that a sensory-based (visual, auditory, and kinesthetic) format helps our subconscious mind to understand our desires and goals. It is important to define our health goals as specifically as possible and to do it in a sensory-based language.

- ***Visualize*** what you will see in your life that will let you know that you have achieved your goal. If your goal is to be healthy, you might see yourself with a thin body on a scale weighing in at your ideal weight; or you may see yourself being active with an abundance of energy throughout the day. Or you may see yourself laughing and fully enjoying life! Visualize any health problems disappearing. If you do have health challenges, send healing light into the distressed area. Tell your body that you are doing everything that it needs to facilitate its healing. See it whole and healthy. Visualize yourself into your 90's-100's in excellent health!
- ***Feel*** and send love to any organ or system that is having any health challenge. Put your hand on the afflicted area as you are sending the love. Next, focus on how it <u>feels</u> in your body to have vibrant energy and health. How does it <u>feel</u> to be strong and have ease of movement? How does it <u>feel</u> to have an absence of pain? Focus on

a part of your body where you notice the greatest concentration of feeling when you think these positive thoughts. What temperature is it? What does it feel like?

- **Hear**: <u>Tell</u> your body that it is strong and whole and healthy. <u>Tell</u> it that you love it and want to take care of it. Then, imagine what you will <u>*hear*</u> other people saying about your improved health, youthful looks, and vitality. What will you be <u>saying</u> about yourself?

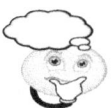

*Exercise 2b: Creating A Health Vision: Short and long term goals for health and wellbeing.* Create your personal health goals and vision. See yourself as healthy and energetic. Write down your vision. Examples: improved digestion; improved blood sugar levels; improved energy levels; a healthy body composition; off of meds; able to walk 10,000 steps; able to do a yoga posture; improved mood or cognitive function; a health challenge reversal etc. Really use all of your senses, as mentioned above. Visualize your goals for a few minutes daily. Try to practice sensory-based meditations often to support your health goals.

___

*In addition*, we can strengthen our immune system and enhance our body's healing process by replacing anxious emotions and negative thought patterns with………………………

*Gratitude–Joy–Laughter–Forgiveness–Love.*

The benefits of having a gratitude practice are well researched. Expressing gratitude lifts our outlook and puts us in the habit of looking for the good in life. Science has proven that people who regularly think grateful thoughts report fewer illnesses, sleep better, are less depressed, and have less stress, headaches, sore muscles, and stomach pain. They also exercise more and generally feel better about their lives.

Here are a few other practices to support emotional wellbeing.

- Practice observing unconstructive thoughts throughout the day, and reframe them.
- Try thinking of 5 things you are **grateful** for before going to sleep each night, and when waking up in the morning, or any other time of day when you need to lift your spirit. Some people write in a gratitude journal daily.
- Try doing something that gives you **joy** every day; something that feeds your soul. Revitalize some forgotten interest or hobby. Walk in nature. Dance around your house. Sing to your favorite songs etc.

- Practice **belly breathing** to promote relaxation. Start in a sitting position. Close your eyes and breathe in slowly through your nose - slowly count to 4 as you feel your belly expand, then slowly exhale out your nose to a count of 4; feeling your belly contract into your back. As you breathe in imagine that you are filling up with peace (let go of any resistance); as you exhale see all negativity and stress leaving your body out your nose. After doing eight repetitions your nervous system will begin to relax and you should start to feel more peaceful. Deep breathing also keeps our respiratory system healthy and our lung cartilage flexible. As we age our lung cartilage may stiffen; this can make our lungs weak and more prone to infections and pneumonia. Deep breathing can minimize this likelihood. This also can be done standing up, and with shorter repetitions when you just need to calm yourself -if stressed or angry.
- Take up a **meditation practice**. Developing or deepening an inner life is a beneficial practice in midlife. Studies have found that meditators have higher levels of the youth hormone DHEA, than non-meditators; and that meditators age more slowly. (approximately 5-12 years younger) Meditation also supports hormone balance and improved sleep. In addition, it helps us to discern deeper meaning and purpose in our lives; very important as we age. The book, *The Relaxation Response,* by Herbert Benson is a great "how to" book on meditation. *Inner Balance by HeartMath* is also a useful meditation i Phone app. that is very helpful for beginning meditators.
- Having a **forgiveness practice** is also very important to quality aging; as holding on to resentments can block the flow of life-enhancing energy. Michael Bernard Beckwith, author of *Spiritual Liberation-Fulfilling Your Soul's Potential,* has a very effective and elegant forgiveness exercise that helps to soften our heart so that we can move beyond anger and bitterness.

## Positive Affirmations

Positive affirmations are also a helpful tool to reprogram our subconscious mind; especially if we find ourselves repetitively thinking pessimistic thoughts about our health. Affirmations help us to focus our attention and energies on achieving a particular positive outcome. Restating positive affirmations can also curb the stress hormone cortisol and can help us to feel calm and in-control. The idea is to make positive assertions of what we want to see manifest in the present, (not the future) and repeat them enough so that they are a part of our belief system and mode of perceiving. However, be sure that your affirmations are realistic; otherwise your inner judge may step in and negate the affirmations. The next page includes some examples. Replace negative thoughts immediately (see them float away like clouds) with these positive ones.

- Today, instead of focusing on what's wrong, I will focus on what's right!
- I do not allow my biological age to define or restrict me.
- I gently relinquish any fears I may have about the aging process.
- My body heals itself naturally and quickly.
- My body is whole and healthy.
- I accept health as a natural part of my life.
- I love and accept my body as it is, and as it changes.
- I am a good person and I deserve to be healthy.
- No one and nothing can disturb the calm peace of my soul.
- I love my body. My body is precious to me.
- There are a lot of ways to improve my health (or sleep, fitness, body composition, etc.) and I can figure out which one works for me.
- I am being guided to find what I need to support my healing.
- I am doing all that I can do to support my healing.
- I can start healthy habits.
- I can stay calm under pressure. Stress is leaving my body.
- I can create positive change.
- All things are working together for the highest and best outcome.
- I choose to be kind and loving to myself.
- I am growing stronger every day.
- My happiness comes from within.
- I am never too old to set another goal or dream a new dream!
- I am guided this day in making right choices.
- I am happy, healthy, peaceful and prosperous.
- Every cell in my body is being renewed.
- Every day in every way I feel better and better.
- I am filled with health and the joy of living!
- There is sunshine in my soul today!
- I can overcome anything with the greatest of ease. I feel wonderful!
- I feel in harmony with myself, with the universe, and with everything around me!
- It is natural for me to enjoy health and well-being.
- I let go of any feelings of lack or limitation.
- I can handle the tasks I have ahead of me. I have just the right amount of work.
- I can find balance in my life.
- Challenge helps me grow. I can handle whatever comes.
- No one and nothing can make me feel bad about myself
- No one and nothing can take away my good.
- I forgive myself and my body for my health challenges. I am now taking corrective action to support my healing.

- I want to feel good. I can change my mood for the better.
- I express my anger openly and honestly.
- I am well-balanced and whole; physically, emotionally, and spiritually.
- I am becoming the person that I always wanted to be!
- I can grow beyond any self-imposed limits.
- I choose to be an overcomer rather than a victim.
- My thoughts are calm and under my control.
- My past no longer has any power over me.
- What I perceive and believe I will achieve.
- I open my heart to love.
- I accept what is.
- I look for the best in life.

## Feel to Heal

*Positive* affirmations, although useful, should not be used to stuff our true emotions, such as anger, grief, vulnerability, hurt, pain, guilt and sadness. Our feelings are "energy in motion" and need to be acknowledged, accepted and expressed in healthy ways; not bottled up inside. Numerous conditions both psychological and physical can be traced back to suppressed and unresolved emotional issues; often stemming from as far back as childhood. Expressing our grief through crying, and releasing our buried anger through safe anger release activities can often be very cathartic. Freeing up painful feelings can help to soften our heart and bring about renewed energy levels, reversal of health problems, and peace. Bodywork is often a helpful tool to tap into and free-up blocked emotions. *Rosen Method* bodywork is especially effective for this purpose.

## Obstacles to Positive Change

*Some of us* have tried positive thinking and affirmations, but somehow aren't able to transform our bad habits, reach our goals or keep an optimistic disposition. This is because in many instances we have acquired strong programming in childhood that has led to dysfunctional belief systems (about ourselves or the world) which can sabotage our attempts at change.

If you feel that all your efforts to change have failed, it is possible that subconscious negative programming is the culprit. The following therapies may help:

- *Psych-K muscle testing is a beneficial therapy to help neutralize negative programming. Consider going to the website psych-k.com for a list of certified instructors in your area that can help you to release the conditioning that is holding you back.
- Biofeedback, hypnotherapy, Emotional Freedom Technique, Cognitive Behavioral or Cognitive Restructuring Therapy, or Dialectical Behavioral Therapy are also useful therapies to help manage subconscious obstacles to change.

- Self-defeating thought patterns and a negative outlook can also be due to a deficiency of the "feel-good" brain chemicals serotonin and/or dopamine. Try boosting these chemicals with omega-3 fats, vitamin D, B-complex vitamins, daily exercise, going outdoors in nature; taking a 20 minute sun bath when the sun is at its peak (light therapy); and ensuring that you have adequate down-time. A very common genetic stress-induced anxiety condition known as pyroluria may also be restricting positive emotions. It may be helpful to go to an integrative/functional psychiatrist or naturopath who can help you balance your brain chemicals naturally.

---

Research also shows that humor and laughter have remarkable health benefits. They can reduce the levels of damaging stress hormones, and increase the levels of health enhancing endorphin hormones. Laughter also increases pain tolerance and strengthens the immune system. Try to laugh more to improve your overall well-being: watch comedies, go to comedy clubs, close your eyes and smile inwardly; even fake laughing is beneficial- as the body can't distinguish between real and fake laughter- the benefits are the same. We all need to laugh more!

Lastly, music has been shown to have restorative qualities. Certain types of music have been found to reduce irritability and agitation. Music also has been shown to improve memory, lower blood pressure, and shorten recovery time after surgery. Below are some suggestions of music that can help calm and soothe the soul.

- Don Campbell, *Mozart as Healer; Classical Healing for the New Millennium.*
- Northsound, *The Wellness Series-Healing Mind-Body-Spirit*
- Nadama, *Healing Touch*
- Shastro, *Shambala*
- David Lanz, *Beloved*
- Andrew Weil, *Self- Healing with Sound and Music*
- Ralph Vaughan Williams, *Inner Peace for Busy People: Music to Relax and Renew*
- Dean Evenson has a number of relaxing C.D.'s
- Gary Stadler has a series of calming C.D.'s

---

*All symptoms and health challenges offer a message to us, and can alert us that something is out of balance in our lives either spiritually, emotionally or physically. Meditation and contemplation can help us to discern the message!*

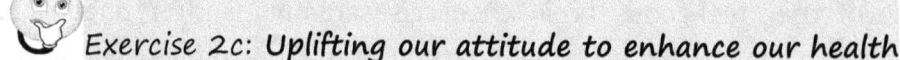

### Exercise 2c: Uplifting our attitude to enhance our health

Set an intention every day to care for your physical, emotional and spiritual wellbeing. Take a little time each day to uplift your mind and spirit!

- Observe your thoughts throughout the day, and reframe them if necessary.
- Write down 5 affirmations that you can repeat daily (in the morning etc.) to uplift your attitude and enhance your health.
- Practice gratitude exercises daily.
- Listen to peaceful music
- Consider doing something that gives you joy on a daily basis.
- Perform belly breathing, meditation or prayer to unwind before bed or any time you are stressed.
- Start a forgiveness practice, if necessary.
- And don't forget to laugh!

Chapter Three

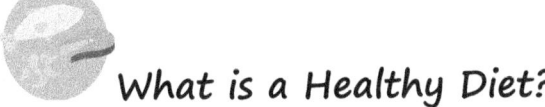 What is a Healthy Diet?

## Nutrient Density and Healthy Aging

Although there are several factors that contribute to enhanced health and longevity, our diet is a major aspect. We have all heard the adage that "you are what you eat," and research has proven that food is the primary promoter of health and disease protection. Studies confirm that food is 300-400% more important than even exercise for optimal health.

As we age, our need for many nutrients increases; thus boosting our consumption of "nutrient-dense foods." is vital to maintaining optimal functioning in our later years. Nutrient-dense foods, as opposed to empty calorie filler-foods, give us the most nutrients possible with the fewest number of calories. They deliver a complete nutritional package of everything we need to stay well nourished: vitamins, minerals, phytonutrients, fatty acids, and essential amino acids. In essence, they give us the biggest bang for our buck! The greater the nutritional value of our food, the more optimally our cells and body will function; which in turn will support the restoration of our energy levels, and increase our resistance to age-related diseases.

While nutritional advice about the ideal diet changes yearly with new scientific findings, there are some nutritional fundamentals that are constant. Eating natural fresh whole foods with a large intake of vegetables and minimizing sugar and refined foods is a basic tenet of good nutrition that never changes. A diet rich in whole plant foods is protective against all diseases. There's an extensive amount of data that proves that deviating from the primarily whole plant-based diet of our hunter-gatherer ancestors is a chief factor in the development of heart disease, cancer, stroke, arthritis, and many other chronic diseases. It is virtually impossible to get our nutritional needs met by consumption of chemical laden, processed foods and sugars, with heaps of poor quality meats, amid sparse quantities of vegetables and fruits.

Due to the fallacy, "better living through chemistry," which stimulated our modern food manufacturing processes; humans today are suffering from many more chronic diseases than ever before. Our bodies were not adapted to absorb synthetic chemicals, and processed foods common in our western diet. These toxins weaken our immune system, and alter our DNA. The addition of fortified and synthetic vitamins and minerals to these foods does nothing to boost their nutrient levels; as these added nutrients are of low quality and poorly absorbed.

Our body identifies the food we eat as either our ally or adversary. Cutting edge science has revealed that our food carries information to our genes to tell them how to express themselves. While nourishing food sends a health-enhancing message to our genes, poor food choices send disease-promoting messages that can alter our DNA. Unfortunately, an abundance of foods available today in the "standard American diet," often called the S.A.D. diet, send incorrect messages to our genes, and are hazardous to our health. Many of the foods we eat for pleasure, or to satisfy our cravings or hunger are "hyper-palatable," nutrient depleted, over-processed, bone depleting, and loaded with harmful food additives. When we allow temporary sensory gratification to override nourishing food choices; it comes at the expense of our health.

*An essential first step to healthy aging is to remove or reduce the C.R.A.P. from our diet.* (Adapted from Bauman, Friedlander, 2011)

| C. | R. | A. | P. |
|---|---|---|---|
| Caffeine, cola, chips, cake, cookies, candy, crackers, cold cereals, cold cuts, cured meats | Refined carbs: white flour, white rice, white sugar, French fries and high fructose corn syrup | Additives, alcohol, allergenic foods, acid promoting foods | Processed, packaged, pesticides, oxidized polyunsaturated oils, and hydrogenated oil |

Making a shift to a nutrient-dense diet entails foregoing empty calories (packaged and refined foods, soft drinks, sugars, bad oils, excess caffeine and alcohol) in favor of life-giving foods. Life-giving foods are phytonutrient rich, vitamin and mineral packed vegetables, fruits, healthy fats, vegetable proteins, and clean animal proteins. Eating with nutrient density in mind increases our body's defenses, and maintains the health of our cells and tissues. Our body will then have nutrient reserves for repair and maintenance, and will be buffered against times of stress, infection, illness or injury. The body draws on these nutrient stores, and if these stores are depleted, the body will struggle, and premature aging and disease can ensue. Eating with a consciousness of nutrient-density will support the regeneration of our body, thus increasing the likelihood of a long and happy "health span."

Every bite of food we eat represents a choice and an opportunity to extract life-enhancing nutrients from our food. The best way to improve our eating habits is to stop and think before we eat anything. It's helpful to ask ourselves: "Is this a food that will strengthen my body or weaken it? " This way of thinking will remind us to eat foods that are packed with nutrients, as opposed to eating filler-foods, that just waste space in our diet. Remember, make every bite count!

Variety is also essential. By eating a moderate and diverse mix of foods we are ensured of receiving a full range of vitamins, minerals, and phytonutrients in our diet, thus avoiding deficiencies.

Improving our diet however is an evolving lifestyle process. Changing our eating habits can be challenging, and sometimes it is hard to prioritize meal planning. We may also have hormone and emotional issues or stress that cause us to overeat or crave carbs and sugar. But, as I mentioned previously, health is a process, and changing the way we approach our daily diet can be done in small incremental steps, thus gently supporting us through the progression.

We also must be careful that our dietary goals are realistic for us. Remember, that we are laying-down new eating routines that should last a lifetime. Trying to make a lot of changes all at once may cause uncomfortable withdrawal and detoxification symptoms; and possibly a rebound effect. This can result-in burn-out and disappointment.

Consider simply accomplishing what is manageable for you each day. Don't dwell on your setbacks; you will probably have some. Just focus on the days that you did well. Use positive self-talk, and visualize yourself eating healthy foods, exercising, and feeling great. Also ensure that you surround yourself with positive health-minded people who can support you through this process. Be patient with yourself; change rarely comes instantly, but by making unhurried gradual improvements, you are more likely to attain your health goals.

It is also helpful to view this process as a journey of self-discovery. I can provide information, and resources to assist you on your journey to high level health, but we are all unique individuals, with distinct dietary requirements (biochemical individuality). It's up to you to test things out to see what works for you, and what doesn't.

Additionally, most people don't connect what they are eating with the way they feel. It is important to pay attention to what your body is telling you, and observe which foods and how much food help you to feel your best. Notice how your body feels when you eat certain foods. Do you feel energized? Do you feel less pain, and stiffness? Does your gut feel less irritation? Do you have less food cravings? Are you more regular in your bowel functions? Is your mind clearer? Do you just feel better emotionally?

Making dietary modifications also does not mean that we have to give up tasty food! Eating a nourishing diet is not about bland food. Fresh, whole, well-seasoned home-cooked food is delicious! Our first step in nutrition consciousness is learning to not only like foods that taste good, but to like foods that are healthy for us, in addition to tasting good.

Incorporating nutrient dense food in our life is also not difficult. It does however call for us to make a mindset shift. It requires us to change our daily focus to nutrition instead of convenience. This means planning ahead and not leaving our food choices to chance. Nourishing our body needs to be front and center in our daily priorities; as it is the most important factor in our body's functioning.

Our earlier ancestors were very aware of this knowledge; and spent a significant part of their day obtaining and preparing their foods in order to support their health. Often when we don't plan our meals ahead of time we end up foraging for food <u>after</u> we have become ravenous; which often leads to draining food selections and over eating. Planning for and preparing good food does not have to be labor intensive however. In the following pages I will share tips on how to prepare foods with minimal effort.

We wouldn't feed our pets food that is not their native diet, and that nature didn't intend. This alien food would be damaging to their functioning. Likewise, it's not self-caring to feed ourselves a foreign diet that will cause poor functioning in our own body.

*Taking the time to nourish ourselves with wholesome food is a self-loving practice.*

---

*Every person* reading this book is at a different starting point in their health journey. Some individuals are just at the beginning, while others have been on the path for a while. I wanted to make the information in this book as easy to put into practice as possible for each person; therefore, I have adapted and individualized the plan. The words "good," "better," and "best" are used to denote different levels of healthy food choices in the following charts.

- o Beginning health-seekers are at <u>level one</u> and should start with "**good**" choices in the charts.
- o Health conscious people who have an interest in nutrition and health (level two and three) can begin with "**better**" or "**best**" choices.

After successfully carrying out your plan for a time, you can move up to the next level (better or best) or continue to stay at your level indefinitely. All levels are health supportive, and will further your wellness.

| Level One Healthy Eating | *"Good"* A nutritional goal that is achievable for level one eating is to eat healthfully 80% of the time, and indulge wisely 20% of the time. In other words, you can eat healthily during the week, and indulge on the weekend, or on special occasions. It is advised to make sure that these indulgent foods are not in your pantry or refrigerator; as they will be too tempting to eat during the week, and only buy enough for the weekend.<br><br>I will also be suggesting alternative foods to substitute for draining foods. Some of these foods may be a new taste sensation for you. Try to keep an open mind, as you try foods out of your comfort zone. Note: avoid trans-fats completely. |
|---|---|
| Level Two | *"Better"* A nutritional goal for level two eating would be to eat healthfully 90 % of the time, and indulge wisely 10% of the time. You can eat healthily during the week, and treat yourself to indulgent foods on one day of the weekend or on special occasions. |
| Level Three | *"Best"* A nutritional goal for level three eating would be to eat healthfully 95% of the time, and to indulge wisely on special occasions. |

**The following page** is a step-by-step guide to help you improve your eating and health habits by substituting poor food and drink choices with healthy choices. Go through these steps at your own pace. Check off the health depleting foods as you remove them from your diet. There is a lot of information here on the health consequences of eating poor quality foods. The object here is not to make you feel guilty or anxious or to be paranoid and fear foods; but to make you an informed shopper and to guide you on providing your body with foods that it needs to thrive. By raising your consciousness about harmful foods, you will strengthen your resolve to eat better. Your body will begin the healing process as soon as you remove the foods from your life.

If you do on occasion eat the following poor food choices- relax and enjoy them without guilt or fear. The important point is to indulge wisely, by not over-consuming; and by making sure to eat foods with some nutritional value. Substituting organic or natural low-sugar treats, and eating these foods after dinner or accompanying them with a protein or fat will lessen the damaging blood sugar spiking impact. Choosing savory protein treats like gourmet cheeses, and flavored nuts are another wise indulgent option. Blue corn or other baked whole-grain/vegetable-based chips; fruit-based snacks; organic low sugar protein bars, and 70% cocoa chocolate bars are some other examples. Antipastos with olives and marinated veggies are also healthy and enjoyable indulgences.

In addition, it is always best to eat peacefully, and chew your food well to support digestion and assimilation, no matter what the food quality is. Remember, it is not the occasional food indiscretion that is harmful to your health, but what you put in your body on an ongoing daily basis that will determine your health status as you age.

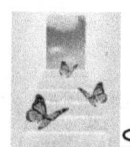 *Step One: Change your beverages*

An important first step toward better health is to change the beverages that we drink. Individuals can improve their health significantly by just eliminating non-nutritive drinks. Pure filtered water is really the only liquid that we need, and the ideal hydration source. Our bodies contain up to 70% water by weight, and our brains contain a little more. Water is important for digestion, temperature control, and transportation of nutrients. It is essential in assisting our body and liver with daily detoxification processes. Additionally, a dehydrated state can lead to skin shrinkage, wrinkles and muscle weakness.

Water also aids appetite control. Many people confuse hunger for thirst; but drinking adequate water throughout the day will fill us up and suppress our hunger. Having a well hydrated body is vital to our over-all health and to prevent disease states in our body.

The rule of thumb is to drink half your weight in ounces of a water-based drink. So, if you weigh 150 lbs. you should drink about 75 oz. (about 9 cups) of a water-based liquid daily: filtered water, green or herbal tea, broth, or diluted fresh vegetable juice (not coffee or alcohol as these are dehydrating.) Try not to drink large amounts of water at one time, it's better to hydrate with small amounts of liquid throughout the entire day. Adding a squeeze of lemon or lime can make water more palatable.

*The Solution to Pollution is Dilution!*   Sherry Rogers

**Exercise 3a: Hydration-** *Drink ½ your weight in ounces of water-based liquids daily. Enter your daily liquid consumption here, and enter it in your wellness plan (8 oz. equals one cup):*

Complete: "Hydration" on your wellness plan ___oz. or ___ cups daily

---

**Unfortunately,** the "Environmental Working Group" has confirmed that there are more than 260 contaminants detected in tap water. Since tap water often has harmful substances (lead, toxic chemicals, pharmaceuticals, chlorination by-products, radioactive contaminants, and petrochemicals) it is a good idea to invest in some kind of water purifier.

The best type of water filter should remove contaminants, but not dissolved minerals. Point-of-use (POU) filters, such as reverse osmosis filters are suggested as they filter the water coming from your pipes as well, which can also leach contaminants; and they filter fluoride additionally. There is a right-to-know law that requires municipal water suppliers to present to their customers yearly water quality reports. It is a good idea to get your free report so that you can find a water filter that can remove contaminants specific to your tap water. Filters that have been independently certified to eliminate particular contaminants are the best. NSF International is the best known organization for setting standards for water filters, and certifying them. (nsr.org) To test your water for lead that may be leaching from your pipes call the EPA water quality hot line to locate a state-certified lab.(1-800-426-4791) or epa.gov/safewater/privatewells/labs.html.

Faucet mounted water purifiers that are sold at a number of stores; although not ideal, are economical and do filter an adequate quantity of contaminants. It's a good idea to also filter water in bathrooms as well; as contaminants can be absorbed through the skin, or inhaled in the steam. Bath tub balls and shower filters exist for this purpose.

Alternately, plastic bottled water is not a good water alternative, as the chemicals in plastic known as phthalates and bisphenol-A (BPA) leach into the water. These plastics are carcinogenic, and disrupt hormone function. Glass bottled water is better than plastic. To hydrate throughout the day fill up a glass or stainless steel large water bottle or thermos, with filtered water. You can add lemon or lime to enhance the flavor.

---

*One of the most important measures* we can take to improve our health is to eliminate or greatly reduce sugar and high fructose corn syrup sweetened beverages (liquid sugar) such as soda, sugary coffees, teas, soft drinks, sports drinks, energy drinks and juices; as these are the single biggest source of sugar calories. Soda, in particular is a poor hydrator, and the phosphoric acid it contains prevents calcium absorption, which can weaken our bones and teeth. The toxic artificial sweeteners in diet soda are also not conducive to good health.

If eliminating sugary drinks will be a hard transition for you: there are other tasty alternatives to these beverages that can help you get over the hump. See next page.

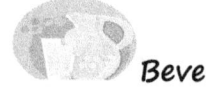 ## Beverage Substitutions:

Level One-Good    Level two-Better    Level three-Best    All levels-All

| Check | Avoid | Use Instead |
|---|---|---|
| | <u>Soda/soft drinks:</u> Full of immune and brain weakening, bone stripping, health depleting sugar, and chemicals | * Good: carbonated juice sweetened drinks/ciders without sugar. (Juice squeeze, Izze, Martinelli etc.) <br> *Better – unsweetened fruit flavored sparkling mineral water, or plain mineral water in glass bottles. You can add a splash of 100% fruit juice at home. <br> *Best- Plain sparkling mineral water with a squeeze of fresh lemon or lime. (You can sweeten it with stevia). |
| | <u>Fruit juice</u>: high in fructose sugar which spikes blood sugar | *Good-Dilute organic 100% fruit juice with pure water (1/3 part juice to 2/3 part filtered water <br> *Better-juice your own organic fruits/than dilute. |
| | <u>Sweetened Iced tea/iced coffee drinks</u>: spikes blood sugar, depletes minerals and vitamins | * Good-Plain iced tea sweetened with stevia <br> *Better-iced green tea or herbal tea sweetened with stevia - don't buy herbal tea w/ "natural flavoring" (code word for MSG) <br> *Best-unsweetened iced green or herbal teas w/lemon squeeze |
| | <u>Coffee with sugar or Flavored coffee drinks:</u> Coffee depletes mineral status, increases stress hormones, dehydrating. | *Good-Plain organic coffee sweetened with stevia (cut down by 1 cup each week until drinking one cup a day) <br> *Better: coffee alternative- Yerba Mate, Teeccino or Pu-erh tea. Add your own stevia. <br> *Best: switch to green tea, rooibus tea, herbal tea, home-made vegetable broths, or a cup of miso soup. (from miso paste or from organic package mix) |
| | <u>Hard liquor, sweetened alcoholic drinks, beer:</u> Leaches minerals from body; liver stressor/toxin, raises blood sugar, pancreas stressor, chemical additives. | *Good-Red wine or red wine spritzer (w/sparkling mineral water) Limit to 1 small drink- daily/or less. (cut down by 1 glass each week until drinking one glass a day) <br> *Better-drink organic red wine 3x/week <br> *Best-drink 1x/wk. or on special occasions or none. Supplementing with resveratrol obtains similar effects |
| | <u>Milk shakes/chocolate milk/hot chocolate</u>: High in sugar; spikes blood sugar, weakens immunity | *Good-Organic unsweetened fruit kefir, or organic milk, or almond milk with unsweetened cocoa or carob powder; add organic stevia sweetener (hot or cold) <br> *Best-Organic plain kefir w/"live and active cultures" on the label. You can blend your own fruit/cocoa into it. Add stevia. |
| | <u>Energy drinks</u>: high in sugar and caffeine, spikes blood sugar | *All- Smoothie blended with spirulina, nutritional yeast, berries and filtered water, or coconut milk or nut milk. Sweeten with stevia. Nutrient packed and energizing! |
| | <u>Sports drinks</u>: high in sugar, and chemicals | *All-Coconut water: hydrating and mineral rich. It should be unsweetened. It is naturally sweet. |

Exercise 3b: Find your health level and write your beverage substitutions in your wellness plan/or print out the chart.

*Step Two: Eliminate Processed Foods and Additives*

A helpful second step in your self-care program is to go through your pantry and refrigerator, and eliminate processed and packaged foods that drain your vitality, and rob nutrients from the body. These foods are often called "food-like" substances because they don't nourish our body as true food does. These foods are toxic to the liver, and overwork our immune system. They inflame our brain, nerves and muscles, and disrupt our digestion.

This step requires that you learn to read ingredient lists on foods; if you don't already. The words-"all natural" on the front labels have no validity; they are just advertising hype. The rule of thumb is to buy foods with **only 5 ingredients or less** on the ingredient label; as products with long lists of ingredients generally have unhealthy chemicals and additives. (The addition of herbs or spices can however add more ingredients; which is fine.) Also if the first ingredient on any package is sugar, high fructose corn sweetener, salt or fat; it is not a wise food choice.

*Note: The following information is given not to scare you, but to raise your consciousness; enabling you to strengthen your resolve to eat better. This information will also help you to be a savvy shopper. Check-off each item as you eliminate them from your diet. You will be substituting higher quality "real food," as shown on the chart for poor quality "food-like" substances. Below is an in depth evaluation of each item. The chart follows the review.

 *Harmful and Draining Foods and Additives: the Worst Offenders*

- o *Eliminate any foods with artificial Trans Fats. These fats cause the most harm. If you find the words "<u>hydrogenated</u>" or "<u>partially hydrogenated</u>", or <u>shortening</u>; these foods contain trans-fats. They are often found in deep fried foods, salad dressings, margarines, crackers, cookies, chips, snack foods, doughnuts, and other baked and fried foods. These oils harm the brain, damage cell membranes, and slow metabolism, and are linked to heart disease, diabetes, and immune impairment. They also deplete HDL- the "good cholesterol."
- o Eliminate refined omega-6 vegetable oils in plastic or glass containers, such as: corn, safflower, sunflower, soy, peanut, and canola. These oils are deficient in nutrients and essential oils. They also are unstable; they become rancid (oxidized) quickly from light and heat. The manufacturers remedy this by adding deodorizers to conceal the smell. These vegetable oils are the main culprit of inflammation and pain. Omega-6 oils also turn on genes that cause heart disease, Alzheimer's, and diabetes.

- Eliminate Mono Sodium Glutamate: **(MSG)** is a very harmful and addictive chemical that was introduced 50 years ago to enhance the flavor of foods. It is linked to Alzheimer's, and Diabetes. Even though the FDA deems that MSG is generally safe, there are over 100 medical studies documented in the National Library of Medicine that prove that MSG is deleterious to health. MSG is a known neurotoxin, and an excitotoxin which causes brain cells to become over-excited and fire uncontrollably; leading to brain cell death. MSG also causes obesity, headaches, burning sensations, heart palpitations, numbness, and sweating. It has been postulated that over 95% of all processed foods contain MSG. It's an ingredient in pre-packaged foods, soups, snack foods, processed meats, drinks, coffee drinks, candy, chewing gum, spices, and in virtually all fast food, and chain restaurants. Even natural and organic food is not immune to this. MSG hides under many names (at least 50). Below is a chart of the most common names documented by the nutrition departments of Bastyr and Vanderbilt University. As you can infer, the safest option is to skip the processed foods, and eat real whole foods. You can consult truthinlabeling.org for more information. Additionally, when at restaurants, request only non-MSG foods, as many Asian restaurants serve MSG laden foods.

*Hidden MSG Terms on Ingredient Labels (code words)*

| Glutamic Acid | Yeast extract, autolyzed yeast, autolyzed plant protein, yeast food or nutrient | Hydrolyzed protein, hydrolyzed oat protein, textured protein, protein fortified | Sodium caseinate, calcium caseinate |
|---|---|---|---|
| Bouillon, broth, stock, seasonings, spices, flavorings | Malt extract, malt flavoring | Natural flavors and natural flavorings, (also in herbal teas) natural beef and chicken flavor. | Soy protein isolate, soy protein concentrate, |
| Whey protein and concentrate, and whey isolate | Fermented | Enzymes, modified enzymes | Ultra-pasteurized |

Harmful and Draining Foods and Additives continued on next page.

- Eliminate **sodium nitrate/nitrite**, often found in processed, cured meats (hot dogs, sausages, bacon) and lunch meats. Nitrite containing foods are considered to be carcinogenic. Organic processed meats will use celery juice as a natural nitrate- which gets converted into nitrites; but some believe has the same harmful effect. Therefore, organic versions should be eaten only occasionally. Smoked fish and meats also contain nitrites/nitrates from the smoking process.
- Eliminate **BHA and BHT**. Found in many packaged foods. This preservative has been found to be a cancer risk.
- Eliminate **Olestra**. Found in many low-fat baked goods, and chips. This fake fat binds with and depletes vitamins A, D E, and K. Cancer and immune health risk.
- Eliminate the artificial sweetener **Sucralose**- which is contained in **Splenda**. It causes blood sugar disturbances, induces DNA damage, and reduces beneficial bacteria. (The first 2 ingredients in Splenda are sugars! Contains one calorie more than sugar.)
- Eliminate the artificial sweetener **Aspartame.** Found in **Equal** and **NutraSweet**, and found in diet sodas-shown to be a neurotoxin (kills brain cells) and carcinogenic. Can lead to obesity (brain can't tell it's not sugar)
- Eliminate **High-Fructose Corn Syrup**-The primary sugar in soft drinks, baked goods, salad dressings and low fat products. A 2004 study published in the *American Journal of Clinical Nutrition* reported that HFCS, and fructose in general metabolize differently than glucose, or sucrose. HFCS short–circuits the hormonal process that signals satiation, and instead goes directly to the liver. The liver than quickly generates new fat cells, and elevated triglyceride levels, causing insulin resistance and rapid weight gain.
- Eliminate **Propylgallate**; carcinogenic
- Eliminate any **food coloring and dye**: FD&C red, blue, yellow etc. Carcinogenic
- Eliminate **refined carbohydrates: white flour, white rice and white sugar**; they are devoid of fiber and nutrients, bone-depleting, and use-up vital nutrients, such as B-vitamins and minerals, while they are being metabolized. These draining foods cause blood sugar imbalances, and overwork the pancreas. White flour, white rice, and sugar are also devoid of fiber, which results in too much glucose entering into the blood stream at too fast a rate; causing a sharp rise in blood sugar (spike) followed by a steep fall. The quick spiking and dropping of blood sugar leads to eventual hypoglycemia, emotional imbalances, diabetes, and obesity. In addition, sugar suppresses the immune system, and can lead to breast, ovarian, prostate, and colon cancer, tooth decay, weak eyesight, kidney damage, arthritis, asthma, gallstones, heart disease, candida albicans yeast infection, and premature aging.

- Eliminate **Genetically Modified foods** (GMO) GMO's are used to enhance certain traits in plants, lengthen shelf life and to increase herbicide/pesticide resistance. Estimates are that 70%-80% of all processed foods are GMO foods. Used in soft drinks, potato chips, corn flakes, cookies, ice cream, ketchup etc. It is in virtually all non-organic **soy** and **corn** products. Genetic modification alters the DNA of the plants that we are consuming. There is little scientific data on the long term safety of GMO foods. However, GMO's are linked to food allergies, cancer, and birth defects. Unfortunately, GMO containing foods don't have to be labeled "GMO," therefore every processed and packaged food is suspect.
- Eliminate **pesticide** containing foods: Pesticides are any substance used to kill or control threats to growing plants.(**vegetables, and fruits**) Pesticides also end up being in commercial animal products: **eggs, milk, fish, poultry and meat**; due their pesticide laden diet. The U.S. and international agencies link pesticides to cancer, hormone disorders, Parkinson's, nervous system disorders, and lung, skin, and eye irritations. Additionally non-organic vegetables and fruits contain significantly less nutrients than organic varieties. Note: grains, beans, and seeds/nuts (except peanut butter) generally contain less pesticide residues than vegetables and fruits; as they are not vigorously sprayed.
- Limit **Commercial Meat and Dairy**. (non-organic) They contain residual hormones and antibiotics, and the animals are fed genetically modified corn and soy. They are also high in omega-6 fatty acids, which cause an omega-3 fatty acid shortage. (inflammation-promoting) Commercial meat and dairy also contain pesticide residues, and may lead to inflammation, sluggish liver, nervous and immune system disorders, and antibiotic resistance.
- Eliminate **processed table salt (not sea-salt)** Processed commercial salt is loaded with additives, aluminum, chemicals, and preservatives. It is also bleached and is devoid of necessary minerals. Alternately, a high quality <u>unbleached sea-salt</u> is mineral rich, which can contain up to 80 alkalinizing trace minerals. This high mineral content can support a neutral pH of 7.2 in the body. Sea Salt and naturally occurring sodium is essential to our health, and according to Dr. David Brownstein, author of *Salt Your Way to Health*; if you are not eating unrefined salt, (sea salt/Himalayan salt) you are salt deficient. He claims that scientific research does not support the flawed advice that a low-salt diet is healthy. Additionally, he states that our human body is designed to ingest salt and that we have salt receptors on our tongue that give us cravings for it. He also states that there are salt receptors in the kidneys, and lining every cell in our body. Unrefined salt is also needed for detoxification and nervous system regulation, and it is important for healthy adrenal and thyroid function. Salt cravings could signal weak adrenals, and mineral

deficiencies; something that natural sea salt can provide. When shopping for sea salt make sure that it is colored and not white. White sea-salt has been bleached and also contains aluminum as an anti-caking agent. In addition, it has less mineral content. If you are not hypertensive, it is fine to salt–to-taste your food. If you are hypertensive and watching your salt intake, according to Dr. Brownstein- you can use small amounts of colored sea salt (1½ teaspoons per day) as it contains 20% less sodium than table salt. The important factor in sodium balance is keeping intake of sodium to potassium at a 1:5 ratio or higher. When you increase your consumption of potassium rich fruits and vegetables, and decrease salt laden processed foods, you will maintain the optimal ratio, and reduce your blood pressure.

**Best unrefined sea salt:** *Celtic sea salt, Himalayan pink salt, Redmond's Real Salt.*
*Note: Most sea salt does not have iodine added to it as conventional table salt does, but the iodine in refined table salt, according to Dr. Brownstein is minimal and poorly absorbed. So, it is better to obtain iodine from iodine rich sea vegetables (nori, wakame, kombu, dulse, kelp, bladderwrack etc.) and seafood or iodine supplements to avoid deficiencies. Dairy and eggs are secondary sources of iodine. Most people suffer from a deficiency of or suboptimal iodine levels; especially those with hypothyroid conditions; or those who have had breast, ovarian, uterine, or prostate cancers. Consuming a large quantity of soy and raw cruciferous vegetables in addition to having excessive exposure to fluoride, bromine, and chlorine will block iodine uptake in the thyroid and other organs. In these cases you will require a higher intake of iodine rich foods or supplements to offset the imbalance.

**Best supplemental iodine**: Iodoral or Lugol's Solution. It is recommended to obtain an Iodine Loading test from a medical professional before attempting iodine supplementation.

---

The harmful food/food additives check-off chart is on the next page.

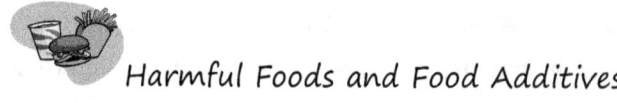

# Harmful Foods and Food Additives

Level One-Good     Level two-Better     Level three-Best    All Levels-All

| Check | AVOID | USE INSTEAD |
|---|---|---|
|  | **Trans fats:** Hydrogenated/partially hydrogenated oils/shortening/cottonseed oils (eliminate completely!) | *All-Cold pressed extra virgin olive oil, organic butter, extra virgin coconut oil, organic red palm oil |
|  | **Refined polyunsaturated oils** in plastic or glass bottles (corn, soy, sunflower, safflower, peanut, canola) | * All-Cold pressed extra virgin olive oil Extra virgin coconut oil, organic butter, and ghee |
|  | **MSG,** autolyzed yeast extract etc. See above. | *Better/Best: sea salt, natural herbs and spices, |
|  | **Sodium nitrate/nitrite** laden meats, sausages, bacon and sandwich meats. Also in smoked fish and meats. Organic varieties (with celery juice) also contain them. | *Good- commercial natural meats with the words "no nitrites or nitrates added" on label. Eat sparingly<br>*Better-Organic meats with no nitrates.<br>*Best: Sliced unprocessed home cooked organic meats, bean and nut spreads, tempeh (fermented soy) |
|  | **Artificial sweeteners** with 0 calories; Splenda, sucralose, aspartame | *Good/Better-Stevia, Lo Han Guo (natural 0 cal. Sweeteners) make sure that it is 100% pure stevia- not with dextrose)<br>* Best: unrefined green powder stevia or try to enjoy the natural taste without any sweetener |
|  | BHA/BHT preservatives | *Good/Better-Natural/organic whole foods<br>*Best: Home-cooked foods |
|  | Olestra | *All-Olive oil, butter, virgin coconut oil |
|  | **Food dyes** (FD&C red, blue etc.)<br>Propygallate | *Good/Better-Food coloring from natural sources listed on the label<br>*Best: choose organic substances |
|  | **High fructose corn sweetener** (HFCS) and **Sugar**<br><br>*If you have intense sugar- cravings; try taking 500 mg. of glutamine up to 3 times per day. It can diminish cravings.<br><br>Gymnema is also known to calm cravings<br><br>Sugar cravings can be due to low blood sugar, or low serotonin levels.<br><br>**Continued on next page.** | *Good-*Fruit Juice concentrate, organic cane sugar (rapadura), date sugar, raw honey, real maple syrup,<br>*Better: 100% organic stevia leaf extract, powder or liquid, xylitol (from birch cellulose), Lo Han Guo (from fruit)<br>*Best: whole stevia leaf (green colored) buy or grow your own<br>*or add banana, raisins or whole dates to sweeten food<br>*or no sweetener (enjoy the real taste)<br>* eat fruits instead |

| Check | AVOID | USE INSTEAD |
|---|---|---|
|  | <u>Refined white flour from wheat</u> (termed semolina) or White rice flour | *Good-Complex carbohydrates: <u>100% whole wheat</u> flour breads and pastas (whole wheat or 100% whole wheat should be the first ingredient on the label, w/ no other wheat ingredients or semolina on it)<br>*Better-use <u>organic</u> 100% whole wheat<br>*Even better- <u>organic sprouted or sourdough</u> whole wheat bread (without any yeast)<br>*Even better--organic <u>non-gluten</u> brown rice, millet, and buckwheat pasta and nut flour breads<br>*Best- minimize breads, and pastas, and eat non-gluten grains in whole form. Also substitute root vegetables, sweet potatoes and winter squash for grains. |
|  | <u>GMO's</u> –typical GMO crops (if not organic)- soy, corn, cottonseed, sugar, canola, zucchini, Hawaiian papaya, yellow squash | *Good/Better-Avoid GMO non organic corn and soy etc.<br>*Better- Avoid all GMO foods<br>*Best- Eat all organic foods |
|  | **Pesticides:**<br>Carcinogenic. The 2013 Environmental Working Groups (EWG) <u>non-organic dirty dozen plus</u>; the worst pesticide offenders with the highest residues:<br>Apples, cherry tomatoes, bell peppers, hot peppers, celery, cucumbers, grapes, strawberries, nectarines, peaches, potatoes, spinach, summer squash, plus lettuce, blueberries, raspberries, green beans, kale, and collard greens.<br>Peanuts (peanut butter) is also heavily sprayed. | *Good-<u>Eat the EWG's "Clean 15"- Low pesticide foods</u>-asparagus, avocado, cabbage, cantaloupe (domestic), eggplant, grapefruit, kiwi, mangoes, mushrooms, onions, pineapples, mangoes, frozen sweet peas, sweet potatoes, watermelon, whole grains, and dry beans,<br>*Better-eat predominantly organic<br>*Best-buy organic Community Supported Agriculture "CSA," or farmers' market produce or grow your own organic produce. |
|  | **Refined salt** | *All-Unrefined/unbleached sea salt (gray Celtic sea salt, pink Himalayan sea salt, Redmond's real salt). |
|  | **Commercial meat and dairy** | *Good/: Organic meats, poultry, eggs, and dairy.<br>*Better: Organic free range<br>*Best: organic 100% grass fed /pastured and finished |

**Exercise 3c: Write your food substitutions on your personal wellness plan/or print out the chart** Affirmation: I treat my body as a temple. It is holy, clean and full of goodness.

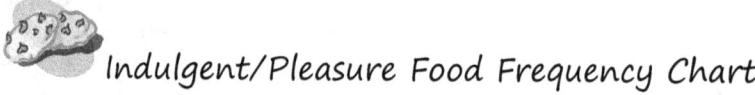 Indulgent/Pleasure Food Frequency Chart.

Remember to indulge wisely

| Food/Drink | Good-level 1 | Better-level 2 | Best-level 3 |
|---|---|---|---|
| Fast Food/chain restaurant food (trans fats/GMO/additives/non-organic, high sugar, refined) | 1-2x/month | 1x every few months | Rarely |
| Junk/snack food: chips, pretzels, crackers, salty refined white flour foods | 1-2x/week | 2x month | Rarely |
| Sweets/candies/pastries/cookies/cakes/ice cream/frozen yogurts | 1-2x/week | 2x/month | 1x/month-rarely |
| Coffee/caf, or decaf | 1 cup/day | 2x/week | 1x month-Rarely |
| Alcohol organic red wine/beer | 1 glass 3-7x/week | 3x/week | 1x/wk.-rarely |
| Restaurant food Food quality is often diminished (non-organic, rancid oils, MSG, GMO's, sugar, additives) | 1-2x/week. Try to find slow-food, farm-to-table restaurants | 1x/ week. Try to find slow-food, farm-to-table restaurants | 2-4x/month-rarely Try to find slow-food, farm-to-table restaurants |

**Exercise 3d: Write your indulgent food frequency level on your plan. Remember to indulge wisely.**

---

**Making changes** to your daily diet however may likely trigger a few withdrawal symptoms, especially if you consume a lot of sugar, refined foods, coffee, alcohol and very few vegetables. These symptoms are nothing to worry about as they indicate that you are eliminating stored toxins, and that your body is rebalancing. The symptoms should abate after a few days. Various symptoms that you may experience are: bad breath, constipation, body odor, nausea, headaches, fatigue, itchy skin, irritability, sleeping problems, and achy, flu-like symptoms. Plan to drink plenty of filtered water to aid detoxification, and take magnesium citrate to clear bowels to prevent headaches and constipation. Consider resting more, and walking daily. Above all be nurturing and kind to yourself as you transition to a healthier diet.

Chapter Four

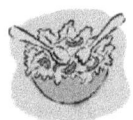

# Macronutrients: Our Primary Food Constituents

## Protein, Fats, and Carbohydrates

Macronutrients are nutrients that provide calories or energy for our bodies. There are three broad classes of macronutrients: protein, fats, and carbohydrates. Macronutrients are required in our body in large amounts; as opposed to vitamins and minerals, which are required in smaller amounts. Macronutrients play a role in promoting growth and development and in regulating our bodily functions.

To facilitate optimal wellness, it is important to select macronutrients in the most favorable proportions for our unique health needs, metabolism, and constitution. The percentage of calories we get from the various macronutrients (macronutrient balance) is the basis for what is known as the "diet direction." There are three distinct health promoting diet directions that we can follow or cycle through in our life: <u>building, cleansing, and balancing</u>. When we follow certain diet directions, we are basically eating more of certain kinds of macronutrients and less of others. Our needs for varying diet directions however may fluctuate throughout our life and should not be rigidly held.

A *Building Diet* focuses on a higher percentage of calories from **fat and proteins** relative to carbohydrates (30-40% from fats, 25-30% from proteins and 30-45% from carbohydrates) The building type of diet is one of **fewer starchy carbs, with more proteins**: (4-6 servings of animal and vegetable proteins) **and fats:** nuts, seeds, avocado, olives, butter etc. Due to its warming and reparative qualities, it is strengthening to pregnant women, laborers, and athletes. It is also very recuperative for individuals who are recovering from illnesses or injuries; have mood problems; or who are under chronic stress. Additionally, those who suffer from immune or endocrine disorders or carb cravings feel healthier on this regime. Individuals who have a fast metabolism benefit from this direction also. However, it is crucial to add leafy greens when adhering to this diet direction in order to keep the system alkaline. The *Paleo Diet* or the *Zone Diet* can be examples of the building diet approach.

A *Balancing Diet* consists of **nearly equal** and **lesser amounts of protein and fats** relative to carbohydrates. This diet supplies about 15-25% of calories from proteins, 15-25% of calories from fats, and 50-70% of calories from complex carbohydrates, such as whole grains, vegetables and fruits. The balancing diet is a maintenance diet that can be adhered to for a long duration. The *Cancer* and *Heart Association Diets,* as well as the *Mediterranean diet* are examples of balanced diets.

A ***Cleansing Diet*** is comprised of a considerable amount **more calories from carbohydrates (vegetables and fruits: 60-80%)** relative to proteins (10-20%) and fats. (10-20%) This cooling diet emphasizes decreased fat consumption; and lower, but adequate vegetable protein consumption. (Beans, nuts, seeds, and marine algae) Dairy and animal proteins are typically eliminated and generous amounts of fresh fruits, vegetables, juices, herbs and algae powders are consumed to restore mineral status. Cleansing diets are therapeutically employed as detoxification cleanses to alkalinize and rid the body of accrued toxins. They can be utilized after a day or week of junk food overindulging, or as a seasonal cleanse. This diet should only be followed for a short duration however, (7-14 days) because it provides too little protein, and can lead to protein deficiencies. *Detox* diets, and often the *Raw,* and *Vegan* diets are examples of cleansing diets.

It is important to note that our nutrient needs can vary yearly, seasonally, daily, and even hourly; therefore, our nutrient requirements and macronutrient balance may need to be modified to support our changing needs. It is a good practice to tune into your body and try to be aware of your cravings and how certain combinations of foods affect you. After you have been making healthy food choices for a while, it will be fairly easy to tell if your body craves and needs more protein or fat one day, or less of them the next.

*Exercise 4a: Determine what diet direction is currently best for you according to your constitution or health conditions. (Be conscious of your changing needs.)*

## Proteins and a Healthy Digestion

Adequate protein is necessary for optimal health. Generally, the typical American SAD diet is too high in protein, especially meat; which places a burden on the kidneys and liver, and increases our risk for osteoporosis, and gout. Conversely, individuals that consume excess starchy carbohydrates, such as breads, pastas, and French fries may be deficient in protein. Dieters and vegans may also not be getting enough protein.

Proteins are the building blocks and primary components of our body, after water. Proteins are necessary for the building and repair of all our tissues and body systems. This is important for keeping our muscles, blood, bones, nails, hair, tendons, and ligaments youthful and strong as we age; and to aid in recovery from illness. Protein is also necessary to synthesize enzymes, hormones, neurotransmitters and our genes. Without sufficient protein, we may suffer from hormone imbalances or mood, and cognitive problems. Protein is also necessary for daily detoxification processes. If we don't consume sufficient amounts of protein, our liver will not be able to complete phase 2 detoxification processes; the phase where toxins are neutralized in the body. Protein is also vital for boosting the immune system; as inadequate protein intake lessens our resistance to infections and viruses. In addition, protein unlike carbohydrates provides us with sustained energy and staying power; necessary for keeping balanced blood sugar levels.

Proteins are made up of building blocks called amino acids. We need 23 amino acids for our bodies to function well, and our body can synthesize some protein itself. There are 9 amino acids that the body cannot make, and these have to be obtained from food. These are known as essential amino acids. The essential amino acids are: histidine (essential during growth) isoleucine, leucine, lysine, methionine, phenylalanine, threonine, tryptophan, and valine. A complete protein consists of all eight essential amino acids. You will find the sources of complete protein in all animal products: meats, poultry, dairy, eggs, and fish. Plant foods often lack one or more amino acids, and thus need to be combined to obtain the required levels of essential amino acids. Grains are limited in lysine; beans are limited in methionine; and nuts and seeds are limited in methionine and lysine. Many foods can be combined to achieve a complete protein profile, however. Examples are: beans with brown rice or quinoa.

Whether or not to eat animal protein is a personal choice. **Nutritionally** speaking, the **quality** of the protein source is more important than whether it comes from animals or plants. We all have individual needs (biochemical individuality) and no one diet fits all people; some people feel better and thrive on animal proteins; while others feel sluggish eating them. Some individuals flourish on eating only vegetable protein, especially those with a slower metabolism; while others, particularly those with a faster metabolism, experience hunger, fatigue and poor immunity without animal protein. And a number of people feel their best on a mix of the two. It's important to experiment and pay attention to your own body's needs; although people with blood sugar imbalances often need to eat high quality animal proteins. (Hyman, 2012)

Consuming animal protein does confer many health advantages owing to its high nutrient-value, however. This allows us to eat less - compared with vegetable proteins. Additionally, animal protein (especially fish, eggs, grass-fed beef, buffalo and game meat) is our best source of DHA; the main constituent of cell membranes in our brain. A deficiency of DHA can leave us vulnerable to brain diseases.

Harvard Medical School's, *Harvard Health Publication,* reported after reviewing the large scale EPIC-Oxford vegetarian study that: "A purely vegetarian diet is not necessarily better than a plant-based diet that also includes poultry and fish." The study also revealed that fish eaters had a lower risk for some cancers. The researchers concluded that there is no scientific validation for eliminating meat from the diet; but that all diets should be well balanced, contain a wide variety of foods, and include plenty of fruits and vegetables.

Many leading authorities believe that previous research studies that reported positive outcomes from a vegetarian diet had to do more with an increased vegetable intake, and a lower protein intake by vegetarians, rather than from excluding meat from the diet. Additionally, many earlier studies on the harmful effects of meat were often confounded by factors such as smoking, BMI, social class and poor animal protein quality.

If you do follow a strict vegetarian or vegan diet, or are interested in doing so, it is important to ensure that you eat adequate protein; as research published in 2012 in the journal *Nutrition* reported that vegetarians and particularly vegans may suffer from subclinical protein malnourishment. The study confirmed that this malnourishment leads to a sulfur deficiency; which can cause many health difficulties- including problems with detoxification, bones, joints, connective tissue, and metabolic processes. The study also discovered that the low sulfur intake by vegetarians and vegans produced damaging high homocysteine levels; which can increase the risk for blood clots and cardiovascular disease.

As we age, our body also may have changing requirements. The diet and protein source that was right for us when we were younger may not be what it needs in middle age. It is always best to listen to our body, and to honor our natural protein cravings. If we are not thriving on a particular diet any longer, than it is not the right diet for us.

Also, climate, and seasons have an impact on the kinds of foods that our body needs. Raw foods and vegetable proteins cleanse and cool the body; while animal foods strengthen and warm the body. In cooler climates and weather our body will feel better with warming and comforting animal proteins. In summer and in warm climates our body may want light cleansing vegetable proteins, and raw vegetables. In addition, our body may crave animal proteins when we are under stress, exercising more or are recuperating from an illness or injury. Our body will also have a natural desire to detoxify of animal proteins in the spring, and therefore may not crave them then. Individuals who suffer from weak stomach acid production can also experience reduced cravings for meat and other animal proteins, due to their difficulty in digesting them.

---

A moderate consumption of organic pastured grass-fed animal protein (3-4 oz.) can be health promoting due to its high nutrient profile. Epidemiological studies singly correlate the consumption of **commercial, non-organic, and nitrate containing meats** with chronic diseases such as cancer, heart disease, arthritis, diabetes, and Alzheimer's disease; not with grass-fed, pastured organic varieties. Adding to their favor, animal proteins are complete proteins, and contain superior quantities of zinc, iron, sulfur, fat-soluble vitamins (A,D,E, and K2) and B-complex vitamins; particularly B12, which is inferior in most vegetable proteins.

As mentioned above, the healthfulness of our diet is determined by the quality of the animal protein we chose to eat. However, making animal protein choices can often be confusing due to the bewildering array of labeling terms. There are so many options to consider today: conventionally-fed (supermarket meats) organic, grass-fed, certified 100% grass-fed, pastured, grain-fed, cage-free, free-range etc. The following information will provide you with the standard to look for on animal protein labels.

**The Top Choice:** (*best*) for selecting red meats and dairy is to buy **Certified 100% grass-fed organic products**, also termed pastured and finished. The pastured cow's sole diet is grass; it hasn't been fattened-up by omega-6 rich soy and corn when it reaches market weight, as some cows are. Conventionally raised animals conversely, are raised in confined feed-lots; are given hormones and antibiotics, and fed non-organic GMO grains. The quality of the protein from 100% grass-fed organic red meats and dairy is far greater than conventional grain-fed varieties. Pastured meat contains a similar beneficial fat profile to wild game. Less than 10% of pastured animal's total fat is saturated fats, compared with conventional grain-fed animals that contain 50% of saturated fats. They also contain 2-4 times the heart healthy omega-3 fat content than grain-fed animal proteins. According to a 2011 study published in *The British Journal of Medicine*, participants who ate moderate amounts of grass-fed meats had healthier levels of omega-3 essential fats in their blood.

Additionally, grass-fed animals possess four times higher levels of vitamin E, and increased vitamin A, B, D, and beta carotene levels. They also provide the crucial bone-building vitamin known as vitamin K2, which is absent in conventionally raised animal protein. Adding to their merit, they are 3 to 5 times higher in the cancer protective and anti-inflammatory conjugated linoleic acid (CLA.) Most importantly, pastured animals don't possess toxic GMO's, pesticides, growth hormones, antibiotic residues, or an imbalanced inflammation promoting omega-6 content. Additionally, they don't contribute to greenhouse gasses as conventionally-fed cows do.

GMO corn and soy, the standard diet that is given to feed lot animals, is not the diet that these animals were evolved to eat. Cows, for instance are ruminants, and their natural diet should be grasses. When animals are fed unsuitable omega-6 rich grains (corn and soy) they incorporate this fat into their flesh. When we eat the meat from them we also integrate this omega-6 fat into our own cell membranes. However, this fat is not necessary for our cells in great amounts and an excess promotes compromised cell function, and inflammation.

**The Top Choice** for selecting **eggs and poultry** is to buy **certified 100% organic pastured;** as opposed to free-range or cage-free labeled varieties. 100% organic pastured chickens roam free most of the time feeding on nutritive grasses, weeds, worms and insects with occasional supplementation of grain; plus they lay their eggs right in the fields where they roam. These chickens and their eggs have much higher levels of vitamin A, vitamin E, vitamin D, and beta-carotenes; with two times more omega-3's. It is easy to tell if chickens have been in the sun and pastured full time or part of the time. Foraging chickens produce bright orange egg yolks, as opposed to chickens that don't forage; which synthesize pale yellow yolks.

**The Second Best Choice: (*better*)** when selecting meats, dairy, eggs and poultry is to purchase products simply labeled **organic.** National Organic Program Standards (NOP) demand that the animals must have been born and raised on a certified organic pasture with unrestricted outdoor access. They also must not have been treated with growth hormones, antibiotics or been given GMO foods. The cows, however are fattened by organic grains when they reach market weight; therefore their omega-3 content will be lower than 100% pastured and finished animals. Organic chickens and their eggs may or may not be foraging for their food in the out-of-doors.

**The Third Best Choice: (*good*)** is labeled **free-range with no hormones or antibiotics.** Free Range labeled eggs and poultry are raised in sheltered facilities with a small door to the outside. However many chickens do not notice the door, and often don't actually go outside. Free-range also doesn't specify the outdoor conditions, it often is a concrete slab that chickens use for 5 minutes a day. These chickens however are not given harmful antibiotics or hormones. The label of **cage-free** on eggs means that chickens are not put in cages, however they still are in an enclosed facility, and it could be small with very little room to run around.

When animals are crowded into tight quarters and are fed an inappropriate diet, they develop health problems. Hence, the need for antibiotics in factory farmed animals. Pastured animals that eat appropriate nutritious foods are healthier animals, and healthy animals make healthier food for us!

Certified 100% pastured meat, dairy and eggs are often not found in supermarkets and frequently are not found in health food stores either. It is a good idea to be your own detective. Don't be afraid to ask questions about the source of the meats in stores. If you can't find pastured products in your stores; you can often find pastured organic eggs at farmers' markets. Additionally, there are websites that offer information on where to find pastured organic animal proteins in your area. The websites: "Eat Wild," "Local Harvest," "American grass-fed.org," and the local "Weston A. Price" chapter can point you to resources and farms in your area that sell and deliver pastured products. These products can be pricey, but if you buy in bulk, or split the cost with friends, the meats can be quite economical.

For those of us on a tight budget, we still can eat healthfully. Choosing economical proteins such as organic eggs, beans, miso, tempeh, canned wild fish, home-made bone stock, and a small amount of organic poultry, or hormone-free and antibiotic-free meats can be a more budget friendly and still healthy option.

With regards to the **quantity** of the meat consumed, it is best not to eat **over-sized portions** of animal proteins. Proteins have high quantities of phosphorous, which can decrease our absorption of calcium. Overindulging in meat protein can also promote an excess of nitrogen waste products, which can overwork our kidneys by its removal. In addition, excessive protein consumption is capable of having a stimulating effect on the mammalian target of rapamycin gene (mTOR) a cancer correlated pathway in our body. The mTOR pathway is held back however, with modest meat consumption. Finally, by consuming less meat you make room for more plants in your diet; which increases your antioxidant protection.

A good rule of thumb is to mix up the types of proteins throughout the day or week; some animal, some vegetable. A number of people need animal protein daily with each meal;

while others only need it several times a week, or not at all. It is important to note that the documented and scientifically studied long-lived cultures of the world have or had a moderate intake of animal proteins.

It is advised to make a mental note to include three servings of mineral rich vegetables (leafy and crunchy) per animal protein serving. Meat is acid-forming, and does exert an acidifying effect on the blood. Adding alkaline forming vegetables neutralizes the acidifying effect that animal proteins generate in the blood.

## Signs of protein deficiency

| Premature skin aging, loss of muscle tone, thin hair, weak nails | Curved spine, low bone-density, slow healing wounds | Tooth/gum decay tingling/numbness blurred vision | Poor immunity, sick often, hormonal imbalances, low sex drive, high toxic load |
|---|---|---|---|
| Low energy, weakness, fatigue, muscle weakness | Anxiety/mood disorders, agitation | Spaciness, brain fog/ confusion/poor concentration | Food cravings, loss of appetite, weight loss, anemia |

## Conditions caused by animal protein excess

| Kidney disease/gout | Heart disease | High blood pressure |
|---|---|---|
| Calcium loss/Osteoporosis Musculoskeletal issues | Cancer | Arthritis |
| Constipation/decay in gut/ammonia in blood | Vitamin B6 depletion | Acidosis and dehydration |

## Protein Requirements

To meet the daily protein requirements: 2-4 servings of protein are generally sufficient. A serving size of animal protein is 3-4 oz.; about the size of the palm of your hand, and the thickness of a deck of cards. A serving size for eggs is 2 to 3. A serving size for a vegetable protein is between 6 oz. to 12 oz. depending on the source. (3/4c. -1 ½ c.) Your protein needs can also vary with age, weight, physical activity and illness. Individuals who lift weights or exercise intensely will need to up their protein intake by 15% or more. Additionally, to prevent burnout during high stress times, consider increasing your protein intake.

## Protein Content:

Note: Grams of proteins are not the same as the total weight of the protein source (proteins sources contain other macronutrients in addition to protein.) Look on packages for protein content.

| Protein Source | Grams Protein |
|---|---|
| Beef | 7 g per ounce |
| Chicken | 9-11g per ounce |
| Fish | 6 g per ounce |
| Large egg | 6 g each |
| Medium cheese (cheddar/swiss) | 7-8 g per oz. |
| Yogurt (1 cup) | 8-12 g per cup |
| Beans (1 cup) cooked<br>lentils-17 g<br>kidney beans-16 g<br>black beans-16 g<br>lima, garbanzo and black-eyed peas-14 g | 14-17 g per cup<br><br>*Needs to be combined with grains for a complete protein |
| Nuts/seeds (1/4 cup) | 4-8 g per ¼ cup |
| Nut butters (2 Tbsp.) | 8 g |
| Whole grains (1/2 c.)<br>quinoa-4.7 g<br>amaranth-4 g<br>steel cut oats- 3.5 g<br>buckwheat-3 g<br>brown rice-2.5 g | 2.5-4.7 g per half cup<br><br>*Needs to be combined with beans/legumes for a complete protein |
| Miso-2 tsp. | 1 g |
| Tempeh- (1 cup) | 31 g per cup |
| Nutritional yeast (1 Tbsp.) | 3 g |
| Spirulina/chlorella: Tbsp. | 4 g (20 % usable) |

**Exercise 4b: Protein Needs Formula.** There is a general formula that you can use to determine your protein needs. Your needs may vary however, according to activity level, state of health, or how you feel (energy-wise.) Most people generally need between 45 to 75 grams of protein per day. (Thirteen to twenty five grams+ per meal)

*Multiply .36 grams by your ideal weight in pounds. (Or .8 grams by your weight in kilograms.) For example: a women who weighs 130 lbs. would need about 46.8 grams of protein daily.*

- Enter your daily protein intake in grams into your Personal Wellness Plan. For several days, try to add up the total amount of protein you are eating each day. Does it total the amount in the protein formula? Observe how you feel. If you feel weak, or still crave protein you may need more.
- Determine if you may have a protein excess or deficiency in your diet. (determine from charts/symptoms)

---

### Protein Sources

*Grass-fed red meat and beef*, when eaten in moderation (2 or less- times a week) is very health promoting, and has no greater effect on cholesterol than poultry. Scientific evidence suggests that it is not the moderate consumption of red meat that may cause cancer and heart disease; but the way that meat is cooked. Research at the University of South Carolina discovered that women who ate well-done red meats had a high risk for developing breast cancer. Carcinogens are formed from high temperature cooking, especially from grilling, charbroiling, and blackening meat. These toxic forms of amino acids (heterocyclic amines) and toxic lipid peroxides damage cell membranes, and cell DNA.

Medium-rare organic or grass-fed red meats are a healthy source of concentrated nutrients; and provide high protein, and an excellent quantity of the cellular supportive B12 and B6 vitamins. 100% organic grass-fed beef is the preferred meat, as the longer the duration the animals ingest grasses; the higher the omega-3 content will be. Organic or grass-fed beef also contains the antioxidants: conjugated linoleic acid (cancer protective), carnitine (brain protective), as well as CoEnzymeQ10 (heart protective.) However, it is suggested to eat red meat in moderation as the high purines that red meat contains can cause gout, and kidney stones in susceptible people.

*Lamb*, another red meat, is lower in fat than conventional red meat, and is an excellent source of vitamin B12 and protein; and a good source of selenium, niacin and zinc. Lamb is a good meat choice in restaurants; as commercial lamb is generally pastured and not given hormones, or antibiotics.

*Poultry*: Organic or pastured chicken and turkey are low fat, high quality proteins that contain two times more omega 3-fatty acids and more vitamin A, D and E then conventional grain-fed chickens. Chicken, especially in chicken bone broth soup, is immune boosting and known to give relief for the common cold. Both chicken and turkey are high in selenium, niacin, and vitamin B6. In addition, chicken, duck and goose include a large quantity of heart healthy mono-unsaturated fat content. However, it is advised to enquire whether the poultry you choose are actually out eating grasses and bugs etc.; as some free-range labeled poultry don't chose to go outdoors; even though they have access to it.

*Ostrich, rabbit, elk, venison, and other game animals* are lower fat beef alternatives. These animal proteins are usually grass-fed, and free-range, and contain high levels of omega-3 fatty acids.

*Buffalo,* typically grass-fed, is especially nutrient dense, low in fat, and contains very high omega-3 fatty acid content. It also has the highest known levels of conjugated linoleic acid; which is valued for reducing the risk of cancer, diabetes, obesity and immune disorders. It also features high quantities of selenium, vitamin E, beta carotene, iron, and vitamin B12.

*Pastured Pork and Ham* are good sources of protein and B vitamins, and have higher levels of omega-3 fats and vitamin D than pigs in confinement. Pork in general however, is associated with worms and parasites. It has been found that pasture rotated pigs who eat alfalfa as forage possess fewer parasites than confined factory farmed pigs. Use your own judgment in making the decision on whether to eat pig meat.

*Fish and Seafood* are high quality nutrient dense proteins with excellent levels of vitamins and minerals. The abundant quantity of heart healthy Omega-3 fatty acids in fish and seafood have garnered them a "super food" status. All seafood, and fish contain some Omega-3 oils, but some have more than others. More than 2,000 scientific studies have concluded that more than sixty different health conditions are prevented by a higher intake of omega-3 fatty acids; especially heart disease, cancer, Alzheimer's, asthma, diabetes, high blood pressure, macular degeneration, multiple sclerosis, and rheumatoid arthritis.

***Seafood Dangers***: Even though the health benefits of eating sea food are considerable, it's consumption can be dangerous to our health and should be limited unfortunately, due to mercury, pesticide contamination, industrial carcinogenic PCB's, and possible radioactive pollutants. Large predator fish concentrate the highest amounts of mercury; such as shark, swordfish, pollock, marlin, grouper, pike, mahi mahi, tile fish and albacore tuna, and should be avoided. In addition, to reduce toxin exposure from fish and seafood, limit fish from inland lakes. Eat only open ocean deep-water fish, and eat smaller, young fish which have less time to accumulate toxins. If you like tuna, and don't want to eliminate it completely; skip jack, and light tuna are smaller sized tuna with less toxic concentrations. See the EWG tuna calculator to calculate how much tuna a week you can eat safely, according to your weight.

***Safe Seafood:*** *The Safe Sustainable Seafood Guide* from the organization- *Green America* lists the fish and seafood that are considered safe to eat in modest amounts. They include: wild anchovies, calamari, clams, crawfish, dungenous crab, stone crab, summer flounder, haddock, hake, herring, king crab, lobster, (spiny and rock) mid Atlantic blue crab, northern U.S. farmed shrimp, and white shrimp; oysters, wild Alaskan salmon, perch, sardines, bay scallops,(farmed) sole, spot prawn, wild tilapia, and whitefish. It is advised to avoid all farmed fish however due to their GMO, omega-6- heavy and toxic diet.

***Highly Recommended Wild Fish*** that contain <u>concentrated quantities</u> of heart healthy omega-3 fatty acids, with less toxin accumulations are: all wild pacific ocean salmon, small sized mackerel, herring, anchovy, and sardines. Eating these fish three to four times a week will supply you with the necessary Omega-3 fats desirable for optimal health. Fish should be wild, (not farmed) small sized and from cold waters. Canned fish with bones offers additional calcium. Try to find BPA free cans to limit toxin exposure. It is essential for our health to obtain adequate levels of omega-3 oils.

If you don't like the taste of fish or are concerned about possible contaminants and still want to obtain the essential omega-3 oils, I suggest "Green Pastures" brand fermented cod liver oil. It is the highest quality, most nutrient-dense cod liver oil on the market today with superior health benefits compared to regular unfermented oils. Regular cod liver all is extracted with high heat, which decreases nutrient content. Fermented cod liver oil however is not heated, therefore the important nutrients are saved. (Vitamins A, D, E and K) Green Pastures also tests its oil for purity from pollutants.

***Dairy*** consumption is a controversial subject. The high heat of modern day dairy pasteurization has rendered most dairy foods enzyme and nutrient depleted. Additionally pasteurization makes dairy very indigestible and highly allergenic. This is the main reason why pasteurized dairy is much more allergenic than raw dairy. Also, the addition of the recombinant bovine growth hormone (r BGH) in most non-organic milks since 1990 is cause for alarm.

However, contrary to flawed dietary advice, dairy is not essential for humans after weaning, nor is it essential to prevent osteoporosis. Asians consume no dairy, but have very low rates of osteoporosis; while Americans who consume excessive quantities of pasteurized dairy, suffer from the highest rates of osteoporosis.

Grass-fed raw milk does, however contain a rich source of protein and nutrients, including cancer protective conjugated linoleic acid (CLA) and health promoting protein fragments- the most noteworthy being lactoferrin. Lactoferrin is cited for its anti-viral and immune boosting effects. Two fatty acids in milk- butyric acid, and sphingomyelin have also been shown to exert anti-cancer effects.

If you enjoy drinking milk, the optimal milk to drink is raw pastured/grass fed whole milk. Raw milk maintains its nutrient and protein profile, and its digestive supporting enzymes. There is very little possibility of bacterial contamination when buying organic grass-fed raw milk. Choose cow, goat or sheep etc.

<u>Reduced-fat</u> dairy though does not provide the necessary natural fat soluble vitamins that whole milk contains or the essential fatty acids. In addition, milk solids and whey proteins are added to low fat varieties for flavor and texture; which increases problematic lactose levels. *The Journal of Clinical Nutrition,* after reviewing studies on whole milk consumption, concluded that the more <u>full-fat</u> (as opposed to reduced-fat) dairy that people consume; the lower the risk of heart attack.

*Cultured plain kefir and yogurt,* made from organic whole milk dairy is an even healthier dairy option. Culturing milk adds probiotics (<u>beneficial bacteria</u>) to it; which aids digestion, immune health, and vitamin synthesis in the body. Countless people in mid-life suffer from a lack of beneficial bacteria, amid an overload of bad bacteria; a condition known as dysbiosis. Years of sugar, stress, antibiotics, poor digestion and medications have resulted in this imbalanced bacterial state. Dysbiosis, and candida fungal overgrowth may be- according to many health professionals, one of the hidden root causes of innumerable ailments, and diseases.

It is suggested, however to make certain to look for the claim "**<u>Live and Active</u>**," on the labels of yogurts and kefirs; otherwise you won't be getting viable beneficial bacteria in the product. It is also advised to not buy sweetened yogurt and kefir because sugar supplies food (sugar) for bad bacteria; which defeats the purpose of eating probiotic-rich foods in the first place. Sweetening your own yogurt with berries, 1/3 mashed banana or stevia is a better idea. Additionally, it is easy to make your own kefir and yogurt at home with a starter culture. If you are casein sensitive, you can still enjoy cultured coconut or almond yogurt with similar probiotic health benefits. Young coconut water kefir is another probiotic-dense option. Consider consuming yogurt and kefir daily for bacterial balance and immune and gut health protection.

Many people as they age become dairy and lactose intolerant due to casein sensitivity, (the former) and lactase enzyme depletion (the latter). Many however, have had the enzyme deficit since childhood and are now feeling the effects more readily. Genetic research confirms that most of our hunter-gatherer ancestors were dairy intolerant after they were weaned from their mothers. Certain ethnic groups however who depended highly on milk developed genetic mutations that allowed them to continue to produce lactase, the enzyme that digests dairy. Scandinavians have the lowest rates of lactose intolerance, while Asians, Native Americans and African-Americans have the highest rates of lactose intolerance.

If you do experience symptoms from dairy, it means that your body can not digest and absorb these foods. As a result, the undigested dairy will build-up and ferment in your gut, thus providing food for bad bacteria and other opportunistic organisms. This can lead to candida albicans overgrowth, immune function weaknesses, leaky gut, iron deficiency, and bone density loss.

*Symptoms of lactose (milk sugar) intolerances are:*

| digestive problems (flatulence, diarrhea, bloating, spasms) | Excess mucous in the sinuses | Mucous in the stools | Needing to clear phlegm from the throat often. |
|---|---|---|---|

*Symptoms of casein (milk protein) sensitivities are:*

| Diarrhea | Constipation | Flatulence, bloating, abdominal cramps | Leaky gut, irritable Bowel Syndrome (IBS) |
|---|---|---|---|
| Joint pain | Fatigue | Behavior issues after consuming dairy | Asthma, rashes, autoimmune conditions |

Some people, depending on their genetic composition and gut health, might do just fine with certain dairy products. Generally, though, many people have problems with it. Consider a dairy-free diet for a month to see if your symptoms abate and you feel better.

You may find that you are in the majority of lactose-intolerant people of the world. Coconut milk, rice milk, and nut milks are tasty alternatives. If you do eliminate dairy from your diet, make sure to increase your consumption of calcium rich foods such as: dark leafy greens, soaked almonds, sunflower seeds, and sesame seeds, bone broth soup, canned sardines and salmon (with bones) and sea vegetables- to substitute for the dairy.

Also, if you suffer from lactose intolerance, taking supplemental <u>lactase digestive enzymes</u> with dairy may help with its absorption. Raw dairy also may help, due to its natural enzyme component. Cultured dairy is another food you can try, as it contains no lactose if it has been cultured for 24 hours or more. (Many yogurts are only cultured for 4-6 hours) Some organic yogurts are labeled lactose-free, however. Goat milk is also a possible alternative. Goat milk has a different lactose and protein profile than cow milk and is closer in structure to human milk. Also try goat milk whey, cheese, and yogurt. Butter and cream have only traces of lactose, and some lactose intolerant individuals can tolerate them. Ghee (similar to butter) is totally free of casein, and lactose. Limit dairy to one to two times a day.

Note: As of 2014, raw milk, especially grass-fed cow, goat and sheep milk from California may contain some amounts of radioactive contaminants from the nuclear fallout from Fukishima, Japan. It is suggested to enquire if ranchers are spraying radiation-absorbing boron on the pastures to protect their herds.

## *Proteins with High Biological Value*

When a protein contains the essential amino acids in the optimal proportion, it is considered to have a high biological value. It is the "gold standard" of proteins. Eggs and non-denatured whey protein powder are considered to have the highest biological value of any other protein.

***Organic non-denatured whey protein powder*** is a great high quality protein sourced from dairy and made from the process of separating the solid curds from the liquid whey. Adding a scoopful to a breakfast smoothie can be a great start to your day. Whey contains very little lactose, and very small amounts of casein. Whey is also supportive of muscle growth and repair, detoxification and immunity due to its high levels of branch chained amino acids, and lactoferrin. Whey also synthesizes our own internal master-antioxidant known as glutathione. Make sure the whey is un-denatured, and preferably grass-fed. Note: whey may contain radioactive contaminants from the Fukishima, Japan radioactive fallout, if from California grass-fed cows and goats. Check whether the pastures are sprayed with boron to protect the herds.

***Eggs, particularly egg yolks*** have an exceptional nutritional profile. Eggs are mineral and vitamin B rich and are nourishing for your brain, thyroid, and hormones. They are the richest source of the eye-protective lutein and zeaxanthin. Several recent studies have debunked the theory that eggs promote high cholesterol. In *The Journal of the American Medical Association,* it was reported that individuals who ate four eggs a week had lower serum cholesterol levels than people who ate only one egg a week. Additionally, the egg consumers were shown to have increased nutritional intake from the egg consumption. Eggs are also an excellent source of choline. Choline synthesizes one of the brain's chief neurotransmitters- acetylcholine. Acetylcholine is exceedingly important for brain function. Eggs also contain betaine, a nutrient which is recognized for decreasing blood vessel damaging homocysteine levels.

The upshot from these research findings is that most individuals can eat up to three eggs a day safely. (12 a week.) The highest quality eggs are 100% pasture raised. These chickens have received their nourishment from foraging. Pastured eggs are 30% richer in vitamin E and are higher in vitamin D, vitamin A, vitamin K2, folic acid and B12. You can tell if a hen is foraging outside by the color of the egg yolk; if it is orangey (and not light yellow) it has been feeding outdoors. Eggs should be cooked quickly, as B-vitamins are heat sensitive. Organic eggs can be eaten raw; but the egg white must be removed to maintain biotin content due to the fact that raw egg whites bind with biotin and interfere with its absorption.

*Legumes* (green peas, lentils, and dried beans etc.) are an excellent source of fiber and protein; having more than two to four times as much protein as grains. They also are a good source of folic acid, molybdenum, iron, magnesium, manganese and potassium. The major health benefits that they provide come from their cholesterol and blood sugar lowering high-fiber content. They also contribute to heart health. Eating beans, and lentils two or more times a week was associated in a Nurses' Health Study with a 24% reduced risk for breast cancer. In addition, beans are a featured protein in healthy Mediterranean diets. According to studies conducted by the *U.S. Department of Agriculture*; richly colored beans are extremely high in antioxidants. Small red beans are rated as having one of the highest antioxidant values. For optimal health; eat four or more cups per week. Soak for 12 hours or more in water with a little vinegar to release anti-nutrient phytates that hinder mineral absorption and digestion. Note: In order to get the required grams of protein; you will have to eat 3/4 cup-1 ½ cups of beans/legumes per meal; as beans contain between 14 to 17 g. of protein per cup. Garbanzo bean flour is a healthy low-carb substitute for grain flours in cooking and baking.

*Aduki* beans are one of the most nutrient-dense beans, as they are packed with trace minerals. A one half cup of aduki beans provide almost 200% of the daily recommended intake of molybdenum, which is very important for liver detoxification. A shortage of this mineral is associated with Parkinson's, Alzheimer's, arthritis, delayed food sensitivity, and chemical sensitivity.

Note: Some individuals have difficulty digesting beans. Cooking the beans with the sea vegetable- kombu can support its digestion. The product known as "Beano" can also be used. Additionally, sprouting beans can increase their nutritional value, and can improve digestibility. Sprouting beans at home is easy and economical. Lentils, garbanzo beans, alfalfa, and mung beans are commonly sprouted. There are sprouting jars and trays available for easy sprouting.

*Nuts/seeds* are good fiber and protein sources; and have important monounsaturated fats and phytonutrients. They are also the best source of the amino acid arginine; which plays an important role in blood vessel and cardiovascular health. Two large scale studies including the *Nurses' Health Study*, and the *Physicians' Health Study*, found that nut consumption is linked to a decreased risk for heart disease. In other large scale studies, people who ate the most nuts were found to have less obesity, possibly due to the satiety effect of nuts. In addition, studies show that nuts protect against diabetes. Substituting nuts for an equivalent amount of starchy carbohydrates is a good approach to enhance weight loss, and your health. Cashews are an exception however; as they contain a higher amount of carbohydrates. It's best to choose other lower carb nuts for your snacking, especially if you suffer from obesity, or diabetes, as cashews often promote overeating.

*Flax seeds* are the most plentiful source of health-giving plant lignans. Lignans wield important anti-cancer effects. In research studies, it was revealed that women who ingested flax seeds had reduced levels of cancer-promoting excess estrogen in their blood. Reducing estrogen diminishes breast cancer risk. It was also found in studies that consuming two Tbsp. of flaxseed meal daily was effective in preventing prostate cancer. In addition, flax seed meal was discovered to improve cholesterol, and triglyceride levels. Flax seeds contain the highest levels of alpha linolenic acid; an omega-3 precursor. It is advised to <u>grind the flax seed into a meal</u>; as the seed coat is too hard to digest properly. It's also recommended to grind flax seeds at home in a coffee grinder once a week to keep the seeds from going rancid, and store them in the freezer. (No need to soak)

*Almonds* are also chock-full of nutrients. They have a reputation as an anti-cancer food due to their high concentrations of antioxidant flavonoids. They also are high sources of potassium, magnesium, calcium, iron, zinc, vitamin E, and fiber. Almonds have demonstrated beneficial effects at lowering cholesterol, and reversing heart disease. Choose raw (best) or dry roasted forms. You can salt your own nuts with sea salt. Almond flour is also widely used as a low carb substitute for grain flours.

Consider soaking nuts and large seeds in water with a little vinegar for 12+ hours- to release the anti-nutrient "phytic acid." Phytic acid binds minerals, and blocks their absorption in the body. After soaking the seeds and nuts; dry nuts in a dehydrator, or on a cookie sheet on the lowest setting on the oven. Refrigerate or freeze.

*Hemp, rice, and yellow pea protein powders* are also excellent vegetarian alternative high-protein powders that can be prepared into morning shakes or afternoon energy drinks. (Mix rice protein powder with hemp or pea for complete protein.) Hemp protein powder contains the fatty acid GLA; which is recognized to prevent inflammation.

*Unfermented high-heat processed soy foods* such as soy cheese, veggie meat substitutes, T.V.P. and soy protein isolates are **not a healthful meat alternative**; as they contain high salt levels, and are sourced from GMO soy, if not labeled organic. Additionally, the high (protein-damaging) temperatures used in the processing of soy, render soy low in nutritional value. Moreover, processed soy contains high amounts of aluminum, and M.S.G. (formed during the high heat processing) which has been shown to weaken cognitive function. Finally, regular consumption of soy, tofu, soy protein powder, and soy milk block thyroid function due to their high goitrogenic anti-nutrients; and goitrogens block iodine uptake in the thyroid. Lastly, soy contains phytic acid; an anti-nutrient which reduces mineral absorption in the body. Sprouted tofu is a better option, as its phytic acid content is neutralized. Small quantities of tofu; as in miso soup seem to be tolerated in Asian cultures. Note: Soy is a common food allergen, and <u>tofu</u> is most commonly associated with food allergies.

*Organic, Non-GMO Fermented Soy* in miso paste, tempeh, tamari, and natto, on the other hand, has been in traditional health enhancing Asian diets for thousands of years. Fermented soy is thought to be one of the major reasons for the low rates of breast and colon cancer in Japan and China. The fermentation process breaks down the difficult to digest proteins, and sugars, which enhances digestion, and the nutritive value of the soy; and lessens the possible allergenic properties. Fermented soy is an excellent source of complete vegetable protein, and is considered almost equal to animal foods in protein. It is also high in molybdenum, calcium, iron, and B and E vitamins. Tamari, another soy product made from fermented soybeans, also offers some nutritional benefits; being a good source of B vitamins, and minerals. Tamari does contain sodium, but because of its sharp flavor, one uses less of it compared to salt. There is a reduced sodium form also.

The phytoestrogenic antioxidant compounds known as isoflavones in fermented soy have been well researched. Phytoestrogens, known as "estrogen mimics" are structurally similar to estrogen, and have an estrogenic effect on the body. Estrogen has a positive and negative side, however; as excess estrogen in the body can be potentially dangerous. Alternately, low estrogen levels in the body can be problematic. Soy isoflavones have the capability to attach to estrogen receptors, and block excess harmful estrogen from affixing to the receptors, thus lowering estrogen levels. However, when estrogen levels are too low, as in menopause, the isoflavone compounds can bind too estrogen receptor sites, and increase estrogen levels.

Soy isoflavones (estrogen mimics) have also been demonstrated to prevent cancer, osteoporosis, and menopausal hot flashes in certain age groups. It has been postulated that

Japanese women have fewer hot flashes, due to their regular soy and seaweed consumption. The most comprehensive study to date on menopause and soy consumption was published in *"Menopause: The Journal of the North American Menopause Association* in 2012. Researchers at the University of Delaware reviewed 19 studies that examined 1,200 women who suffered from menopausal symptoms. The researchers sought to determine the effects of soy on menopausal hot flashes. The researchers concluded that consuming two daily small servings of soy for six weeks reduced the frequency and severity of hot flashes by up to 26 percent. Additionally, women who consumed soy for 12 weeks or more, had decreases in hot flash frequency approximately three-fold greater. However, fermented soy products (miso, tamari, natto, and tempeh) are recommended.

In some studies, Isoflavones have been found to be particularly protective against breast, colon and prostate cancers in humans. In a study published in *Science Daily* in May, 2013, it was shown that eating soy foods significantly reduced prostate cancer. When participants consumed one to two small servings of soy daily, and included three to four servings of tomato-based foods weekly, the benefits were even more amplified. Studies on animals have shown that those animals whose diets were composed of as little as 5 percent soy had dramatically repressed chemically induced cancers.

Ito Watanabe, a Japanese developmental biology researcher, and cancer expert demonstrated through studies that fermented miso soup dramatically lowered the risk of breast cancer for women, and also had been shown to reverse it. Moreover, natto, due to its high bone forming vitamin K2 content, was shown to be osteoporosis protective. Women who suffer from osteoporosis have been known to have low levels of vitamin K2 in their blood. Natto also possesses anti-wrinkle attributes due to its high vitamin E, and lecithin content; which is evidenced by the youthful skin of Japanese women. Natto is also available as a supplement.

The amount of fermented soy isoflavones found to be cancer, osteoporosis, and hot flash protective is between 25-100 mg per day. A 4 oz. serving of tempeh, or natto contains about 40 mg of isoflavones. Miso is eaten in smaller servings (about 2 tsp-2 Tbsp.) Only moderate consumption of fermented soy is recommended however. (One or two ½ cup servings daily.)

It's important to remember that a large consumption of soy may affect hormone levels detrimentally, and possibly effect fertility. Additionally, even fermented and cooked soy still contain some amount of goitrogens, which block thyroid function. It is best to consume high iodine rich seaweed or seafood when ingesting soy in order to counteract the goitrogenic effect. Those individuals with hypothyroid, or thyroiditis should probably restrict soy consumption altogether. A significant point to remember is that the traditional Asian diet is not composed of excessive quantities of soy (at one sitting) and soy's goitrogenic effects are offset by the regular inclusion of seaweed with meals.

**Estrogen sensitivity warning**. Soy consumption is controversial; as soy exerts effects on hormones in both men and women in moderate amounts. High levels of estrogen have been linked to estrogen dominance and cancer. Yet, generally human studies show that low to moderate consumption of soy foods do not increase risk, and in some cases may lower it. More large scale soy studies are needed. Therefore for the present it is advised that premenopausal women, and women who have estrogen sensitive breast tumors, and younger men should restrict their soy intake.

- If you are a menopausal woman and soy is too controversial or not a healthy option for you, herbalist Susan Weed recommends drinking red clover infusions, as red clover has been shown to have 10x more phytoestrogens than soy.

*Chlorella and Spirulina* are nutrient-dense microalgae that offer a wealth of health promoting constituents. They are a complete protein, and contain essential fatty acids, and chlorophyll. They are so nutritive that they are considered "super foods." Consuming these super foods is one of the best anti-aging strategies.

- *Spirulina* is a freshwater microscopic algae which hales from Lake Chad, Africa, and Central and South America. Aztecs revered the health promoting and strengthening properties of spirulina, and mixed it with chocolate. Spirulina is a very high protein food, and is one of the best sources of Gamma Linolenic Acid (GLA), an essential fatty acid which is known for its anti-inflammatory effects, and for imparting youthful, strong skin and hair; as well as supporting arthritic conditions. Spirulina is also widely recognized for its detoxifying properties. Its abundant quantity of chlorophyll contributes to its blood building, and purifying assets. Its high sulfur content supports the liver and nervous system in detoxifying poisons and toxic heavy metals. It also aids liver and pancreas function. In addition, spirulina contains a superior antioxidant profile which can protect us from ultraviolet radiation. Spirulina's antioxidant mix includes: immune boosting beta-carotenes, vision enhancing zeaxanthin, and anti-aging Super-Oxide Dismutase. (SOD.)
- *Consuming Chlorella* is another way to advance your health. It contains the widest spectrum of nutrients of any other food. In fact only 1 tsp. contains the nutritional value equal to several servings of dark leafy greens. Chlorella also boosts the immune system and alkalinizes the blood. Additionally, it aids in regulating our blood sugar, and exerts beneficial effects on our brain function. Due to its rich GLA content, it also has anti-inflammatory and skin disorder healing properties.

Amazingly, chlorella contains "Chlorella Growth Factor;" (CGF) which offers many of the same benefits found in our body's own anti-aging natural "human growth hormone." Chlorella's claim to fame is its great detoxifying properties. It has been used to aid in detoxifying heavy metals, prescription drugs, PCB's, plastic compounds, flame retardants, and pesticides that are stored in our fat. Additionally, chlorella stimulates the growth of friendly bacteria four times the normal rate! The highest quality chlorella is termed "broken cell wall" chlorella. This is a process in which the tough, indigestible cell wall is broken apart which optimizes absorbability.

o  Making a smoothie is an easy way to add spirulina or chlorella to your diet. In a base of raw milk, coconut or almond milk, (1 cup) add ½ tsp-to 1 Tbsp. spirulina or chlorella; add a non-denatured whey protein powder; include ½-1 cup berries, and two Tbsp. of flax meal and nutritional yeast. You can also add 1/3 banana or stevia to sweeten it. It's a nutrient packed way to start your day!

## High Anti-Nutrient Phytate Diet:

### (Grains, Nuts, Seeds, Legumes and Soy)

Un-soaked grains, legumes, soy, nuts and seeds possess a type of anti-nutrient termed phytic acid or phytate. Phytates aren't digestible by humans and non-ruminants (non-cud chewers) because we lack the enzyme phyase to break them down. Phytates interfere with the mineral absorption of grains, legumes, nuts, seeds, and soy by binding to zinc, iron, magnesium, and calcium in our intestines; and excreting them from our body. As a result, individuals who have a high phytate-containing diet may experience mineral deficiencies.

Conditions that reflect mineral deficiencies such as iron deficiency anemia, PMS, anxiety, insomnia, muscle cramps, poor immunity, and weak bones could possibly be the result of an over consumption of un-soaked phytate-rich foods. The good news is that the minerals in phytate rich foods can still be absorbed if they are sprouted, fermented or soaked and covered with water using an acid such as apple cider vinegar or lemon juice. (One Tbsp. of acid per cup of grain etc.) You can also make your own phytate-free nut and seed butter with this process using a powerful blender. Sprouted grains are also beginning to be sold in health food stores now.

Enzyme inhibitors are another anti-nutrient common to these foods, wherein the digestion of proteins is inhibited. Soaking will remedy this problem as well. If you think that soaking all of your anti-nutrient containing foods is a daunting prospect, you can avoid this almost completely by choosing grain-alternative carbohydrates such as: cooked root veggies (carrots, beets etc.) winter squash, sweet potatoes, yams, and small red and purple potatoes etc.

## Protein Tips

- When shopping for organic or grass-fed meat, choose bright red or purple colored meat. Brown meat indicates a lack of freshness.
- Persistent environmental toxins (dioxins and PCB's) can be concentrated in the fat of animal proteins. These toxins, due to their hazardous nature get sequestered into the animal's fat cells in order to be removed from the blood stream. For this reason, buy lean meats or trim off excess animal fat from meats (even grass-fed meats) to lessen your toxic load. However, leave a little fat on to obtain fat soluble vitamins, omega-3s, and other fatty-acids.
- Fish should be cooked rare-to avoid fat oxidation. If you want to eat raw sushi-grade fish; first freeze it for at least 48 hours to destroy possible parasites and bacteria.
- Brining poultry in salt and water for ½ hour–to 45 min. will render it more tender and digestible.
- Make sure to eat a protein packed breakfast within an hour of rising to support blood sugar balance, and to rev-up your metabolism. (fat burning) It should be 1/3 or more of your daily protein intake.
- Add three servings of vegetables (leafy/crunchy) for every animal protein serving you eat to alkalinize your blood.
- You may expect temporary digestive problems (gas) when you are making a change in your protein choice, especially vegetable proteins; as your internal microflora (beneficial bacteria) will need to adjust to the new food. You also may need to support HCL production if you have been a vegetarian, and want to introduce animal proteins to your diet. (See digestion section on the next page.)
- Minimize grilling meats/fish due to the carcinogenic by-products (heterocyclic amines and toxic lipid peroxides) that grilling creates. If you must grill; use a spice or herbal marinade with vinegar to protect the meat. Avoid eating the blackened parts of meat.
- Limit cooking meats at high temperatures above 250 degrees. When meats and other foods are exposed to high temperatures; sugars react with fats or proteins causing a process known as **glycation**. Glycation is involved in accelerated aging and in many degenerative diseases. Glycation in essence reduces tissue flexibility and effects organs where suppleness is critical, such as the heart, eyes, kidneys, skin, and the brain. Several studies have revealed that restricting glycation can lead to a lengthened lifespan. Consider cooking most of your food on low to moderate heat if you can. More healthful ways of cooking animal proteins are steaming, simmering, stewing, braising, and using a slow cooker. Try to limit broiling, boiling, frying, and roasting.

## Nutrients that have been shown to prevent glycation:

| Green tea | Cinnamon | Ginger |
|---|---|---|
| Cumin | Black pepper | The supplements carnosine, benfotiamine, and alpha lipoic acid |

### Exercise 4c: Protein Information

- Add some healthy protein sources to your wellness plan. Input some protein tips, cooking guidelines and glycation reduction information.
- Determine whether you may be lactose intolerant, or casein sensitive. Input dairy options/substitutions/enzymes if needed.

---

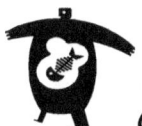

## Compromised Protein Digestion in Middle Age

A healthy digestive system is vital to vibrant aging as it is the basis for a healthy immune system and energy production. Overall good health in midlife is not possible without being able to properly break down, digest and assimilate the foods that we take in. When we don't adequately digest and assimilate our foods; we won't be able to obtain the nutrients from them, and the undigested food can decay, build-up and become food for opportunistic health-impairing microbes.

The first step to optimal digestion is chewing food well. Slow, thorough and relaxed chewing calms us and activates our digestive enzymes to begin the digestive process. Unhurried chewing also allows time for our stomach to register fullness.

When you sit down to eat, consider taking a deep breath before you place food in your mouth. This will promote calmness. Then try to really taste the food you are eating. Chew slowly until the food starts to turn soupy in your mouth. This simple process often reverses a number of digestive issues. You will also find that you don't need to eat as much!

Digestive problems are very common as we hit middle-age. Our digestion and assimilation of proteins can be especially compromised due to a slowing down of gut function. (Low hydrochloric stomach acids and pancreatic enzymes.) As a result, it is possible that we can be protein deficient even though we are eating sufficient amounts of it. About 50% of individuals over 60 suffer from low stomach acid production; and if we have a stress-filled life, it is more than likely that we have low acid levels. Additionally, when we do not take-in enough essential vitamins and minerals; our body will not be able to make sufficient stomach acids.

Without sufficient stomach acidity, we won't be able to digest proteins well; and we will have difficulty separating minerals from the foods that bind them. We will also have problems extracting other nutrients from our foods, especially vitamin B12. Also, with a lack of acid in our stomach we may not be able to kill harmful microorganisms that travel down into the digestive tract from our mouth or from our food. For this reason the most important thing we can do as we age is to make sure that we have sufficient stomach acidity; otherwise we will suffer from nutritional shortfalls and possibly bad bacteria overgrowth and low immunity. Signs of low stomach acid are gas, burping and bloating immediately after meals; a feeling of heaviness in the stomach post meals; and feeling nauseous when taking supplements. Signs of low pancreatic enzyme function are: gas, and flatulence an hour and a half or more after eating.

➡ *Baking Soda Stomach Acid (HCL Test)*: Upon rising, drink ¼ tsp. baking soda with 1 cup water; then time yourself. A burp should come up within 1-5 if you have adequate HCL levels. (Due to the reaction between an acid and an alkaline compound) if a loud burp comes within 3 minutes: optimal stomach acid levels are indicated. If a burp comes between 3 and 5 minutes: adequate HCL levels are indicated. If a late burp, or no burp: **poor HCL** levels are indicated; and supplemental HCL capsules are suggested.

Note: individuals with GERD (reflux and indigestion) may have **excess** stomach acid production, or ill placed acid in the esophagus and will burp immediately. An **excess** of stomach acid is also not optimal. To test if you have excessive stomach acid production while having reflux symptoms: take 1 tsp. baking soda with 1 cup water; If your GERD is resolved with baking soda then excessive or ill placed stomach acids are indicated. If it is resolved with 1 tsp. of apple cider vinegar and 1 cup water; it may indicate low stomach acid levels. Test for H. Pylori antibodies and high histamines when suffering from GERD.

---

*Tips to aid weak digestion in middle age and increase "digestive fire."*

| Inadequate HCL Levels |
|---|
| **For very low HCL stomach acid levels:** (flatulence immediately after meals) Take Betaine HCL with Pepsin: Take 1-4 betaine HCL capsules before meals. Start with one capsule before your first meal and build up by one capsule until a slight burning sensation is felt, then back-off by one. This should be the optimal dose to support protein digestion. Stomach acid levels may improve with stress management and improved nutrition. Some people need to take 4 capsules, and others only one. For very poor or no HCL production; puree animal proteins into a pate to aid digestion. |

| |
|---|
| **Option one- for mild HCL support**: Drink 1 tsp.-3 Tbsp. apple cider vinegar with one cup water shortly before meals. (stimulates HCL) |
| **Or option two-for mild HCL support**: Drink the juice of 1 lemon in 6 oz. of water shortly before meals. (stimulates HCL) |
| **Eat bitter foods**; such as arugula, dandelion, and parsley 15 min. before eating, to help stimulate stomach acid production. |
| **Drink home-made bone stock** to improve HCL production long-term (glycine-rich) |
| **Avoid drinking liquids with meals**, (except lemon or vinegar water) Liquids dilute stomach acids. |
| **To increase "digestive fire"**: Drink ginger tea before meals, or eat hot peppers, black pepper and other spicy foods with meals. |
| **To repair acid-secreting cells in the stomach/increase HCL**: Drink bone stock. Take supplemental L-glutamine, vitamin B5, zinc, glycine, and DGL-licorice or *Gastromend*. |

| |
|---|
| **Pancreatic digestive enzyme support**. If gas, and bloating occur an hour and a half or more after meals; low pancreatic enzymes are probably indicated. Take 1-3 digestive enzymes with each meal. Make sure that the supplement contains amylase, lipase, and protease enzymes to support carbohydrate, fat, and protein digestion, and absorption. |
| **For GERD and Indigestion**: Take DGL with meals (a form of licorice) and sea vegetables daily to support the thyroid and esophageal sphincter (valve between the esophagus and stomach). Slow, relaxed eating and stress reduction are also essential to remedy the problem |
| **For Constipation**: Less than one bowel movement per day. Eat cultured yogurts, kefir and fermented vegetables. Constipation is common as we age. When we are constipated, we reabsorb the toxins back into our blood. This is damaging to the liver, and other organs. To facilitate regularity, we need to correct dysbiosis with probiotics; particularly with bifidobacterium from yogurt or supplements. Bifidobacterium Longum BB536 in particular has been the subject of numerous clinical studies, and has demonstrated immense improvements for constipation. Probiotic populations decline as we age, and are replaced overtime by E. coli, and streptococci lactobacilli.<br>**Other constipation recommendations**: Put feet up on a small stool and lean forward when defecating. (simulates squatting) Increase fiber, water, and exercise, and take magnesium citrate to bowel tolerance.(very effective) Rule-out hypothyroid. |

*Exercise 4d Determine possible compromised digestive status* with symptom list and baking soda test. If needed, add to your wellness plan foods/supplements to support your HCL, digestive fire, pancreatic enzymes, GERD and constipation

Chapter Five

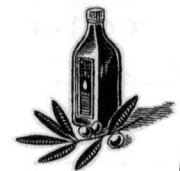

# Fats and Healthy Aging

Fat is not an evil word! There are many flawed assumptions about fats, but healthy fats are essential to our health, and everyone needs them. There is no need at all to be afraid of fats; and it is absolutely harmful to abstain from them. It has been demonstrated that individuals who restrict fats from their diet create a fatty acid deficiency and often end up binging on fatty foods. This is the body's way of alerting a person of a fat imbalance. However, it is equally detrimental to ingest an excess of the wrong kinds of fat.

Fats and oils provide essential fatty acids (EFA's) which play a major role in our immune and cell health. Without healthy fats in our cell membranes, we increase our risk for heart disease, diabetes and neurodegenerative diseases. Fats support menopause and aid in our hormone and anti-inflammatory prostaglandin production. They also nourish and moisturize dry skin, hair, and mucous membranes.

Our brain is made up of a whopping 60% fat. Fat also has a role in our body's eye, cognitive, and cardio vascular function, and it is the primary source of energy for the heart. Fats also transport our fat soluble vitamins A, D, E, and K and are needed to convert beta carotene rich foods (carrots, leafy greens etc.) to vitamin A. Without consuming enough healthful fats we can suffer from vitamin deficiencies, fatigue, poor concentration, bipolar disorder and depression.

Additionally, fats slow down the absorption of our food, increasing satiation; thus helping us to go longer without feeling hungry. The danger in consuming low fat meals is that they cause us to feel constant hunger; which ultimately leads to over eating. Additionally, many manufacturers replace fat in a product with added sugars, high fructose corn syrup, or salt to make the food more palatable. This substitution ultimately degrades the product.

Cholesterol, a beneficial waxy substance found in our blood, is often maligned, but it too is essential for our health. According to integrative cardiologist Dr. Stephen Sinatra and nutritionist Jonny Bowden, authors of the book *The Great Cholesterol Myth*, our body uses cholesterol for producing sex hormones, and adrenal stress hormones. Cholesterol is also responsible for cell wall maintenance, producing vitamin D from sunlight, and synthesizing bile salts for fat digestion. It also has numerous health applications for memory and learning. In fact, research studies have confirmed that low cholesterol levels (often induced by cholesterol lowering drugs) can lead to cognitive decline; as the organs that are especially rich in cholesterol are the brain and nervous system.

It also has been scientifically proven that cholesterol in certain foods such as eggs is completely safe, and not the cause of high lipid cholesterol levels. Additionally, contrary to cholesterol misinformation, research has revealed that high blood cholesterol levels can sometimes be a <u>symptom</u> of heart disease, but are not the <u>cause</u> of heart disease. Scientific studies have discovered that cholesterol acts as a protective antioxidant to defend the body against damaging free-radicals in the arteries. It also has a role in repairing inflammation. When high cholesterol levels are reported from lab tests it may indicate that the body is using cholesterol to protect itself from high levels of free-radicals and oxidized/damaged fat.

Additionally, contrary to outdated medical advice, numerous research studies have found that it is not the level of cholesterol in our blood that is detrimental to health, but whether the cholesterol is **<u>oxidized.</u>** When cholesterol is oxidized, it is very dangerous. Cholesterol ought to be large and fluffy; but when it is in a small and hard oxidized form, it can lead to arteriosclerosis (hardening and thickening of the arteries), atherosclerosis (arterial plaque), high blood pressure, blood clotting risk, and cardio vascular disease.

## Causes of Oxidized Cholesterol

- Chronic stress
- Smoking
- Diet lacking in plant foods
- Nutrient deficiencies
- Regular ingestion of refined sugar/carbs
- Regular use of refined polyunsaturated vegetable oils- (canola, soy, corn, peanut, safflower, sunflower) trans-fat use, fried foods. (check package labels for oil content)
- Excess coffee (more than once daily)
- Excess alcohol (more than once daily)
- Fats and meats heated to high temperatures (BBQ etc.)

## Nutrients and activities that reduce high oxidized cholesterol in the blood

| Avoid alcohol and smoking | Omega-3 fatty acids: fish and seafood | Lecithin: which is found in eggs peas, soy and beans | Vitamin E: found in avocados, nuts, seeds |
|---|---|---|---|
| Vitamin C: found in citrus (and their pith) sprouts, cabbage, parsley, kiwi, and peppers. | *Most important: Lower insulin resistance and high insulin levels by reducing/eliminating refined carbohydrates (sugar, pastas, chips, grains etc.) | Include plenty of high fiber foods & vegetables. Consume eggs, grass-fed meats, and coconut oils | Exercise regularly and support low thyroid conditions with sea weed and vitamins A, D, K. |

➡ Lab Test: Cholesterol Particle Size test

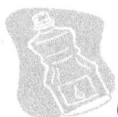 ## Unhealthful Fats

There are however toxic "unhealthful fats" that we want to stay away from. There are really only two types of fats that are harmful for us. These are polyunsaturated refined vegetable oils, (and reheated vegetable oils used in frying) and trans-fats. These fats are oxidized (rancid) due to high heat processing. These damaging fats are vitamin E deficient, and contain lipid compounds that are destructive to our cells due to their high free-radical content. Examples are:

- **Partially hydrogenated fats and oils/trans-fatty acids (TFA):** These unnatural, altered "fake fats" are the worst fat offenders, as they clog up our cell membranes. These synthetic fats were created to offer increased shelf life and intense flavor; but contain no nutritional benefits. The documented adverse effects of TFA's are many: lowered HDL (good cholesterol), and higher oxidized LDL, (bad cholesterol) increased heart disease incidence; impaired blood vessel function; impaired cell membranes; increased diabetes risk; lowered testosterone levels, and impaired immunity. In addition they displace and interfere with our body's ability to use other important essential fatty acids. Tran-fats are found in: packaged foods, fast foods, French fries, doughnuts, baked goods, snack foods, margarine/vegetable shortening, and cottonseed oil. Avoid completely, very deadly!
- **Refined polyunsaturated vegetable oils** (omega-6) (soy, corn, safflower, sunflower, canola, peanut oil etc.) These oils are very unstable with heat, light, and oxygen, and

become oxidized and rancid quite quickly. Manufacturers are knowledgeable of this fact, and add deodorizers to their bottled oils to conceal the odor. These poor quality fats are also used to make fried foods- where they are reheated over and over again causing more oxidation. Furthermore an excessive intake of omega-6 fatty acids can disrupt our body's ability to manufacture the anti-inflammatory compounds that omega-3 fats provide. Additionally, vegetable oils promote inflammation, pain, and heart disease. Lastly, consuming an overload of refined vegetables oils contributes to a fatty acid deficiency in the body. Avoid cooking or eating packaged foods with polyunsaturated vegetable oils (corn, sunflower, safflower, canola, peanut and soy). O-6 fats are also contained in salad dressings, mayonnaise, and spreads. Additionally, processed and fast foods, grain fed (not grass fed) beef, dairy, poultry, and farmed fish have an inordinate amount of O-6.

*Exercise 5a: Note Bad fats in your diet* and whether you may have a lifestyle that is contributing to possible oxidized cholesterol. Mark on your wellness plan.

---

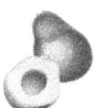 Healthy Fats:

All fat containing foods are a mix of several different fats. Most animal proteins and plants are a blend of saturated, polyunsaturated (omega-3 and omega-6) and monounsaturated fats. Two fats are considered to be essential fatty acids owing to the fact that they are vital to our well-being, and our bodies can't make them. These are the **omega-6 and omega-3** fats. These essential fats are essential for healthy cell membrane function, but they need to be balanced for healthy functioning. Scientific research has determined that if the ratio of omega-6 fats to omega-3 fats exceeds 4 parts O-6 to 1 part O-3 fats- individuals begin to suffer from health problems. The typical SAD diet has a ratio of about 20:1 (O-6 to O-3). Most experts suggest that a healthy ratio of omega-6 to omega-3 fats should be between: a 1:1 to 1:3 ratio. (O-6: O-3.)

As mentioned above, refined polyunsaturated oils are a source of free radicals due to their instability to heat, light, and air. When we consume these fats we are ingesting the free-radicals they contain. **Monounsaturated fats** are more stable, while **saturated fats** are the most stable. It is always important to buy oils in dark bottles, and to store oils in cool dark places or the refrigerator to avoid rancidity and free-radical formation.

**Omega-3s/Alpha Linolenic Acid (ALA):** It has been estimated that over 90% of adults in the U.S. may be deficient in omega-3 fatty acids due to diets low in fish and sea food. Omega-3 oils are vital for our heart, brain and nervous system health. Our body uses essential fatty acids for building tissues and for the production of hormone-like prostaglandins that play a role in inflammation control and immune health. Omega-3 is highly regarded for other nutritional and health benefits including; optimizing our defenses against heart disease, cancer, autoimmune diseases, and arthritis. Omega-3 fats (DHA) also support cognitive and mood health, as our brain is made of DHA. There are over 50 health conditions related to an insufficiency of omega-3 fatty acids; and a deficiency may be the underlying cause of hundreds of thousands of premature deaths per year.

Note: Those individuals who are carriers of the ApoE4 genotype must take care when ingesting omega-3s in food or supplement form, as DHA is more readily oxidized (damaged) with this variant. However, when the diet is centered on whole-foods (not packaged) and ample vegetables, the oxidation is held back.

Although many people are deficient in omega-3s, some health conscious people may have an excess due to over-consumption. An excess can lead to hair loss, rashes on arms or thighs, and joint aches. If you experience these symptoms from over-use, cut back on your omega-3 supplements or eliminate them. Simply eating 3-4 servings a week of fish is often enough to gain the O-3 benefits- especially for those who have been supplementing for a while.

**Omega-3s (DHA and EPA) found in:**

1. Oily fish (pre-formed DHA/EPA): choose wild salmon, sardines, mackerel, anchovy, herring - cook lightly to avoid oxidation. Eat 3-4 times a week.
2. Molecularly distilled cold-pressed Antarctic krill oil (supplements that are free from mercury or PCB's) or fermented cod liver or skate liver oil (fermented is best due to increased nutrient density/absorption) Fermented cod liver oil is also helpful to take in winter for its Vitamin D3 content. Krill oil has been found in many studies to be far superior to fish oil. (Daily dosage: 1-2 tsp. cod liver oil or 1,000 mg krill oil)
3. Algae: (spirulina/chlorella) High in minerals and B vitamins. Use raw in smoothies or in energy snacks
4. Seeds of flax, chia, hemp, pumpkin, and walnut contain the fatty acid alpha-linolenic acid (ALA) which is converted to EPA/DHA in our bodies, albeit

somewhat inefficiently as they are not preformed. Flax is the best source of ALA; however, diabetes, vitamin deficiencies, and medications are known to prevent the conversion to DHA/EPA. Additionally, not every ethnic group has the necessary enzyme activity to convert ALA to DHA/EPA. Native Americans, Scandinavians, Welsh, Scottish, Irish and Inuit peoples are not genetically programmed to do so. For these ethnic groups it is not an adequate substitute for fish. Alpha linolenic acid is very unstable to air, heat and light. Make fresh flax meal using a coffee grinder to avoid oxidation. Refrigerate or freeze all seeds and nuts to avoid oxidation. Use 2-4 Tbsp. flax meal daily for cancer prevention. Flax meal is preferred over flax oil. Note: not all people can synthesize EPA and DHA from plant oils.

5. <u>Grass fed</u> free-range meat, poultry and game meat (very high in o-3s)
6. Raw milk/cheeses from grass fed cows and goats contain omega-3s (not found in feed lot animals)
7. Free-range pastured eggs or eggs w/ omega-3 printed on the label
8. Leafy vegetables contain alpha linolenic acid. Eat a wide variety
9. For Vegans/Vegetarians: algae containing preformed DHA
10. You may need to add an omega-3 supplement if you haven't been consuming omega-3s. Antarctic cold-pressed Krill oil or *Green Pastures* brand fermented cod liver or skate liver oil are recommended omega-3 supplements.

<u>Omega-6s/Polyunsaturated fats</u>: These are necessary pro-inflammatory fats to help the immune system respond to injuries, but can cause inflammation when over consumed. SAD diet contains too much. It's best to consume omega-6 oils in raw **nuts and seeds**, not in bottled oils. Try pecans, almonds, walnuts, Brazil nuts, sunflower seeds, cashews, hazel nuts, and sesame seeds. Keep refrigerated to avoid oxidation/rancidity. Smell nuts, and nut butters to ensure freshness. If they smell similar to oil paint, they are oxidized. Must be in moderation and balanced with omega-3s. Keep omega-6 to omega-3 at a 1:1 to a 3:1 ratio.

* **<u>You can keep a healthy ratio of omega-6 to omega-3s in your cells by:</u>**

    o Limiting polyunsaturated vegetable oils and eliminating trans-fats
    o Eating some fresh raw nuts and seeds daily. (omega-6) Keep refrigerated.
    o Adding walnuts, chia or flax meal daily. (ALA) Keep refrigerated.
    o Eating 3-4 oz. of wild, small cold-water fish or seafood 3-4 times a week (omega-3)
    o Eating 100% grass-fed or pastured meats/eggs
    o You may need to add an omega-3 supplement if you haven't been consuming omega-3s on a regular basis.

*Omega-9: Oleic acid/monounsaturated fats* (MUFA's): Very important for heart health. MUFA's lessen the risk for heart disease and stroke. *The American Heart Association* recommends consuming MUFA's to improve cholesterol levels. Omega-9s also decrease the risk for breast cancer and reduce pain and stiffness in rheumatoid arthritis sufferers. Studies demonstrate that switching to MUFA's resulted in weight loss and reduced belly fat. These oils have been a central part of healthful diets of many cultures for centuries, especially the Mediterranean cultures. High in the antioxidant vitamin E. Eat in abundance!

*Monounsaturated Fats Sources*

| Extra Virgin Olive Oil- olive oil contains anti-oxidant rich phenols, and vitamin E | Olives | Avocados-contains high fiber and potassium |
|---|---|---|
| Raw almonds, almond butter-(high in vitamin E, and antioxidant flavonoids) | Raw macadamia nuts (very high level of MUFA's and vitamin E) | Other raw nuts: hazel nuts, pecans, cashews, walnuts, peanuts, and their nut butters. |
| Sesame seeds/oil | Tea Seed oil- from the tea plant | Duck, goose, and goose liver pate; chicken |

*Gamma-Linolenic Acid (GLA):* An omega-6 fatty acid that is downstream in the omega-6 metabolic pathway. We convert this fatty acid from linoleic acid (previously mentioned). It then is converted into anti-inflammatory hormone like-substances called prostaglandins. GLA has many vital anti-inflammatory applications. It aids in the treatment of asthma, allergies, rheumatoid arthritis, heart disease, premature aging, PMS, platelet sticking, weight loss and healthy immune function. It also provides flexibility and moisture retention to skin. Several health conditions such as diabetes, pyroluria, (an anxiety disorder) and viral infections can interfere with its conversion, causing a GLA deficiency. Excess alcohol and sugar, aging and vitamin deficiencies can also interfere with its necessary conversion. We can however supplement with foods and dietary supplements to make up the difference. GLA is found in spirulina, chlorella, evening primrose oil, borage oil, red current oil, hemp seed oil, and in organ meats.

*Saturated fats*: Our body can't function without saturated fats. In fact if we don't get sufficient saturated fats in our diet, our body will synthesize them. Saturated fats constitute 50% of our cell membranes, which gives it necessary stiffness and structure. Saturated fats are essential for the health of our liver, heart, and immune system; and are also an excellent fuel source. Additionally, they are brain-nourishing, and are necessary for supporting our hormones and nervous system. Saturated fats are also necessary for the absorption of calcium for our bones, and contain high quantities of our fat soluble vitamins. (A, D, E, and K2) Saturated fat containing foods richest in fat soluble vitamins are: eggs, butter, fish, shellfish, fish eggs, dairy, and organ meats.

According to integrative cardiologist, Dr. Stephen Sinatra, co-author of the book: *Reverse Heart Disease Now,* there is no scientific evidence to support the argument put forth by proponents of the *Lipid Hypothesis Theory*, that so called "artery clogging" saturated fats cause heart disease, and that low saturated fat diets reduce death from heart disease.

There are numerous studies debunking this heart disease/saturated fat myth. A meta-analysis published in 2010 pooled data from 21 studies and included 348,000 adults. It found no difference in the risk of heart disease and stroke between people with the lowest intake of saturated fats and with people who had the highest intake of saturated fats.

Another study published in 2010 in *The American Journal of Clinical Nutrition* found that reducing saturated fat in the diet resulted in an <u>increase</u> in obesity, diabetes, triglyceride levels, and insulin resistance; on account of the replacement of saturated fats with added carbohydrates. The journal declared that efforts to aid heart health should stress the limitation of refined carbohydrates (sweets, chips, pastas, breads) and implementing weight reduction strategies instead of limiting saturated fats. Additionally, the *Harvard School of Public Health* announced that low fat dietary recommendations were based on little scientific evidence and may have caused health consequences to the public. They also stated that the amount of saturated fats in the diet has no effect on our heart health, and that saturated fat intake is actually associated with <u>less progression of atherosclerosis.</u>

It is remarkable to note that heart disease was rare in America before the 1920's, and saturated fat consumption in the form of lard, dairy, butter, and meats was very high. Even in the 1950's there were only 500 cardiologists in the U.S. compared to today. The inundation of heart disease today has necessitated 30,000 more cardiologists. The low saturated fat medical advice/dogma that has prevailed for the last 50 years has not held up to the realistic evidence shown by the low heart disease mortality rates of many cultures of the world. The Maasai of Kenya, the Inuit Eskimos of Canada, and the Tokelau of the Atoll Islands in New Zealand all consume 60-75% saturated fat daily in their diets, and maintain low heart disease mortality rates.

In fact, human breast milk is composed of 54% saturated fat; confirming the fact that we are biologically intended to consume saturated fats. Several Mediterranean societies (Crete etc.) have low rates of heart disease even with moderate goat cheese, lamb, and sausage consumption. In Okinawa, individuals eat moderate amounts of pork, goat and seafood, and cook in lard, but still boast the highest centenarian population in the world.

Today, 40% of all U.S. deaths are caused by heart disease. The sharp increase of heart disease since 1920 corresponds not surprisingly with the 400% increase in polyunsaturated vegetable oil consumption, and with the 60% increase in sugar and processed food consumption by Americans. Additionally, contrary to most people's assumptions; saturated fats are only a small component of the fat concentrations of most animal proteins. Almost all animal proteins have higher concentrations of the heart healthy monounsaturated fats then saturated fats; with the exception of dairy products and turkey! Pastured animal meats possess even lower concentrations of saturated fats. (The balance of the fats, the polyunsaturated fats vary with each meat.)

## Fat Concentrations of Certain Foods in Percentages (not pastured)

| Source | Saturated % | Monounsaturated % |
|---|---|---|
| Cheese | 60 | 29 |
| Beef | 33 | 38 |
| Pork | 35 | 44 |
| Ham | 35 | 49 |
| Chicken breast | 29 | 34 |
| Egg yolk | 36 | 44 |
| Turkey | 31 | 20 |
| Duck/Goose | 35 | 52 |
| Salmon | 28 | 33 |
| Butter | 63 | 29 |
| Coconut oil | 86 | 13 |

Nutridata.com/Feinberg School Nutrition Fact Sheet

## Saturated fats found in:

1. Butter: Butter consists of 29 g of monounsaturated fats, in addition to its 63 g of saturated fats. The compound butyric acid in butter is beneficial for healing an inflamed intestinal lining. Raw butter from grass-fed cows is the best butter choice because of its naturally occurring enzymes. It is best not to heat raw butter over 110 degrees, as it will lose its health promoting qualities. Butter contains low lactose levels. Ghee is clarified dairy butter, which lactose intolerant people can eat. It also aids digestion and possesses anti-cancer properties. A small amount of butter, according to Dr. Sinatra is heart-protective.
2. Saturated fat-rich raw dairy contains high amounts of vitamins, minerals and digestive enzymes. Conversely, pasteurized dairy, especially ultra-pasteurized, has

been cooked at very high heat which destroys many of the nutrients and enzymes. However, yogurt and raw cheese contain beneficial bacteria, and vitamin K2; necessary for bone building and osteoporosis prevention. Do not heat over 110 degrees to retain its health supportive qualities.

3. Chicken, duck, and geese contain saturated fats, but have a higher monounsaturated fat profile. Organic pastured poultry also have two times higher levels of omega-3 fats than grain-fed varieties. They are moderately consumed in heart healthy Mediterranean diets

4. Saturated fats in meats and eggs: While there are constant admonitions to avoid saturated fats, the American Journal of Clinical Nutrition published that there is no correlation between saturated fats and heart disease. In the early 1900's heart disease was rare. It was not until the 1950's that heart disease had become a leading cause of death in the U.S., and research indicated that polyunsaturated vegetable oils were implicated with this increase. When enjoying eggs, make sure to eat the whole egg; the egg yolk is rich in antioxidants, brain supportive choline, and eye protective lutein.

5. Coconut, shredded coconut, coconut milk, raw virgin coconut oil, and coconut water contain a health promoting medium chain saturated fat whose only other abundant source in nature is in human breast milk. Raw virgin coconut oil and coconut milk according to research studies increase levels of HDL (good) cholesterol. Contrary to past flawed studies it does not cause an increase in cholesterol. Coconut oil and its milk contain a large amount of medium-chain fatty acids called lauric acid; which are able to destroy a wide variety of disease causing organisms such as bacteria, fungi, protozoan, and viruses. Coconut oil also supports healthy weight management due to its thermogenic (fat burning) properties. In addition, coconut oil protects against heart disease, Alzheimer's disease, and supports healthy immune function. Choose cold-pressed extra virgin coconut oil. It is the optimal oil for high heat cooking.

## Fat Composition Requirements and Tips

Fat requirements can vary or fluctuate with each individual. The season will also have an impact on our fat needs. In winter, we usually need to eat more fats for warmth and comfort. In summer, we often don't need as much. Some individuals in general feel better on a lower-fat diet, while others need a higher fat diet to feel good. Additionally, it is beneficial to supplement the diet with more healthful fats when we are reducing energy generating starchy carbs; as fats are the most concentrated energy food. Fats additionally are excellent for making us feel satiated, as they take the lengthiest time to digest compared to animal proteins and carbohydrates.

No matter what our individual fat needs are, it is important to include a healthy fat with each meal. The most important consideration for cell membrane health, and therefore our overall health is to ensure that we are getting the correct proportion of essential fatty acids in our diet. (Omega-3s and omega-6s) Studies confirm that our cell membranes are more influenced by the essential omega-3 fats, and the ratio of omega-6 to omega-3 fats than they are influenced by saturated and monounsaturated fats, as the latter fats can be made by the body.

However, it is essential to vary all the healthy fats in our diet to receive the myriad of benefits that healthy fats have to offer. Use healthy oils/fats abundantly in foods. Add some olive oil or butter to green and orange vegetables to support beta-carotene absorption. Drizzle some olive oil on salads and steamed veggies. Eat nuts as snacks. Sprinkle seeds on hot cereals, salads and grains. Consume fish and seafood or fermented cod liver oil. Try to eat pastured grass-fed omega-3 rich meats if you can afford them. Add flax meal and chia seeds to shakes and smoothies. Replace omega-6 containing rancid mayonnaise with mashed avocado in your favorite recipes; or make your own mayo with eggs, olive oil, lemon and sea salt. Add olives to salads. Use health enhancing coconut oil for cooking. Make sure to keep oils in cool places in opaque containers to avoid oxidation. Choose organic cold-pressed or expeller-pressed unrefined oils.

## Healthy Fats

| Monounsaturated fats: olive oil, olives, macadamia nut oil, macadamia nuts, avocado, almonds, duck, goose, chicken, sesame seeds, tahini | Polyunsaturated fats-Omega-3: fish, seafood, grass-fed meats/eggs, fermented cod-liver oil, krill oil, flax meal, chia, walnuts, pumpkin seeds |
|---|---|
| Polyunsaturated fats-Omega-6: all raw nuts and seeds, *sesame seed oil, Evening primrose oil, spirulina (GLA) | Saturated fats: pastured/organic animal meats, raw cow or goat milk, raw cheese, yogurt, kefir, eggs, coconut oil, shredded coconut |

*Note: a few drops of cold-pressed toasted sesame seed oil can be used in moderation; as it contains many antioxidants that hinder oxidation. (Add after cooking.)

The quantity of fat that feels right for us varies greatly due to our biochemical individuality. Some people do very well consuming an abundance of healthy fats. The quantity tolerated also has to do with the health of our liver and gall bladder, and whether we are making sufficient amounts of digestive enzymes. As we age, we may begin to suffer from fat intolerance. It is advised to take care to not over-consume butter, dairy and oils when suffering from fat intolerance, as an excessive amount of fat may slow down liver function. A small amount of unrefined raw coconut oil should not be a problem however. Limiting fat in the evening (especially from dairy) is also suggested, even when not suffering from fat intolerance; to avoid overwhelming the liver while we sleep.

Consuming fermented foods, and taking fat digesting enzymes such as lipase, pancreatin, and ox bile can boost fat digestion. Taking herbal cholegogues such as artichoke, dandelion root, gentian, yellow dock, rosemary, milk thistle and sage stimulate the flow of bile from the liver; which can facilitates fat digestion, and aid in strengthening the liver.

## Symptoms of Fat Intolerance

| Feeling tired just after eating | Neck and shoulder pain | Upper-right abdominal discomfort. Spasms in the large and small intestines; nausea |
|---|---|---|
| Gall bladder problems | Flatulence, belching, indigestion, bloating an hour and a half or more after meals | Gray or pale stools, oily stools, hard stools |

- ➡ Other conditions that reduce the body's ability to absorb fat: Chrone's disease, celiac, cystic fibrosis, pancreatic insufficiency, liver disease, and surgical removal of the stomach.
- ➡ Individuals will also have difficulty in absorbing fats if the lining of their intestines has gotten thin and porous, also known as "leaky gut." Leaky gut becomes increasingly common as we age, especially with chronic stress. See Food Allergy section in Chapter 7 for more details.

## Cooking Fats/Oils

It is important when cooking with oils and fats to not let them smoke, and to choose fats that possess high heat-stability. Heat-stable oils and fats produce less free-radicals in the cooking process. Oils that smoke and have poor heat-stability become oxidized and produce rancid by-products known as lipid peroxides. This oxidation damages our DNA, cells, and tissues and can promote heart disease and cancer. Use assorted oils/fats for various temperatures while cooking. Do not heat flax oil, and other cold-pressed organic polyunsaturated oils- due to their instability to heat.

Use these oils for the following temperatures:

| High Temperature (Frying, over 375 degrees F.) Do sparingly | Medium temperature (Sautéing, baking, up to 375 degrees F.) Do moderately | Low Temperature (Up to 250 degrees F.) Cooking foods at low temperatures is the best way to protect our health. |
|---|---|---|
| Ghee | Butter | Extra virgin olive oil (high in antioxidants) |
| Untoasted sesame oil/grape seed oil, tea seed oil | Cold pressed virgin coconut oil | Cold pressed virgin coconut oil (high in lauric acid) |
| Grass-fed animal fats (lard) | Macadamia nut oil | Macadamia nut oil (very high in vitamin E) |
| Virgin red palm oil | Virgin red palm oil (50% sat. fat) | Virgin red palm fruit oil: Beta-carotene and vitamin E rich |

*Restrict microwave usage- as it has been shown to deplete nutrient content in foods.

**Exercise 5b: Healthy Fats.** Add some Omega-3, Omega-6, monounsaturated fats, GLA and saturated fat sources to your Personal Wellness Plan.

**Exercise. 5c:** Note possible conversion difficulties with GLA/ALA and problems with fat intolerance.

**Exercise 5d:** Add fat tips and cooking temperatures to your plan

➡ Lab testing for Omega 3-fatty acids is useful to determine if you have a balanced fatty acid profile.

Chapter Six

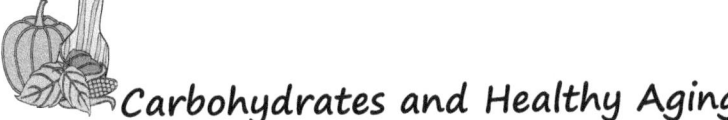

# Carbohydrates and Healthy Aging

As with fats, there are healthy carbohydrates, and there are unhealthy carbohydrates. Carbohydrates are mainly in plant foods, such as fruits, vegetables, grains, beans, nuts, and seeds; and also are in sugars and dairy foods. Carbohydrates are an essential macronutrient that supplies the body and brain with a quick source of energy, thus supporting physical activity and thinking. Carbohydrates are also important for immunity, blood clotting, and detoxification. They also form the structure of DNA, RNA and cell walls.

The quality of the carbohydrate determines the healthfulness of it. So called "bad carbohydrates" digest quickly; which produce hazardous blood sugar spikes. Blood sugar spikes lead to inflammation, and a whole host of health impairing conditions.

**Refined carbohydrates;** these "bad carbohydrates" are stripped of nutrients (sugars, white flours, white rice, refined corn products, etc.) and are the primary cause of premature aging, and many chronic diseases. The SAD diet, with its high refined grain and sugar emphasis results in vitamin B, vitamin E, mineral and fiber deficiencies. These deficiencies cause poor elimination, blood sugar imbalances and toxic conditions in the body.

## Refined Grains

| **Refined corn**: corn flour, pasta, cornstarch, grits, hominy, masa harina, enriched corn | **Refined barley**: pearled barley | **Refined oats**: instant oatmeal | **Refined rice**: rice, converted rice, instant rice, polished rice, partially milled brown rice, white basmati rice, rice flour |
|---|---|---|---|
| **Refined wheat**: all-purpose flour, bleached flour, couscous, durum, enriched wheat, farina, semolina, gluten, nine grain flour, orzo, seitan, unbleached flour. | **Refined potatoes**: peeled mashed potatoes, peeled whole potato, potato flour, potato chips, potato starch, French fries, | **Modified food starch** and maltodextrin | **Refined sugar**: cane sugar, cane syrup, caramel coloring and flavoring, corn syrup, dextrose, fructose, glucose, lactose, maltose, sorbitol, rice syrup, sorghum, sucrose, words ending in "ol", and "ose." |

## Conditions caused by an excess of refined carbs and a deficiency of fiber

| Hypoglycemia | Insulin resistance | Diabetes |
|---|---|---|
| Heart disease | Cancer | Obesity |
| Colon dysfunctions/diseases | Hemorrhoids | Hiatal hernia |

**Exercise 6a: Carbohydrates: Input any refined grains** (from chart) that you can begin to cut out of your diet

_____

## The "Healthful Carbohydrates"

A youth enhancing diet emphasizes the "healthful carbohydrates," otherwise known as complex carbohydrates. Complex carbohydrates are the whole plant instead of parts or fragments of the plant. They are not stripped of their bran or germ or processed in a factory. Complex carbohydrates come from vegetables, fruits, whole grains, beans, legumes, and nuts and seeds. Complex carbohydrates are slow digesting, and support our energy levels, mood, and cognitive function.

The *Center for Disease Control and Prevention* (CDC) reported in 2010 that one of the chief problems with many of Americans' diets is that they are not consuming enough fruits and vegetables. In their surveys they discovered that only 26% of Americans ate vegetables 3 or more times a day, and only 32.5% of Americans consumed fruit two or more times a day.

*Organic Vegetables* are one of the most important sources of carbohydrates, and are the defining factor for optimal health. Vegetables contain the broadest range of nutrients of any other class of food. A reduced intake of vegetables is linked to cancer, and other chronic diseases. Conversely, people with the highest intake of vegetables (especially leafy greens) had the lowest cancer and heart disease rates. Vegetables also are low in calories and high in fiber; which aids colon cleansing and digestion. Vegetables are detoxifiers; green leafy vegetables are especially beneficial because of the chlorophyll that they possess. Chlorophyll contains blood building and detoxifying properties, and is soothing to the nervous system. In addition, green leafy vegetables are excellent sources of calcium, magnesium, iron and vitamin B6.

Starchy vegetables, such as winter squash, cooked corn, peas, roots, and tubers, (carrots, red skinned potatoes, sweet potatoes, garnet yams, beets, and turnips etc.) although higher in starch and sugar, contain high quality minerals and carotenes. They provide the body with energy, strength and warmth.

Many people have concerns about whether to eat their veggies raw or cooked. However, it is wise to combine both <u>cooked and raw vegetables</u> to the daily diet, as each has health giving qualities. Raw vegetables <u>retain more</u> of their vitamin C, folic acid, phenolic antioxidants and enzyme content. While <u>cooking some vegetables,</u> especially carrots, spinach, mushrooms and tomatoes, <u>increases their antioxidant numbers and the absorption of their nutrients</u>; especially when cooked with fats. It is also not wise to eat raw cruciferous vegetables, as they contain thyroid weakening goitrogens. Cruciferous vegetables include: bok choy, broccoli, broccolini, Brussels sprouts, cabbage, cauliflower, Chinese cabbage, choy sum, collard greens, kai lan, kale, kohlrabi, mizuna, mustard greens, radishes, rapini, rutabaga, tatsoi, and turnips. Eating a small quantity of raw cruciferous occasionally should not be a problem however. Raw food can also be harder to digest for some people, especially those who suffer from HCL deficiency, weak digestion, loose bowels or a micro flora imbalance; or those who run cold.

Optimally, it is beneficial to consume a large daily salad with crunchy and leafy vegetables- which will ensure an adequate supply of health-enhancing nutrients. Consider shopping at a farmers' market or join a CSA (Community Supported Agriculture farm) for your veggies, as most produce from stores lack freshness. They are shipped from far off locations, and sit in the store for a time; which accelerates the nutrient loss. Vitamin C, folate and vitamin E are often highly depleted in store produce. Conversely, farmers' market and CSA produce are often harvested that day or the day before, and have much higher nutrient content. To locate a CSA farm near you go to localharvest.org/csa.

If vegetables are difficult for you to eat, consider receiving your vegetables in the form of fresh vegetable juices or organic green powders such as *Paleo Greens* powder *by Designs for Health*.

A *vegetable* that is chock full of nutritional value is the artichoke. Globe artichokes are an exceptionally high source of fiber, magnesium, and chromium, but are especially respected for their liver-protective, and liver-regenerating effects. Artichokes decongest a sluggish liver by promoting the flow of bile and fat to and from the liver. This is especially useful as we get older, as liver function slows down. Artichokes have also been shown to lower blood cholesterol and triglyceride levels, and combat atherosclerosis. Artichokes also are appreciated for aiding blood sugar control; which makes it a great veggie for pre-diabetics/ diabetics.

***As with dairy, fermenting vegetables*** adds to their nutritional value, owing to the fact that the vegetables have been pre-digested by the friendly flora. This process enhances their nutrient bio-availability, and probiotic status. Buy fermented sauerkraut and other fermented vegetables in the refrigerated section of grocery stores, as non-refrigerated sauerkraut does not supply probiotics. A better option is to make your own fermented sauerkraut and vegetables with a culture starter. This is an easy and inexpensive way to ensure that you are inoculating yourself with beneficial bacteria on a daily basis. See Recipe.

---

***Fruits***, especially citrus, apples, and deeply colored berries are also health-promoting carbohydrates which provide high sources of vitamin C, potassium, and anti-inflammatory and anti-oxidant rich nutrients. Fruits are known to offer protection against cancer, heart disease, cataracts and strokes. Drinking the juice of ½ a lemon in water each morning is an alkalinizing start to the day; and also helps to cleanse the liver. Due to their low sugar status, limes and lemons can be used unlimitedly in the diet to increase vitamin C status. Sip on diluted lemon and lime juice throughout the day. Squeeze their juice on your veggies. Eat the pulp and zest for added antioxidants. It is suggested to use a straw or rinse your mouth after consuming lemons and limes to avoid stripping your tooth enamel. Limit all other fruits to three or less a day for blood sugar balance.

***Blueberries*** are widely extolled for their health benefits, mainly due to a combination of extremely powerful antioxidants known as anthocyanin and pterostilbene. Blueberries have been widely studied, and researchers have concluded that blueberries activate our longevity genes, (sirtuins) and protect the brain from oxidative stress and other age-related brain function declines. Consuming one cup of blueberries daily was found to improve memory, learning and motor skills. The most acknowledged therapeutic use of blueberries is for vision protection, especially against macular degeneration, cataracts, and glaucoma. Blueberries also have a host of other health benefits including offering cancer protection, heart protection, and stabilizing blood sugar. Wild blueberries contain still higher levels of flavonoids. Enjoy frozen blueberries in your morning smoothie. Put fresh blueberries in your hot breakfast cereal. Eat them as a snack.

---

***Nuts and Seeds*** are another beneficial type of carbohydrate, but they are actually composed of all three macronutrients- proteins, carbohydrates, and fats. Nuts and seeds promote satiation more than grains due to their higher fat content. Large population studies in America show that people who consumed the most nuts were less obese. Nuts are also a healthy grain-alternative.

***Whole grains*** (that have been soaked) are an additional group of nutritious carbohydrates. They are rich in fiber, protein, minerals, and vitamins. (Especially the B vitamins.) Diets rich in whole grains, as opposed to refined grains, are known to protect against heart disease, cancer, diabetes, varicose veins, and colon diseases. Grains however are currently a controversial topic. The consumption of gluten containing grains is of particular concern. Grains that are comprised of gluten are: wheat, rye, barley, spelt, kamut, bulgur, and oats. (If not labeled gluten- free.)

Today's wheat in particular contains up to 40 times the gluten as grains cultivated decades ago due to selective breeding and genetic modification. This disproportionate quantity of gluten can be acid-forming, inflammatory, hard to digest for many people; and can lead to allergies, gut disturbances and gut impairments. It has been speculated that one out of 133 Americans have negative reactions to gluten. (gluten sensitivity) Gluten is also known to cause brain fog, joint pain, and extremity numbness in susceptible individuals. Mounting studies are also verifying the link between gluten sensitivity and autoimmune conditions and neurological dysfunctions. This is true even for people who have no problems (apparent symptoms) digesting gluten. Researchers are finding that gluten is one of the main stimulators of inflammation, and inflammation has been shown to be the chief cause of all degenerative conditions- including brain disorders. Various brain disorders that gluten is associated with are: depression, headaches, migraines, seizures, insomnia, anxiety, ADHD, poor memory, and Alzheimer's

## Conditions Linked to Gluten Sensitivity

| Allergies | Gut disturbances, impairments, irritable bowel | Diabetes | Joint pain | Extremity numbness |
|---|---|---|---|---|
| All autoimmune conditions | Bi-polar disorder, schizophrenia | Headaches, migraines, epilepsy | Seizures, movement disorders, Tourette's syndrome | Insomnia |
| Mood disorder's Anxiety, depression | ADHD | Memory problems, brain fog | Alzheimer's disease | Inflammatory skin conditions, arthritis |

***An extreme manifestation*** of gluten sensitivity is a disease known as celiac. It is important to note that there are many individuals who have undiagnosed celiac disease. Celiac is the most common autoimmune disease in the world today; which can cause severe intestinal damage. People of northern European ancestry are particularly susceptible. Adults with celiac are less likely to have digestive symptoms than children; but they will experience symptoms such as unexplained iron deficiency, bone and joint pain, arthritis, bone loss, depression, anxiety, canker sores, missed periods, migraine, and dermatitis.

## Celiac Associated Conditions/Symptoms

| Iron deficiency | Bone and joint pain | Arthritis |
|---|---|---|
| Bone loss | Depression and anxiety | Canker sores |
| Missed periods | Migraine | Dermatitis. |

Some experts believe that gluten is also an addictive substance that has an opioid affect. A 2005 study published in *The Journal Life Sciences found* that gliadorphins formed during the digestion of gluten grains can stimulate the same hormone (prolactin) which opioid drugs stimulate; inducing a pleasurable high.

Consider testing for gluten sensitivity if you have any of the conditions correlated with sensitivity to gluten. It is also recommended to reduce or eliminate consumption of gluten-containing grains to prevent digestive and neurological disturbances, as well as over-acidity and inflammation. It is common however for people to go through a withdrawal period when giving up gluten, wheat in particular. Don't give up! There are plenty of healthy gluten-free foods to substitute with. If you do eliminate or reduce gluten, make sure that you do it healthily by avoiding so-called "gluten-free" foods made of poor ingredients such as: refined white rice flour, rice starch, cornmeal, corn starch, or potato and tapioca starch. Brown rice or another whole grain should be the first ingredient on the label. No other refined rice or grain or starch should be listed.

## Wheat Sources

| Alcohol, beer | Breaded foods, bread crumbs | Candy | Canned meat | Chewing gum | Communion wafers |
|---|---|---|---|---|---|
| Cous cous | Stamps, lipstick | Denture adhesives | Dextrin | White and grain vinegar | Dried fruit |
| Farina, Semolina | Ketchup | Mayonnaise | Self-rising corn meal | Instant coffee | Frozen turkey |
| Hydrolyzed plant protein (HPP) | Hydrolyzed vegetable protein (HVP) | Immitation cheese/ | Luncheon meat | Malt | Maltodextrin |
| Medicine | Modified food starch | Soy sauce | Starch thickener | Vegetable gum | Immitation seafoods |

➡ Gluten Sensitivity Testing: *Cyrex array 3*-most comprehensive marker of gluten sensitivity, or Anti-tissue *transglutaminase* (tTG-IgA), *anti-endomysial antibodies* (EMA), and *total serum IgA*

*Cyrex array 4* (optional) Measures sensitivity to 24 "cross-reactive" foods to which a gluten-sensitive person may also react to.

**Exercise 6b: Determine whether you may have Celiac disease or a gluten/wheat sensitivity** by noting symptoms and condition charts. Note healthful gluten-free features and print out wheat sources chart. Consider a gluten sensitivity test. Input any info into your wellness plan.

It's a good idea to always vary the selections of grains in your diet, whether you go gluten-free or not; as consuming the same grains can cause reactivity in our immune system from overexposure. This can create health concerns for us.

There are numerous types of "ancient grains" that are gluten-free, hypoallergenic, and can be a part of a health-promoting diet. These grains are easier to digest for most people; and have a lower level of anti-nutrient phytates than gluten containing grains. The ancient grains buckwheat, amaranth, millet, and quinoa are rich in nutrients, high in protein; and less likely to be inflammatory. These grains are more seed-like than the gluten cereal grains. Wild rice, teff and organic corn meal are other gluten-free options. These gluten-free grains may however be-cross reactive for grain sensitive individuals. Additionally, whole grains may trigger the onset or worsening of autoimmune diseases. Those individuals who suffer from autoimmunity or diabetes may be able to improve their conditions if they eliminate all grains from their diets for several months to a year. (Hyman, 2014) However, it is always suggested to eat all grains in moderation to avoid blood sugar spikes. (1/2 cup servings)

*Quinoa's* protein quality and quantity is the highest of all grains, and is considered a complete protein. It is higher in calcium, magnesium, potassium, copper, manganese, and zinc than wheat or rice. Quinoa is also a hypo-allergenic grain. Quinoa supports endurance and strength, and is excellent for bone health- due to its high mineral content. It is also useful for blood sugar control, migraine headaches, and healthy blood pressure.

*Oats* are technically gluten-free, but they are often grown in close proximity to other gluten-containing grains; which can cause cross-contamination. For this reason it is important to buy certified gluten-free oats if you have gluten sensitivities. Oats in the form of old fashioned oat meal, steel cut oats and oat groats are all whole grains with similar nutrient profiles. They are a good source of heart healthy fiber, B vitamins, potassium, magnesium, and iron. Adding nuts, flax meal, raw milk, almond milk or protein powder to the oatmeal increases their protein status. Sweeten with berries, stevia, ½ mashed banana, or dates. Savory oatmeal with salt and pepper- instead of toast is also a tasty accompaniment with eggs.

***Corn***, in the form of polenta or stone ground tortillas is also gluten-free. However, non-organic corn is almost exclusively genetically modified (GMO). For this reason it is advised to purchase organic corn products. Corn can be inflammatory for some people, though.

***Brown rice*** is also gluten-free and a hypo-allergenic grain. It contains high amounts of B vitamins, as well as manganese, iron, selenium, and magnesium. It also contains a good supply of fiber, proteins and gamma-oryzanol- a rice bran extract that is supportive of menopause and cholesterol problems. Brown basmati rice is a lower-glycemic rice choice.

***Spelt***, also commonly called farro is a distant cousin to wheat and although it does contain gluten, the gluten is more fragile; which makes it easier to digest and less likely to cause allergic reaction in wheat sensitive people. However individuals with celiac should not consume it. To its merit, it has high levels of B vitamins, and minerals and higher protein and fiber content than wheat. Kamut is another ancient wheat cousin that is also high in protein, and may be tolerated by wheat sensitive people, but not with people suffering from celiac.

*Note: It is recommended to soak and cover whole grains for 7-12 hours, or overnight, and add a Tbsp. of vinegar or lemon juice for each cup of grain. This process removes the anti-nutrient mineral-binding phytates that all grains possess, thus supporting the full absorption of minerals into our blood stream.

## Daily carbohydrate servings

| Food | Serving size | Servings per day |
|---|---|---|
| Fruits: (low glycemic) berries, cranberries, apples, acai, kiwi etc. (lemons and limes are unlimited ) | ½ cup or 1 medium fruit | 1-3 |
| Leafy vegetables: lettuce, mustard greens, kale, spinach, collards, swiss chard, bok choy etc. | 1 cup raw<br>½ cup cooked | 2-5 |
| Crunchy vegetables: broccoli, carrots, celery, cauliflower, green beans, beets etc. | ½ cup | 2-5 |
| Unrefined starches: Beans, sweet potatoes, yams small red potatoes, winter squash, buckwheat, quinoa etc. | ½ cup | 1-3 |

# Dietary Fiber

An important component of carbohydrates is the fiber they contain. Fiber comes from the plant cell wall, and its indigestible residues. Animal products do not contain fiber. There are two types of fiber, soluble and insoluble fiber. Soluble Fiber helps to slow down digestion, absorb nutrients, and bind excess cholesterol and sugar. Insoluble fiber moves waste through the intestinal tract. Most plant foods have both soluble and insoluble fibers.

Consuming sufficient amounts of fiber, **between 35-50 grams** daily keeps our triglyceride and cholesterol levels optimal; and supports toxin and heavy metal removal. Fiber rich foods also slow down the release of glucose into the bloodstream; vital for preventing blood sugar spikes and insulin surges, and pre-diabetic conditions. Increasing fiber will also help us feel full, lose weight, and keep our bowels cleansed and regular.

A high fiber diet also contributes to a healthy thriving beneficial bacteria population in the colon. Fiber increases the formation of short chain fatty acids, which are instrumental in reducing the colon pH. (Acidity) Acid conditions in the colon help acid-loving friendly bacteria to thrive.

However, it is advised to get fiber from foods, as fiber supplements can cause gas, bloating, blockages, and can reduce absorption of certain minerals. They also lack vitamins, minerals, and antioxidants that come from eating whole fiber-rich foods. Beans are a very rich and inexpensive form of fiber. Shredded dried coconut is also very high in fiber. Consider adding fiber-rich chia seeds or flax seed meal to smoothies, salads, and yogurt to increase your daily fiber intake. Chia seeds can be eaten whole; while flax seeds need to be freshly ground to be digested well. Flax meal oxidizes quickly, so it should be refrigerated immediately after it is ground.

Incorporate high fiber foods gradually into your diet- as your body, and your microflora will need to adjust to the change. Otherwise you may experience gas and bloating.

## Conditions Caused By a Low Fiber Diet

| Colon/Gastrointestinal Disorders: | Heart Disease | Diabetes | Obesity |
|---|---|---|---|
| Constipation, colon cancer, irritable bowel syndrome, diverticulitis, ulcerative colitis, hiatal hernia, hemorrhoids, appendicitis | High fiber diets reduce oxidized cholesterol, reduce triglycerides, and improve low HDL levels | Soluble fiber has therapeutic benefits for diabetics | Fiber increases chewing time, promotes satiety, fecal calorie loss, and blood sugar control |

Fiber chart on the next page.

## High Fiber Foods

This chart lists foods high in fiber, with approximate quantity in grams. <u>Note</u> if a snack doesn't provide at least 1-2 grams of fiber, it is not a good selection.

| Beans/legumes 1/2 cup | Vegetables 1/2 cup | Fruits 1 cup or medium | Grain 1/2 cup | Nuts/seeds-1/4 cup |
|---|---|---|---|---|
| Split peas-8 | Avocado-whole/12 | Raspberries-8 | Amaranth-2 | Peanuts-6 |
| Pinto-8 | Kale-7 Spinach-3 Collard greens-2.5 | Apple/med-6 | Quinoa-2.5 | Pumpkin seeds- 4 |
| Black bean7.5 Lentils-6.5 Kidney beans-6 Navy-5.5 | Artichoke- 6 Baked red potato-5 Mushrooms-1.5 Baked sweet potato w/skin-3 | Pear/med-6 Figs/dry-5 Blueberries-4 Strawberries-3 | Oats/oatmeal-2 Buckwheat-2 Brown rice-2 Millet-1.5 | Sesame seeds- 4 Almonds-4 Pumpkin seeds-4 Sunflower seeds-4 |
| Lima-4.3 | Winter squash/yam 2.5 Carrots-2.5 | Kiwi/med -3 | Corn-1.5 | Walnuts-2 Coconut (1 oz. dried)-5 |
| Green peas-4.5 | Asparagus-2.5 Green beans-2 | Banana (1/2)-2 | Popcorn/1 cup-1 | Flax seed meal: (2 T.)- 6 (choline, lignan and folate rich) |
| Aduki beans-8 | Sea weed-1 | Apricot-1 | Barley-6.5 | Chia : 2T -10 |

**Exercise 6c: Print out the daily carb serving sizes chart.** Make note of some healthful carbs and add some healthy fiber-rich carbohydrates from each category to your wellness plan or print a copy of the chart. (Write down fiber content) Try to get 35-50+ g. in daily. Consider counting fiber quantities up for one day. Soak carbs to remove mineral-binding phytates.

_____

## Carbohydrates and the Glycemic Response

One of the biggest health problems created by our modern diet today are blood sugar imbalances. However, balanced blood sugar levels are vital for optimal functioning of our brains, and for calm and happy moods, especially as we age. Blood Sugar balance is also essential for the healthy operation of our hearts, and for efficient energy metabolism.

When we eat carbohydrate containing foods, our body breaks them down into sugar. (Glucose) These sugars are absorbed into the blood stream, and carried by the hormone-insulin into the cells where they are used as fuel for energy. Insulin is the primary hormone that controls our blood sugar balance. But this system often becomes disturbed.

In order to effectively keep our blood sugar balanced, it is important to know the difference between rapidly digesting carbs and slow digesting carbs. Foods that are rapidly digested and absorbed (refined carbohydrates and simple sugars) cause blood sugar to increase quickly, or spike. This spike supplies instant, but not long lasting energy, causing eventual fatigue. These foods also don't contribute to satiation and trigger weight gain, inflammation and high triglyceride levels.

Foods that are digested and absorbed more slowly (complex carbohydrates) allow blood sugar to be released more slowly and steadily; which provides satiation, and longer lasting energy. These carbohydrates improve bowel function, lower cholesterol, support weight loss, and prevent inflammation.

Keeping our blood sugar stable is the secret to high quality aging and longevity. Our body works best when our blood sugar levels are kept low and even. The effect that food has on our blood sugar levels after we have eaten is known as the "glycemic response." The glycemic response is dependent on the **amount** and **type** of the carbohydrate that is eaten, and the amount of fiber that food has. Carbohydrates higher in starch and sugar and low in fiber produce a higher glycemic response; while carbohydrates lower in starchy carbs and high in fiber produce a lower glycemic response.

High glycemic starchy and sugary foods are the snack of choice for most people and are the most over-indulged foods. Sugar and refined grain ingestion can be addictive because of the instant energetic blood sugar "lift" that is produced from them. These starchy carbs also activate feel-good chemicals and reward centers in the brain, including neurotransmitters like: dopamine, serotonin, and beta endorphin. However, this carb "high" will cause us to over-eat.

Having an excess of high glycemic foods in our daily diet will not further our health, and will promote inflammation and accelerate the aging process. An excess can also lead to weight management difficulties, mood problems, after lunch fatigue, adrenal stress, low blood sugar, and pre-diabetes. Carb-associated blood sugar surges also deplete B vitamins and mood normalizing neurotransmitters such as serotonin, GABA, epinephrine, nor epinephrine, and dopamine.

*The ideal nutritional approach is to keep our conversion of carbohydrates to blood sugar-even and slow.*

## Glycemic Control Tips:

- Leafy and crunchy vegetables can be eaten without restraint as these digest slowly, and don't cause any blood sugar imbalances.
- Low sugar fruits such as lemons, limes, berries, green apples, grapefruit, acai, and fresh cranberries cause very little glycemic response, and should be the most prominent fruits in your diet.
- The remainder of the fruits and starchy carbohydrates (beans, peas, sweet potatoes, potatoes, winter squashes, corn and whole grains), look different under a microscope, as they have a different carbohydrate profile than non-starchy vegetables. These digest slightly quicker, and therefore cause a slight glycemic response. These should be eaten in moderation, although beans and legumes have been found to be a good choice for diabetics and those who want to achieve stable blood sugar levels.
- Refined carbohydrates digest the quickest, and should be eaten only occasionally, or not at all
- It is best to combine starchy carbohydrates or high sugar foods together with protein or fat, to slow down the digestive process; and therefore the glycemic impact. This will result in a slower absorption of glucose into the blood stream; and therefore a more controlled blood sugar increase; thus preventing inflammation. For example, when you eat a high sugar fruit such as a banana- it is best to eat it with some kind of protein or fat to delay its absorption; maybe with some nuts. High fiber foods will also slow down sugar absorption. Eating the fiber rich skin of vegetables and fruits also lessons the glycemic impact. In addition, when eating tubers such as red skinned potatoes- chose two or three small potatoes, as opposed to one large one. The extra skin will increase the fiber load, and lesson the blood sugar surge.

*Carbohydrate rule: Avoid "naked carbs." Always add fiber, protein, and/or fat to each starchy snack and meal to stabilize blood sugar levels.*

---

As mentioned above different carbs affect blood sugar levels differently. The ranking system known as the Glycemic Load is a relatively new and more comprehensive way to measure the effect that a food has on blood sugar levels based on the <u>quantity</u> of carbohydrates in a serving. The higher the number, the greater the blood sugar response. Any moderate serving of food that is mostly water, (watermelon) fiber, (beets or carrots) or air (popcorn), will not cause a blood sugar spike. As long as you eat a sensible portion of a low glycemic-load food, the effect on blood sugar is negligible. (One cup or less) However, if you take the fiber out of a carb-dense food, such as when you juice carrots or fruit, blood sugar levels will become elevated.

Considering the glycemic impact of our foods is the best way to solve many personal health challenges. Being attentive to the glycemic-load of our food choice is particularly crucial if we suffer from conditions such as: overeating, sugar and carb cravings, mood disorders, memory problems, blood sugar disorders or cholesterol problems.

Limiting the body's glycemic response to foods has a profound influence on many aspects of our health; particularly on energy levels, digestion, cholesterol levels, and memory. It is the key to long term health for anyone who wants to avoid age-related chronic diseases.

The following page shows a chart of the glycemic load of selected whole unprocessed foods.

*Note: The load values are an approximation, due to variations in selected food products. There are also variations in glycemic and insulin responses from person to person. Additionally, differences in glycemic responses can occur from one time of the day to another. Be mindful of how you feel throughout the day to determine the quantity of carb-dense foods that feels right for you. You may need more servings of a complex starchy carb if you suffer from insomnia or depression.

Cashews are a bit higher in carbs than most nuts, which can set-off overeating. Consider selecting lower carb nuts. Red skin potatoes contain a lower glycemic load than tan skinned varieties. I noted both on the next chart to show the difference.

## Low Glycemic foods – Try to emphasize foods that don't spike blood sugar

Rating: High GL: 20+ (dramatic spike)   Medium GL: 11-19   *Low GL (best): 10 or less

| Vegetables<br>1 cup or medium | Fruits<br>1 cup or whole fruit | Grains<br>½ cup | Beans<br>½ cup | Nuts/Dairy<br>One ounce (2 T.) |
|---|---|---|---|---|
| Leafy greens: 2-3<br>Above ground veggies: 2-4 | Lemons/limes: 1-2<br>Sour green apples: 3<br>Large fresh fig: 4 | Quinoa-9<br>Buckwheat-7 | Black beans: 7<br>Garbanzo beans: 8.5 | Almonds: 0<br>Brazil nuts: 0<br>Pecans: 0 |
| Med. sweet potato w/ skin: 10<br>Med Red potato with skin: 15<br>White potato: 17<br>Green peas: 7 | <u>Berries</u><br>Strawberries: 3<br>Black berries: 4<br>Raspberries: 3<br>Cranberries: 2<br>Blueberries: 6 | Brown basmati rice/wild rice-10 | Lima beans: 7<br>Split peas: 6.5 | Walnuts: 0<br>Macadamias: 0 |
| Spaghetti squash: 7<br>Kabocha squash: 7<br>Butternut squash: 8<br>Canned or baked pumpkin: 6 | Watermelon: 8<br>Cherries: 5<br>Kiwi (small): 6 | Oatmeal: 6<br>Steel cut oats: 6 | Pinto beans: 7.5 | Cashews: 3<br>Peanuts: 1 |
| Carrots, turnips: 2<br>Beets: 6 | Thompson grapes: 9<br>Lg. grapefruit (1/2): 3<br>Medium apricot: 5 | Spelt: 6 | Lentils: 6.5 | 1/2 cup yogurt: 8 |
| Bean sprouts: 1 | Small plum: 4.5<br>Med. feijoa: 2<br>Acai: 2 | Amaranth- 10<br>Millet-10 | Kidney beans: 7.5 | 2 cups Popcorn: 7 |

*Note: Canned beans have a higher GL than dry beans. *GL values: nutritiondata.self.com

Note: I refer you to a pocket guide for more glycemic load values: *The Glycemic Load Counter: A pocket guide to GL and GI Values for Over 800 foods.* Berkeley: Ulysses Press

*Exercise 6d: Input/print out glycemic control tips and glycemic values* on your plan. Try to emphasize foods with a glycemic load of 10 or less. Be mindful of how you feel to determine the quantity of carbs that feel right for you. Consider Purchasing the book: *The Glycemic Load Counter.*

---

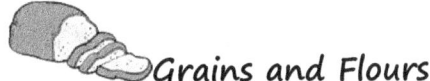Grains and Flours

Our modern culture has an over-dependence on grains, especially from flours made from grains. Flours are considered by some experts to be another form of sugar; as they act more like sugar when being digested. Pasta, bread, chips and cereals, a favorite of many individuals, are the chief culprits that drive our food cravings and trigger overeating.

Many of us over-eat **whole grain flours** as well. Whole grains contain more fiber, which slows down the release of sugars; but they still are high in carbohydrates- especially when eaten in a flour form, such as whole grain pasta or breads. Flour, even whole grain flours are considered to be refined, and are mucous and acid forming. They contribute to constipation and raise blood sugar levels; increasing sugar cravings and weight gain. Most flours sit in warehouses for a long time; losing nutrients, and collecting molds, and causing possible allergic reactions in some people. Additionally, whole wheat breads have the same glycemic load as white breads.

For these reasons it is wise to cut down on flour products for long-term wellness. Try to have <u>several</u> or <u>all</u> flour-free days during the week. Grain flours are not beneficial for sugar sensitive individuals especially, and for these people it is best to avoid flour products. Removing flours from the diet is also an effective strategy for weight loss.

According to the renowned neurologist, Dr. David Perlmutter, author of *Grain Brain,* and *The Better Brain Book;* "Our culture is eating far more grain (especially wheat) than our great grandparents or our early ancestors ate." Dr. Perlmutter states that our hominid ancestors' access to carb rich starchy food was rare, seasonal, and limited, and that their diet was low in starchy carbs, but high in fats, and proteins. Dr. Perlmutter contends that modern grains have no chemical likeness to what our "hunter-gatherers" ancestors ate.

This over consumption, he believes is challenging our physiology with substances that we are not genetically equipped to deal with. He makes the case that glucose-elevating, grain-heavy diets promote protein glycation and inflammation; which can impair our brains, and cause dementia. Dr. Perlmutter affirms as well that excess grain consumption, especially gluten containing grains, trigger brain cell inflammation, mitochondrial dysfunction, and formation of Alzheimer's related amyloid plaques.

A Mayo study confirmed this finding, by noting that individuals eating the highest quantity of carbohydrates had four times the risk of mild cognitive impairment. Another study revealed that impaired glucose tolerance (IGT) among participants in their 60's, doubled the risk for them developing Alzheimer's disease.

It is suggested that when eating whole grain processed products to make certain that the whole grains or parts of the grain are visible in the product. The optimal grain containing foods should also take some time to chew, the longer the better. There are several cracker, and bread products that have these characteristics; especially sprouted breads. Also, many low-glycemic grain alternative flours are available containing almond, coconut, chestnut, hazelnut or garbanzo bean flours. These don't increase blood sugar levels, and can be used in cooking and baking.

If it will be difficult to give up whole grain flours; a better option is to soak your own grains, dry them and then mill them in a coffee grinder or high powered blender. There is no mold or phytate problem, and the nutrient content is higher. Partially sprouting grains at home is an additional way to increase enzyme and mineral content of grains, increase their digestibility, and lower their glycemic impact. Simply soak them, and rinse them for several days until a tiny 1/10 of an inch sprout appears. Then dry the sprouted grains in a dehydrator or the lowest setting of the oven. These sprouted grains can be run into a coffee grinder, grain mill or high powered blender to make your own super healthy whole grain sprouted flour. Many health food stores are beginning to sell sprouted-grain flour as well.

There are other dense sources of carbohydrates that can serve as satisfying and nutrient-rich grain alternatives. Fiber-rich root vegetables, tubers; and orange and yellow vegetables such as: sweet potatoes, garnet yams, and winter squashes (kabocha, acorn, butternut, spaghetti, pumpkin etc.) are very high sources of vitamin A, B6, potassium, manganese and carotenoids. They don't have anti-nutrients, as grains do; and are a common feature in extremely healthy cultures. Small red and purple potatoes, peas, fresh corn, parsnips, lotus root, taro, turnips, jicama, daikon radish, burdock root, rutabaga, Jerusalem artichoke, celeriac; and cooked onions, leeks, and beets can also be a gratifying substitute for grains. Legumes and beans are also a nutritious grain-alternative. It is recommended to substitute these foods for grains for part or all of your dense carbohydrate needs.

New medical evidence has also revealed that being on a carbohydrate restrictive diet has been shown to mimic the longevity enhancing biological effects of calorie restriction. Calorie restriction has been shown in studies to activate our anti-aging gene, known as SIRT1 (sirtuin) and can extend one's life span by limiting calories. However evidence reveals that restricting starchy carbs, especially grains can now offer the same benefits of calorie restriction, without actually cutting calories.

The bottom line is that there is abundant scientific evidence suggesting that foods with the highest correlation of resistance against disease and a longer life are not grains, but vegetables, low glycemic fruits, raw seeds, nuts, legumes, and pastured animal proteins. Eating grains in moderation or eliminating them entirely is a good anti-aging strategy. Emphasizing higher carb foods at the end of the day (beans with quinoa etc.) however can support the synthesis of "sleep chemicals" serotonin and melatonin; promoting a good night's sleep. Additionally, individuals with mood problems such as depression or anxiety may need to eat a moderate amount of a complex starchy carb at each meal to facilitate the synthesis of the feel-good chemical serotonin.

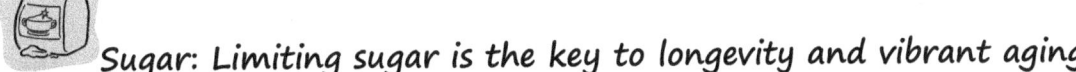

## Sugar: Limiting sugar is the key to longevity and vibrant aging

An essential part of healthy aging is reducing our sugar consumption. Many leading experts have made pronouncements about the damaging consequences of sugar. Endocrinologist Dr. Robert Lustig, a leading expert on obesity and the author of the book *Fat Chance*, believes that foods made with sugar are toxic to our bodies. He states, "Evolutionarily, sugar was available to our ancestors as fruit for only a few months out of the year or as honey; which was guarded by bees." He adds, "But in recent years, sugar has been added to nearly all processed foods, limiting consumer choice." "Nature made sugar hard to get; man made it easy," proclaims Lustig.

After decades of research on the damaging effects of sugar on our health, Dr. Mark Hyman, author of numerous books on blood sugar imbalances, asserts that it is <u>sugar,</u> not fat that causes heart attacks, weight gain, and other chronic diseases. He and other experts believe that 50 years of government eating guidelines and doctors' advice have been wrong. He contends that the guidance to swap sugary processed cereal for eggs is flawed and dangerous. A rigorous new sugar study published in the *Journal of the American Medical Association* of *Internal Medicine* involved 40,000 participants. The study showed that those participants with the highest intake of sugar had a four-fold increase in their risk for heart attacks, compared to those with the lowest intakes of sugar.

Sugar is a vitamin robber, and also weakens our immune system; causing us to catch colds and flues more often. Excess sugar consumption also leads to mood problems, such as depression, and anxiety. Additionally, research has shown that over consumption of sugar has a direct relationship with the development of diabetes, liver failure, dementia and cancer.

There is an abundance of scientific evidence that demonstrates that sugar feeds cancer cells, as tumors take up sugar at a faster rate than other healthy cells. This is owing to the fact that cancer cells require glucose for their energy and growth. Studies have established that there is an especially strong correlation between sugar consumption and breast cancer. Medical specialists have recognized for many years that sugar promotes cancer by employing the use of current medical PET scans. These PET scans use radioactive glucose (sugar) to find tumors. This injected glucose from PET scans goes directly to these tumor sites, where it has increased absorption and usage of it.

## Sugar and Endogenous Glycation

Excessive sugar consumption accelerates the aging process by promoting an abnormal reaction between sugars and proteins in the body. This reaction is known as endogenous glycation. Glycation, as mentioned earlier, also accounts for the browning of foods, and the caramelizing of sugars when cooking. Glycation occurs in our body when sugar molecules bind with protein molecules. This reaction creates pro-inflammatory products otherwise known as "Advanced Glycation End Products" or AGES. AGES promote protein damage called "cross linking." This makes our tissues become hard and stiff. Glycation can occur in our organs or even our skin; causing wrinkles and age spots. When proteins are glycated, the amount of free-radical damage formed is increased 50 fold- which leads to a loss of cell function and cell death. Many-age related diseases such as hardening of the arteries, cataracts, diabetes, autoimmune diseases, osteoarthritis and neurological impairment are attributed to glycation.

### Other sugar related ailments are listed as follows:

| Adrenal gland exhaustion | Anxiety, depression | Bone loss | Candida overgrowth | Flatulence, and bloating | Eczema |
|---|---|---|---|---|---|
| Fatigue | Gallstones | Gout | Hormonal problems | Hypertension | Insomnia |
| Kidney stones | Liver dysfunction | Low HDL cholesterol | Hormonal imbalances; PMS, polycystic ovaries | Decrease in life span. | Mental fogginess, headaches |

It is important to read ingredient labels carefully, as sugar is hidden in almost all processed foods. If a label says sucrose, glucose, maltose, lactose, fructose, corn syrup, evaporated cane juice or white grape juice concentrate; than sugar has been added to the product. Fruit yogurt has high sugar levels, as well as tomato sauce. Most breakfast cereals- even whole grain, are loaded with sugar. Highly processed breakfast cereals, including puffed cereals are a poor start to the day, and can wreak havoc on our blood sugar and insulin levels as well. In addition, breakfast cereals go through a high heat extrusion process that damages the proteins in the cereal; rendering them nutrient depleted.

Generally, it is always recommended to try to purchase foods without sweeteners. You can always add a little of your own 0 calorie natural sweeteners such as: stevia, lo han guo, or birch bark xylitol to the food at home. If you don't like the taste of 0 calorie natural sweeteners, you can add 1/3 banana, (mashed) or a couple of chopped fresh dates or figs, or a Tbsp. or two of raisins.

Additionally, you can drizzle a bit of raw antioxidant-rich buckwheat, manuka or tupelo honey or dark maple syrup (Grade B or C) to lightly sweeten it at home. (Level 1) However, many of us can't stop eating sugar once we start. Therefore, it is best just to avoid any natural sweeteners if we have this problem, and stick to only low glycemic fruit and 0 calorie natural sweeteners.

Try substituting unsweetened gluten-free muesli or unsweetened granola for your morning cold cereals; or forego the grains and use instead: ground nuts/seeds, protein powder and coconut flakes with raw milk, coconut milk or almond milk. Top with berries or chopped green apples.

Note: If you do buy products with added sugar- try not to buy anything with more than 8-10 grams per serving of sugar on the label.

### Glycemic load of Nutritious Natural Sweeteners (keep under 10)

| Raw honey: 1 Tbsp.- GL 10 | Dark Maple Syrup: 1 Tbsp.-GL 8 | Molasses: 1 Tbsp.-GL 9 |
|---|---|---|
| Small banana: 6"- GL 7 | Raisins: 25 raisins (.5 oz.)- GL 6 | Dates: One deglet noor-GL 3 One medjool-GL 9 |

From Nutritiondata.self.com

Health-conscious individuals tend to over-consume fruits thinking that they are healthier than sweets. But many fruits have high sugar content, and can raise blood sugar levels too rapidly. With the exception of lemons and limes, it is best to limit fruit from 1- 3 servings daily, with emphasis on the low sugar/low glycemic fruits. (Berries, green apples, cranberries, acai, feijoa, and grapefruit)

*In summary:* the likelihood of us developing heart disease, diabetes, dementia, Alzheimer's disease, and other chronic diseases can be greatly minimized by reducing our sugar and starchy carbohydrate consumption.

## Sugar Cravings and Addiction.

According to the scientific literature, sugar is physiologically addictive as it stimulates excessive reward signals in the brain. In fact, it has been found to be 8 times more addictive than cocaine. The food industry also contributes to this addiction by hiring "craving experts" to create the "bliss point" of junk food that can pull in "heavy users."

Uncontrollable sugar cravings additionally can be driven by several hormonal, bacterial, fungal and neurotransmitter imbalances. Blood sugar highs and lows are particularly at the root of our food cravings and propel us to eat carb dense foods. Indulging in sugar promotes a blood sugar rollercoaster effect. When we treat ourselves to our favorite sweet treats; we experience blood sugar, serotonin, and endorphin surges. These treats make us feel good! They give us more energy, and a euphoric mood; but are followed by insulin spikes for blood sugar regulation. The subsequent insulin upswing leads to a draining- low blood sugar state; causing fatigue and mental fogginess. This ensuing low energy and mood trigger carb and sugar cravings again to re-bolster our energy; which starts the vicious cycle all over again. This recurring cycle disrupts our equilibrium; resulting in weight gain, hormone imbalances, hypoglycemia, and eventual insulin resistance. The potential health risks of habitual sugar consumption could cost our body in the long run; as sugar drives multiple disease processes, particularly cardiovascular disease, Alzheimer's, cancer and diabetes.

One of the mainstays of blood sugar stability is **protein**. When we experience blood sugar plunges we often become ravenous and lose control of our eating. This shows us that we didn't eat enough protein or eat it frequently enough. Protein stabilizes our blood sugar and mood and decreases our carb and sugar cravings. Protein is the key!

*Consuming adequate protein is the key to reducing sugar and food cravings, and keeping blood sugar levels stable:*

- Eat a large protein packed breakfast within an hour of waking;
- Have protein rich snacks every 3 or 4 hours;
- And a protein rich lunch and dinner of fish, poultry, grass-fed beef, game animals, tempeh, or beans and quinoa etc.

## Breakfast Examples

| |
|---|
| 2 eggs with spinach on a bed of savory cooked steel cut oats and 1/2 grapefruit or 3 eggs sautéed with garlic, kale, tomatoes and mushrooms w/ a side of berries |
| Protein powder shake with almond milk, berries, flax seed meal, spinach, nutritional yeast & spirulina, |
| Nut butter sandwich with sprouted grain bread, with a celery stick and green apple |
| Whole milk yogurt with berries, flax meal and walnuts- with a carrot stick on the side |
| Steel cut oats or buckwheat hot cereal with nuts/seeds, protein powder and berries |
| Sprouted buckwheat granola or muesli with raw milk, chopped apple, protein powder and almonds; with a small breakfast salad. (tomatoes, cucumber, sprouts) |

## Snack Examples

| |
|---|
| Nuts/seeds with shredded coconut or some raisins |
| Humus or almond butter spread on celery sticks |
| Sea weed, topped with avocado, sesame seed, cucumbers and tamari |
| Bean dip with carrot and jicama sticks |
| "Live and active" yogurt with seeds and berries |
| Raw cheese with small green apple |
| Organic low-sugar *Paleo protein bars* |
| Olives or olive tapenade with *Mary's Gone Crackers* crackers or veggie sticks |

## Supplements that support cravings and balanced blood sugar levels

- **Sugar craving support:** L- glutamine: 500 mg.-up to 3 times a day or chromium piccolinate 200 mg./3x daily
- **Sugar, chocolate and fat cravings support:** Gymnema Sylvestre fluid extract. Put 4-6 drops of the fluid on your tongue to eliminate cravings and use before meals to lesson hunger. Gymnema makes it difficult to taste sweetness for hours. Sugar and chocolate taste like putty. Good for weight loss.
- **Blood sugar stabilizing minerals:** Chromium Picolinate: (200-600 mg) Manganese: (10-30 mg)/zinc: (30-50 mg) daily.
- **Blood sugar stabilizing spice:** Cinnamon-Sprinkle generously in your shakes, smoothies, yogurts, fruits, squashes, and yams. 1 tsp. a day.

*Intense sugar cravings* are also often triggered by a fungal overgrowth in the gut known as candida albicans. This is owing to the fact that sugar feeds and fuels candida. By ingesting probiotic-rich cultured vegetables, yogurts and kefirs daily, you will be able to crowd-out and facilitate their elimination, thus rebalancing microflora/yeast populations. As an additional benefit, eating sour-tasting fermented foods daily actually lessens sugar cravings.

- **Dysbiosis/candida control:** Eating a low-sugar diet; consuming cultured foods or taking a professional strength multiple strain probiotic supplement daily; and using powerful herbal antifungals such as: Pau D'arco, oil of oregano, grapefruit seed extract, and caprylic acid (also found in coconut oil) is effective at eliminating the overgrowth. *Thorne Research's Formula SF 722* (undecylenic acid) has been shown to be especially powerful for candida eradication. Refer to candidadiet.com, or *The Candida Cure* book for more information; and always consult a doctor before starting a course of antifungals.

*Extreme sugar cravings* can also be attributed to inadequate levels of our serotonin neurotransmitters. Serotonin's role is to produce a sense of satiety (satisfaction and fullness) after eating. When serotonin levels are optimal, we have reduced food cravings. If low levels predominate- we often suffer from overeating, food cravings, and eating disorders. It is important to note that stress is a contributing factor in declining serotonin production.

**Serotonin neurotransmitter production support:**

- High quality animal proteins (60 g+ per day) with healthy fats.
- Eat a modest amount (1/2-3/4 cup) of low glycemic complex carbohydrates with each meal:
  Tubers, winter squash, root vegetables, and whole grains support serotonin synthesis by aiding tryptophan (an amino acid responsible for serotonin production) to gain entry into the blood brain barrier.
- Supplements: HCL with meals- (if low HCL) vitamin C (1,000-3,000 mg/day) Vitamin D3 w/ vitamin K2 (2,000-5000 mg D3) B complex vitamins (50-100 mg/day) 5HTP (50-300 mg/day in divided doses- for mood/serotonin support) Multi-minerals and fermented cod liver oil/ or krill oil.
- It might be wise to get checked for vitamin D & B6 levels, hormone imbalances, and adrenal stress/insufficiency; which can play a role in suboptimal serotonin levels.
- Give yourself sweetness through pleasurable experiences that don't revolve around foods, such as: taking a fragrant bath; getting a massage; reading a relaxing book of fiction; communing with nature; giving yourself a home spa-like treatment; and listening to uplifting music.

---

*It is a good idea to slowly begin to substitute low glycemic carb options for your typical high glycemic carb fare.*

On the following page is a food swap chart that will help you to switch-out high carb selections for healthier low-carb ones.

# Carb Food Swap Chart.

## The cornerstone of Healthy Aging and a Healthy Body Composition

| Instead of This | Eat This |
|---|---|
| **Processed hot/and cold breakfast cereals**- These extruded cereals (even organic) are processed with high heat and pressure, and stripped of nutrients. Hard to digest (even the organic kinds), blood sugar spiking | - Buckwheat cereal w/ cinnamon and stevia (*Pocono* brand) w/ unsweetened almond milk<br>- *Food for life Ezekiel* Sprouted grain granolas<br>- Soaked buckwheat or steel cut oat hot cereal<br>- Protein powder shake with spirulina- (helps blood return to alkaline state after sleeping.)<br>- Eggs<br>- Quinoa flakes from *Ancient Harvest* or in bulk section of health food store<br>- High quality sugar-free granola or muesli w/ raw milk |
| **Breads, bagels**- all breads are highly processed, acid forming, difficult to digest, and clog your intestines. Sprouted whole grain bread and authentic whole grain sourdough bread is a better choice. | - Choose whole grain sprouted bread. Do not eat bread daily, and try to mix up the types of grains in the bread. (Brown rice, millet, buckwheat etc.) *Food for Life Ezekiel* and *Alvarado Street Bakery* are 2 sprouted grain brands<br>- Eat whole grain sourdough bread w/o yeast<br>- *Paleo Bread*: made w/o grains (almond meal)<br>- Romaine lettuce leaf or nori seaweed wrap with hummus, salmon salad, or turkey etc.<br>- Add hummus to "Mary's Gone Crackers" crackers<br>- Baked eggplant slices can substitute for pizza crust or bread sticks. Use with a dipping sauce.<br>- Portobello mushrooms can take the place of a bun. Broil/bake to soften.<br>- Put spreads on tomato slices |
| **Pasta**- any grain (even whole grain) that has been processed into flour is a high glycemic food. It also loses some of its health promoting nutrients and causes acidity. Pasta generally makes you want to overeat. | - Sprouted or whole grain quinoa, buckwheat or brown rice pasta-eat infrequently<br>- Shirataki (*Miracle*) noodles- a soluble fiber made from unrefined Japanese yams used for centuries to enhance health. Expands in belly to give sense of fullness. Takes on flavor of sauce.<br>- Spaghetti squash-Cook in oven, then scrape out inside; spaghetti-like strands form.<br>- Cut long strips of cabbage |

| Instead of This | Eat This |
|---|---|
| Pasta continued | • Sea palm strips (sea weed)<br>• Kelp noodles-nice in salads and soups<br>• Winter squash and sweet potatoes are very satisfying replacements |
| French Fries/Home fries-High glycemic, full of oxidized oils, low in nutrients; weight gain promoting | • Thinly sliced small red potatoes or yams brushed with coconut oil and baked at 370 degrees F. for 10-15 minutes until brown.<br>• Savory oatmeal or steel cut oats with salt and pepper topped w/eggs -instead of home fries |
| Ice cream/frozen yogurt-Loaded with sugar | • Frozen blueberries w/ plain yogurt or coconut milk blended together w/stevia<br>• ½ frozen banana coated with crushed walnut pieces<br>• Chilled full fat coconut milk blended with 1-2 tbsp. cocoa powder and stevia<br>• Fruit and plain yogurt smoothie<br>• Cranberry or strawberry sorbet w/ stevia |
| Chips/crisps/microwave popcorn-loaded with refined salt, trans fats, and bad oils.<br><br>Salt cravings can be caused by stress and weak adrenal function or a mineral depletion. | • Kale chips<br>• Toasted nori seaweed sheets w/ olive oil<br>• Cassava chips w/ palm oil (*Arico* foods)<br>• Homemade veggie chips w/ coconut oil<br>• A handful of raw nuts sprinkled with sea salt<br>• Flax seed crackers (*Mary's Gone Crackers*) with hummus or avocado guacamole<br>• Celery, tomatoes, or cucumber sprinkled with sea salt and pepper<br>• Pan or air popped popcorn w/ a little sea salt, butter or olive oil added |
| Sweets/candy:<br>Filled with chemicals and made with an excess of sugars. | • Celery sticks with almond butter<br>• Shredded coconut with nuts and raisins<br>• Sliced apples with almond butter and cinnamon<br>• berries<br>• Low sugar *Paleo protein* bars<br>• 70+% cacao square (w/stevia or lo han guo) |

**Exercise 6e: Input some blood sugar/glycation stabilizing meals/supplements.** Input some grain alternatives into your wellness plan. Try to have flour-free and grain-free days in your week. Write down some strategies to reduce your sugar consumption and sugar/carb cravings. Print out the carb food swap chart

*Chapter Seven*

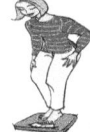

# Carbs, Middle-Aged Weight-Gain and a Dysfunctional Metabolism

It is very common to gain weight as we age. This is because we have more hormone imbalances and metabolic dysfunctions that promote middle age fat accumulation. More than 61% of Americans are overweight; but being overweight in midlife is not conducive to quality aging.

It has been estimated that excessive weight takes nine years off the life of the average person, and makes our heart work two to three times harder than it normally would. It also limits our vitality and mobility. What's more, obesity causes an inflammatory state in which our fat cells stimulate the release of damaging cytokines (chemicals that cause aching muscles and joints, and arterial damage) As a result, obesity increases our risk for many illnesses; including heart disease, stroke, diabetes, gall bladder disease, and osteoarthritis.

Obesity is also correlated with erectile dysfunction, sleep apnea, depression and fatigue. Recent research has also revealed that it is highly associated with colon, prostate, and female organ cancers. It is surprising to note that obesity may well now be the leading cause of preventable death in America; even surpassing smoking!

Weight loss plans for many of us in midlife have not achieved encouraging outcomes. This is because there are other obstacles that can interfere with our maintaining an optimal body composition. Weight-loss is not just about calories in and calories out. There are other factors that need to be addressed in order to manage our weight such as: behavioral issues, emotional difficulties, nutritional issues and metabolic concerns.

## Emotional Eating

Research shows that most of our food preferences and current eating habits began while we were in our mother's womb and throughout our childhood. (Following our family's cultural preferences and eating behaviors.) Unfortunately, this early conditioning subconsciously affects our eating behaviors as adults, and is usually the root cause of emotional eating. Nearly all people experience emotional eating from time-to-time. It is universal to try to comfort ourselves with food. But when this becomes the only coping mechanism to deal with uncomfortable feelings; than a person is over-using food to deal with their problems. This is not a healthy or productive approach. Dr. Roger Gould, one of the world's leading authorities on emotional eating believes that emotional eating is the reason that 95% of diets fail.

Awareness is the key to managing emotional eating. It is best to try to discern what emotions trigger our emotional eating. It could be anger, shame, lonliness, guilt, anxiousness; a feeling of not belonging, or a sense of a void that we have to fill up. Situations can also set-off emotional eating. Certain situations can be especially triggering such as: stress, boredom, procrastination; or not standing up for ourselves or expressing our anger. Journaling can be a helpful way to gain consciousness about what emotional triggers are causing our emotional eating. Once we know our triggers, we can start to address them in other more therapeutic ways instead.

When feeling an uncontrollable desire to overeat or indulge in danger foods- consider taking a minute to go within to try to determine if you are really hungry; and if not- what feelings are coming up for you? Ask yourself, "What am I feeling right now?" and "Where did this feeling come from?" It is also good to ask yourself "How will I feel after I eat this food?" By asking these questions, you just might get enough insight and strength to calm yourself and control your impulses. Additional ways to restrain yourself from emotional overeating might be to practice deep breathing and positive affirmations. Joining an emotional eaters' support group or seeking counseling can also be very therapeutic.

Dr. Gould, mentioned above, is the author of *Shrink Yourself*; and the shrink yourself online program where he outlines the 12 types of emotional eating. The following chart reveals some examples of emotional eating issues gleaned from his website *diet.com and other sources*. If you identify with any of these emotional eating triggers and issues, than it is an important dynamic to address if you struggle with losing weight.

## *Emotional Eating Signs/I Use Food to:*

| Pacify myself when I'm angry, lonely, bored, depressed, stressed, frustrated, shamed or anxious | Avoid confrontation when others make me feel bad. | Avoid feelings of the pain of rejection or anger in current close relationships | Stuff down self-hatred and inner-criticism |
|---|---|---|---|
| Fill up on love, trust and security which I'm not getting in my relationships. Not feeling a sense of belonging. | Forget the past, and make up for the deprivation I felt as a child | Assert my independence, and to rebel. I don't want anyone to tell me what to do! | Avoid taking a risk when facing new challenges; to protect myself from a fear of failure. |
| To avoid intimacy and my sexuality | To work out resentments and get revenge; or control anger from old hurts | To keep myself from facing the challenges of growing up; to feel carefree. | To avoid the fear of change; To avoid the fear of becoming thin. |
| My hunger comes on very fast; as opposed to growing gradually, and I feel a desperate need to eat right away. | I binge eat. I am secretive about my eating habits. I hide food to eat at a later time. | I have feelings of guilt and defeat after I indulge in comfort foods. | I Always feel too fat no matter how much I weigh. I feel jealous of models/actresses. I am a chronic dieter. |

As you read through this chart ask yourself how many of the emotional eating signs or feelings apply to you. It is recommended to seek professional help if you are dealing with traumatic issues.

*Exercise 7a: Is emotional eating causing your weight gain?* What signs or emotional triggers apply to you? Input healthful strategies to address this in your wellness plan.

---

Given that we all have unique metabolic, biochemical and genetic differences, there is no single one-size-fits-all diet that works for everyone. Additionally, many individuals don't have the genetic makeup or metabolism to be successful with the conventional practice of rationing calories. This is due to the fact that many of us suffer from what has been recently dubbed a *"switched metabolism."*

A switched metabolism is an impaired metabolism in which a person is preferentially storing calories as fat instead of burning them. Stress and our modern "SAD" diet is often the main trigger for this dysregulated metabolism which sets off a signal to store everything as fat. If we want to be successful at weight-loss, we need to reset and rebalance our metabolic signals. There are five metabolic groups that cause an impaired metabolism.

1. Carbohyrate sensitivity
2. Insulin resistance/metabolic syndrome
3. Food hypersensitivites and addictions
4. Hormone imbalances (leptin, adrenal, estrogen, thyroid)
5. Impaired liver detoxification/chronic exposure to environmental toxins

## Carbohydrate Sensitivity and Weight Management

Carbohydrate sensitivity is a condition in which our body receives the signal to store, not burn fat. It involves the hormone insulin, which is often called the fat storage hormone. A carbohyrate sensitive person, after consuming a high glycemic food will have an <u>exaggerated</u> blood sugar and insulin response. Insulin's job is to carry glucose (sugar) to our cells for fuel. But, if our cells are saturated and don't need glucose the body will receive the signal to store fat. This amplified surge in insulin will then result in a rapid drop in blood sugar; which typically stimulates cravings for more carbohydrates to remedy the uncomfortable symptoms of irritability, fatigue, and brain fog that it triggers. The combination of genetics; a diet high in sugar and carbs; and a lack of exercise combine to form carbohydrate sensitivity. Research reveals that the carbohyrate sensitive person is much more sensitive to carbs than the average person, and does not have the genes to handle the high glycemic grains and starches that are present in our modern diet today. Carbohydrate sensitivity usually develops over a long period of time however, and If not kept in check will most often progress to insulin resistance, metabolic syndrome, and possibly diabetes.

---

## Insulin Resistance and Weight Management

Heart disease is the number one cause of death in America for both men and women. A major predictor of cardiovascular disease, even more than just being overweight, is the amount of fat we carry in our mid-section, and our <u>waist-size</u>. When our waist size is over <u>35" for a women</u> and <u>over 40" for a man</u>, (apple-shaped figure) a health condition known as insulin resistance is most likely indicated. Suffering from insulin resistance can speed up our aging process and will put us at risk for heart disease and diabetes.

Belly fat or visceral fat, dubbed the *"killing* fat," is dangerous not only because of its association with insulin resistance, but because the fat in our midsection releases damaging proinflammatory cytokines. These cytokines are involved in many age-related degenerative conditions such as: cancer, stroke, heart disease, diabetes and dementia. Just losing a few inches off of our waist can help us to maintain healthy insulin levels; which can promote the longevity of our cells. This alone can lower our blood pressure, and cholesterol levels; improve our heart health, and lower other health risks. Interestingly enough, having extra weight on our hips and thighs, also referred to as a "pear-shaped figure," is not considered dangerous.

Food quality is a strong factor in insulin resistance. The dietary underpinnings that produce insulin resistance are a diet of excessive sugar and carbohydrates. Insulin is like a key that unlocks the cells to let sugar in. When we eat an excessive amount of carbohydrates our body pumps more and more insulin into our blood to try to keep blood sugar levels in check. Eventually our body's cells, which act like cellular locks, get warn and become numb to insulin's efforts to bring sugar into the cells. This ultimately leads to damaging high insulin levels in our blood. Insulin resistance is the prime factor in belly fat, high blood pressure, cholesterol imbalances, infertility, low sex drive, depression, fatigue, dementia, and a higher probability of diabetes and cancer.

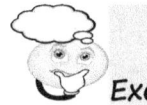

## Exercise 7b: Healthy Body Composition/Waist Circumference

Measure your bare waist circumference with a tape measurer. Make sure the tape is at the level of the belly button. If your waist size is over 35" for a women, and over 40" for a man; insulin resistance is probably indicated. Record your waist size on your health plan.

---

### Metabolic Syndrome and Weight Management

Genetic factors predispose many people to develop a newly diagnosed condition known as "metabolic syndrome." Metabolic syndrome is a condition which is characterized by a combination of insulin resistance, elevated blood sugar levels and excessive overproduction of insulin. It is estimated that 23% of the U.S. population suffer from it. Overeating; consuming refined carbohydrates, plus a lack of physical activity promote metabolic syndrome; and put us at risk for diabetes. Many people with metabolic syndrome are impacted by midafternoon energy crashes, mood swings, and intense irresistible food cravings; along with the tendency to gain weight easily. (especially the telltale abdominal weight gain.) In addition, there are five other features of metabolic synrome; three of which must be present to define the syndrome. The criteria are:

1. Elevated waist circumference (40+ in.- men/35+ in.- female)
2. Triglycerides levels above 150 mg/dl
3. Decreased HDL Less than 40 mg/dl for men and less than 50mg/dl women
4. Blood pressure above 130/85
5. Fasting blood sugar above 100 mg/dl
6. Lab test: Glucose Tolerance Test (To verify if you are a heavy insulin secretor)

As a consequence of their genetics, individuals who suffer from metabolic syndrome have enough insulin to process blood sugar, but they posses <u>excessive insulin levels</u> in order to compensate for their insulin resistance. Excess insulin release causes an abrupt plummeting of blood sugar levels, which creates symptoms of headaches, hunger, anxiety, fatigue, and irritability. The overproduction of insulin (2 or 3 times the normal amount) eventually leads to burnout of the pancreas, and diabetes ultimately develops. Other conditions associated with metabolic syndrome are: breast cancer, stroke, sleep apnea, gout, hypertension, heart disease, polycystic ovary syndrome, and high cholesterol.

*In order to be successful at attaining a healthy body composition, inividuals with carbohydrate sensitivity, insulin resistantnce, and metabolic syndrome need to consistently choose low glycemic foods.*

Note: Diabetes, often an asymptomatic disease early on is highly underdiagnosed, and many Americans who have it don't know it. According to a new study reported in the *Annals of Internal Medicine*, about 12% of U.S. adults had diabetes in 2012; and nearly 30% of Americans today don't realize that they have it. Diabetes is a very serious and life-threatening disease, and it is highly advised to seek diabetes testing if you are overweight and have a family history of diabetes; as early intervention can avert its disabling complications. (kidney disease, blindness, amputations, death.)

**Support for Insulin Resistance and Metabolic Syndrome:**

These supplements will aid in promoting weight loss, curb cravings, support fullness, balance blood sugar, and improve insulin function.

- *Metabolic Synergy*: multivitamin/mineral by *Designs for Health*. Glycation control.
- Ultraglycem X *(by Metagenics)*, a medical food to support insulin resistance and diabetes.
- Or Natural Factors Well Bet X PGX products: Meal replacement; multivitamin; *PGX w/ mullberry*; (appetite suppresant, blood sugar stabilizer); and *Well Bet X Glucose Balancer.*(supports metabolism, energy, and balances glucose.) *Well Bet X cinnamon extract* (potentiates insulin action) *PGX* is a fiber blend that studies have shown has a thickness and expansion quality greater than any other fiber. Research presented at the 64$^{th}$ Annual Scientific Session of the *American Diabetes Association* showed that in overweight insulin resistant subjects *PGX* lowered after meal blood glucose by 20% and also lowered insulin secretion by 40%. It also optimized cholesterol levels. If used regularly- hypoglycemic cravings are eliminated. Can't be taken with meds. *Well Bet X* must be taken 1 hour before or 2 hours after taking medication.
- Or For improved blood-sugar and insulin regulation Glucose Tolerance Factor Chromium: 200 mcg./2 times daily. Lipoic acid: 200 mg./2 times daily.
- *Green Pastures* Unfermented cod liver oil or EPA/DHA rich Krill oil: 1-2 tsp.
- Magnesium glycinate,
- Vanadyl sulfate
- Conjugated linoleic acid (CLA),
- Biotin, inositol, and vitamin E

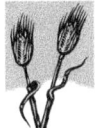
# Food Hypersensitivities, Food Addictions and Weight-Loss Resistance

Delayed food hypersensitivity is a common problem as we get older. It is also a frequent component of an impaired metabolism; especially if a person has a history of lifelong allergic tendencies. A food sensitivity occurs when the immune system identifies a food as foreign and sets out to destroy it.

Food sensitivities promote weight gain due to several mechanisms. Toxic chemicals known as inflammatory cytokines are discharged into our bloodstream to mitigate adverse reactions to specific foods that disagree with us; but these chemicals damage our cells by causing swelling and inflammation. Our body responds to these inflammatory chemicals by causing allergic symptoms; and releasing a flood of water into our cells to dilute and lessen the unfavorable effects of the toxins. This reaction is the source of water weight gain and fluid retention in many individuals with an impaired metabolism.

Some foods cause an immediate and dangerous allergic reaction that can result in throat swelling, a response known as as anaphylaxis. But, there is another more common form of allergy that generates a delayed immune response to reactive foods. It is known as an immune IgG antibody response, and it is often overlooked as it is subtle, and may not be apparent for 24 to 72 hours after the trigger food has been ingested. The damaging immune chemicals that are released to neutralize the threatening food may build up after years of recurrent daily exposure and impair our fat cells; disrupting our fat metabolism. These immune toxins may also get deposited from the bloodstream into our skin tissues, joints, respiratory tract, and our gut, causing allergic symptoms to appear in these areas.

Science has proven that we are addicted to foods that we are allergic to. Compounds in grains and dairy called exorphins weakly stimulate the same receptors activated by heroin and morphine. Exorphins are similar to our own internal endorphins and can heighten our cravings for offending foods; which can trigger us to overeat. Exorphins are toxic chemicals resulting from the battle between our immune antibodies and the reactive food. This conflict releases breakdown products from partially digested reactive foods which bind to certain areas of the brain (opioid receptors) that trigger addictive behavior. We feel temporarily better when we eat these foods, and worse when we don't.

Food sensitivites can also sometimes cause gas, bloating, and constipation. In addition they raise our stress hormones. The most common reactive and addictive foods for many of us are wheat, and dairy. Other reactive trigger foods are soy, eggs, corn, peanuts, tree nuts, shellfish and sugar.

All IgG delayed food hypersensitivites cause persistant, ongoing symptoms; which may involve many foods, and often are accompanied by a damaged small intestine lining, termed increased intestinal permeability or "leaky gut syndrome." This is when the intestinal lining becomes so thin and porous that undigested food particles leak into our bloodstream- triggering an upturn in our immune defense system. The best approach to reverse food allergies, and leaky gut syndrome is to eliminate the reactive or "danger food" from the diet for 90 days. After the elimination period, it is often possible to re-introduce the offending food without the negative immune reaction; as long as the reactive food is not eaten daily. (1-3 times a week/not consecutively).

Over the first 30 days of the elimination program the antibody levels are drastically reduced due to the discontinued immune provocation. During the second 30 day period, there is noticeable relief from allergic symptoms (brain fog, aches, rashes, gut issues etc.) and considerable weight loss. The last 30 day interval allows the memory component of the immune system to "reset" so that it will in the majority of cases be able to allow small amounts of the offending food, especially if it is not eaten daily. Eliminating the food for four months or more is needed if a moderate or severe reaction is noted. (Cooper, 2007)

Lab tests that can determine IgG food reactions/allergies are the *ALCAT* and *ELISA*. Other tests for delayed food allergies are *MRT* lab testing and *muscle testing*. Another method is to simply eliminate suspect foods for three months, and observe if there are improvements in health and weight loss.

After the elimination program, the next step is to systematically reintroduce the trigger foods back into your diet. It is important to only introduce one food at a time; and to eat it two or three times in that day with each meal. (wheat bread, tortillas, pasta etc) Then, for the next 48-72 hours, you will need to observe your body and look for symptoms. Fluid retention, headaches, brain fog, fatigue, or other symptoms concerning your gut, skin, or upper respiratory tract may appear. If you have negative symptoms after you introduce the food, continue with another 30 days of abstinence; and then test again. If you do not notice any symptoms within the alotted period; you will be able to reintroduce the food, but eat only one serving one to three times a week. (not consecutivelly) After the 72 hour period, you can try the next offending food, and note symptoms. It is suggested to undertake a leaky gut repair program while undergoing the food elimination protocol, as reactive foods often damage our gut lining; impairing our gastrointestinal and immune systems.

## Leaky Gut Repairing Nutraceuticals and Foods

- L-glutamine: 2,500 mg with vitamin B-6 morning and evening on an empty stomach
- Aloe vera: 200-400 mg capsule, or drink 2oz. twice a day
- Deglycyrrhizinated Licorice Extract (DGL): 500-1000 mg
- Slippery elm tea
- Home-made bone broth soup
- *Apex Energetics* makes a very good professional dietary supplement powder that combines L-glutamine, aloe vera, DGL, and slippery elm together to support leaky gut lining repair.
- *Designs for Health's- GI Revive* is also very effective for repairing the gut lining.

➡ It is best to support and repair "leaky gut" under the guidance of a nutrition or experienced health professional.

If you do decide to eliminate wheat; it is improtant to know that wheat is in many sources. The following chart lists many of them. Brown rice, quinoa, millet, buckwheat, teff, tubers, tapioca, or arrowroot are good wheat substitutes.. If you decide to eliminate dairy avoid milk products derived from casein also.

### Wheat Sources

| Alcohol, beer | Breaded foods, bread crumbs | Candy | Canned meat | Chewing gum | Communion wafers |
|---|---|---|---|---|---|
| Cous cous | Stamps, lipstick | Denture adhesives | Dextrin | White and grain vinegar | Dried fruit |
| Farina, Semolina | Ketchup | Mayonnaise | Self-rising corn meal | Instant coffee | Frozen turkey |
| Hydrolyzed plant protein (HPP) | Hyrolyzed vegetable protein (HVP) | Immitation cheese/ | Luncheon meat | Malt | Maltodextrin |
| Medicine | Modified food starch | Soy sauce | Starch thickener | Vegetable gum | Immitation seafoods |

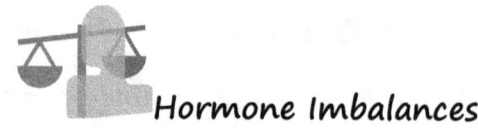 **Hormone Imbalances**

## The "I'm Full" Hormone: Leptin and Weight-Loss Resistance

Leptin is our appetite control hormone made by our fat cells, and it is the key to maintaining lean body composition. The leptin hormone, discovered in 1994, tells our brain that our body is satisfied and full, and can stop eating. It also functions as a regulator of body weight. However, chronic over-eating and stress increases our fat cells; and an overload of fat cells leads to a surplus of leptin and a condition known as leptin resistance.

When an individual suffers from leptin resistance their brain stops recognizing that it is full. Chronically high levels of leptin trigger the appetite control center in our brain (hypothalmus) to shut down to prevent overload. Essentially, we become intolerant to leptin. This results in excessive levels of leptin circulating in our blood and an inability to feel signals of satiety and fullness. Many individuals in midlife suffer from leptin resistance due to their increased fat deposits, and have difficulty losing weight. It is strongly recommended that leptin resistance be addressed because it is a risk factor for all cancers, especially breast cancer. It is also linked to stroke, and an enlargement of the heart.

**Tips and Supplements to restore leptin sensitivity:**

- Avoid MSG spiked foods; it destroys or binds to leptin receptors.
- Eating slowly allows leptin signals time to kick in; which give signs of fullness and pleasure.
- Reduce inflammation. Leptin resistance is linked to chronic inflammation. Reduce high glycemic load and processed foods. Take omega-3s, ginger, curcumin. (See inflammation chapter.)
- Exercise supports weight loss; which corrects leptin resistance.
- Work with an accountability partner or a buddy to support you in your wieght loss/exercise regimen.
- De-stress
- Conjugated linoleic Acid (CLA) and resveratrol have been shown to reduce leptin secretions.
- Take supplemental Irvingia Gabonensis extract. (African Bush Mango) It reduces carbohydrate absorption, and corrects leptin resistance. Double blind studies performed by research scientist Dr. Julius Oben revealed that overweight patients who took Irvingia Gabonensis lost an average of 28 lbs in ten weeks. In addition waist circumference and body fat percentage decreased. Leptin resistance,

cholesterol levels, inflammation, fasting glucose, and insulin resistance levels were also improved.

Clinical research suggests taking Irvingia Gabonensis: 150 mg. twice a day.
- o Garcinia cambogia is an Asian fruit rind that is found to improve leptin resistance; as well as reduce appetite and burn fat.
- o Fuxoxanthin seaweed extract is revealed to rebalance a dysregulated metabolism and to upregulate fat burning.

---

## 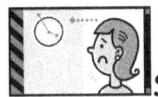Stress, the Cortisol Hormone, and Weight-Loss Resistance

Chronic high stress will cause us to gain weight, and it will also be an obstacle to losing weight. Cortisol, our adrenal stress hormone, is another fat-storage hormone. We produce cortisol when we are experiencing stressful events or emotions. When we are stressed, cortisol raises blood sugar levels to produce energy to handle alleged "threats." But, this excess glucose from incessant blood sugar surges can be rapidly stored as fat around our bellies; encouraging an apple figure and insulin resistance. Stress-induced fat also can be stored in our upper back. Chronic high stress is also responsible for tearing down our muscles. This will thwart our efforts at weight loss; as muscles help us to burn fat.

It is vital to learn to reduce our stress levels; as stress wears out our adrenal glands, and contributes to a condition known as adrenal fatigue. Adrenal fatigue impacts our appetite by causing us to crave sugar. Additionally, worn out adrenal glands decrease our "feel good" neurotransmitter serotonin, and promote low blood sugar; both of which trigger sugar cravings. It also is the causitive factor in a sluggish metabolism and an underactive thyroid. Lastly, chronic stress lowers our own natural fat burning and anti-aging hormone known as DHEA. Limiting our stress levels by implementing stress reduction measures will reduce cortisol-related weight gain, and is an essential component of healthy aging.

### Tips to Strengthen our Adrenal Glands/Nervous System and to Lower Cortisol Levels

- o Implement a stress reduction activity daily: deep breathing, yoga, biofeedback, meditation, prayer, exercise, warm baths etc.
- o It is suggested to work with a professional to learn stress-reduction skills
- o Phosphatidylserine: 600-800 mg in divided doses (lowers cortisol levels)
- o High protein and healthy fats sooth a stressed-out nervous system
- o Drink calming and strengthening herbal teas: tulsi, oat straw, nettle, passion flower, chamomile, and lemon balm

- Eat vitamin B complex and vitamin B5 rich foods: eggs, mushrooms, broccoli, nutritional or brewer's yeast, spirulina, or chlorella
- B-complex: 50 mg/3 times a day
- Vitamin B5: 500 mg.daily
- Eat vitamin C rich foods/supplements: citrus, kiwi, strawberries, peppers, sprouts etc. Ester-C with bioflavonoid: 1000-3000 mg daily in divided doses
- Magnesium citrate or glycinate 400-1000 mg daily in divided doses
- Use adaptogenic herbs to support your body's anti-stress defense mechanism: Ashwaghandha: 500 mg 3x/day
- *Designs for Health*: Adrenotone

**See stress chapter for more information.**

---

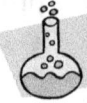 ## Estrogen Dominance, Xenoestrogens and Weight Loss Resistance

Estrogen dominance or estrogen overload is a very widespread problem today affecting both men and women due to our high-stress lifestyles, and our overexposure to estrogen-like chemical substances known as xenoestrogens or endocrine disruptors. These rampant estrogen-mimics go unchecked in our body threatening our health with numerous side effects; most notably weight gain. We absorb these fake estrogens into our blood and they then bind to our estrogen receptors on the cell's surface; taking the place of our real estrogen.

Unfortunately our body does not know that these xenoestrogens attaching to our receptors are not our actual estrogen hormones. In response to these continuous receptor signals, our body gradually retains more estrogen than we need; which overwhelmes our liver, and imbalances our other hormones. Xenoestrogens also compromise our health by altering our DNA and obstructing our cell signaling; potentially contributing to breast cancer.

These rising estrogen levels in our body increase our fat deposition. This occurance is the motivation behind giving feed-lot farm animals hormones. The estrogen hormones given to farm animals fattens them up quickly for slaughter. When our body becomes inundated with these fake estrogens from non-organic animals and dairy; our physique begins to acquire a doughy appearance. Our muscles get replaced with fat and our belly fat increases, along with cellulite in our thighs and rear.

Many estrogen dominant perimenopausal or menopausal women often suffer from food cravings and undue weight gain. Estrogen dominance is also often accompanied by low progesterone levels; as excess estrogen imbalances progesterone. Stress also creates progesterone depleting effects. Women who experience estrogen dominance and therefore progesterone insufficiency often have other related conditions such as: fibroids, fibrocystic breasts, borderline hypothyroid, PMS, and water retention. The good news is that estrogen dominance can be turned around with dietary and lifestyle modifications.

Males are also effected by high estrogen levels and can be inappropriately feminized by them. Xenoestrogens are capable of causing men to lose their virility, confidence and strength as well as turning their muscles into fat. These estrogens also can be the stimulus for eroding prostate health. Reducing xenoestrogen exposure and making dietary adjustments can boost a healthy testosterone to estrogen ratio; thus increasing weight loss, and also help to boost male energy, power, and performance.

Note: The Center for Disease Control tested for the presence of the xenoestrogen PFOA (listed below) in the general population, and discovered that every person that was tested had trace amounts of this poison in their blood.

## Some Sources of Xenoestrogens

| Plastics BPA/pthalates | Unfiltered drinking water | Hormones in dairy and fats | Perfumes | Makeup with parabens |
|---|---|---|---|---|
| Pesticides | Hormones in meat | Perfluorooctanoic acid (PFOA) from teflon and goretex etc. | Deodorants | Body washes |
| Fertilizers | Detergents | Hair spray | Moisturizers | Nail polish |

➡ Check out the *Environmental Working Group's* website "*Skin Deep*" to review more sources of xenoestrogens-such as other personal care products.

**Tips to reverse estrogen dominance**

- 2-4 Tbsp. flax seed meal daily
- Cruciferous vegetables contain estrogen neutralizing compounds (broccoli, cabbage, Brussels sprouts, collard greens, cauliflower, kale etc) cook these thoroughly to neutralize goitrogens.
- Avoid excess sugar, breads, and pastas. (insulin stimulates estrogen production)
- Avoid hormones in meats and diary. (or cut out the fat on meats to reduce exposure)
- Limit all organic dairy to small quantities, as xenoestrogens get stored in dairy fats.

- Moderate amounts of healthy fats can be beneficial
- Estrogen Inhibiting foods to eat: citrus, citrus pith/ peels, grapes, berries, figs, melons, pears, squash, onions, green beans, sesame seeds, and pumpkin seeds
- Moderate exercise (brisk walking)
- Estrogen-dominant women can also benefit from taking bio-identical natural progesterone. (cream or patch)
- The herb chasteberry balances low progesterone levels, caused by excess estrogen.
- The supplements: Indole-3-carbinol (I3C) and DIM (both synthesized from cruciferous vegetables) have been the subject of research studies for many years. *The Journal of Endocrinology and the National Cancer Institute* have reported that these remedies have been shown to convert less desirable estrogen forms to neutral estrogens.
- B vitamins, magnesium citrate, vitamin C, Vitamin E
- Lipoic acid
- Limonene

---

## The Thyroid Gland and Weight Loss Resistance

Our thyroid gland is considered a master gland as it effects every aspect of our health. It specifically controls our metabolism and weight. Thyroid function, like other glands, can become dysregulated as we age. Additionally, if our adrenal glands are not functionally properly due to chronic stress, the thyroid gland will not function appropriately; as they are interrelated. The thyroid gland is also extremely sensitive to the nutritional status of our body. If minerals and vitamins are lacking- our thyroid glands will not work properly. Many of us are unaware that we have a thyroid problem; as an underactive thyroid is the leading unrecognized hormonal imbalance in the U.S. Scientists from the *University of Colorado Medical School* recently reported that 20% of mature women suffer from a mild thyroid disorder. According to Richard Shames, the author of *Thyroid Power*- by age 60, one women out of six is hypothyroid. Many thyroid problems first manifest while in perimenopause.

The thyroid is one of the most vital glands in the body. It is in charge of our energy levels, how well we sleep, our detoxification, our memory, and how we gain and lose weight. A poor functioning thyroid additionally will slow bowel motility; causing constipation. When our thyroid is dysfunctional, we will have difficulty converting beta carotenes (vegetable sources of vitamin A) to retinol vitamin A. (true vitamin A) If this occurs, we may become vitamin A deficient if we don't eat adequate amounts of animal proteins (retinol vitamin A) such as liver, egg yolks, butter, cod liver oil or dairy.

It is also widely known that an underactive thyroid will cause our metabolism (the rate at which we burn our food) to slow down. This will result in weight gain. Even if we eat very little food we still may not lose weight if our thyroid is not functioning optimally. Low thyroid performance is also often to blame for estrogen dominance due to decreased liver detoxification and clearance of surplus estrogen; and as stated earlier, estogen dominance can trigger weight gain.

Stress, and poorly functioning adrenals are a prime factor in low thyroid functioning. Other contributers are sex hormone imbalances; heavy metal toxicities; autoimmune reactions; halogens; and vitamin/mineral deficiencies- particularly iodine. Iodine, a trace mineral, is crucial for healthy thyroid function. Dr.David Brownstein, medical director and author of numerous natural health books estimates that 95% of Americans are deficient in iodine.There are many substances that can block iodine uptake in our body, causing an iodine deficiency.

Overconsumption of foods containing goitrogens- especially from excessive soy and raw cruciferous veggies are one example. Compounds known as hologens such as: chlorine, flouride, and bromine also block iodine absorption in the thyroid. Additionally, if we don't consume adequate seafood or sea vegetables we may have sub-optimal iodine levels. Iodized salt is not a good source of iodine, according to Dr. Brownstein.

Hashimoto's thyroiditis, an autoimmune condition, is the most common form of hypothyroid. If you think that you may have a thyroid imbalance, it's a good idea to see a healthcare provider to get tested. An optimal working thyroid will have a TSH value of under 2.0; yet conventional physicians may deem that levels over 3.0 are diagnostic of hypothyroid. Additionally T3 levels should be checked, as failure to convert T4 effeciently to T3 in the body can result in low thyroid and a swiched metabolism. It's also recommended to take the Hashimoto's thyroiditis antibody tests, as it is a very common condition for women between the ages of 40 to 60.

- Thyroid Lab Testing: TSH (ideal between 1 and 2), Free T4 (ideal 1-1.4 ng/dl), Free T3 (ideal 300-400 ng/dl)
  Thyroid Peroxidase Antibodies (TPO) and Thyroglobulin Antibodies testing for Hashimoto's Thyroiditis. (Autoimmunity)

If it is determined that you do suffer from a hypothyroid condition or thyroiditis through lab testing, ask your doctor for a natural thyroid medicine such as *Nature-Throid*.

Additionally, consuming foods to bolster thyroid function will greatly enhance fat metabolism and weight-loss.

See chart on next page.

## Tips, Foods and Nutraceuticals to Support Thyroid Function

| |
|---|
| High protein foods such as animal proteins and legumes |
| *Iodine rich foods: sea vegetables (kelp, wakame, bladerwrack, dulse, hijiki, nori, arame, kombu) seafood (clams, shrimp, oysters, sardines, salmon) raw dairy, eggs, asparagus, lima beans, mushrooms |
| *Vitamin A rich foods: fermented cod liver oil, liver, egg yolk, butter, organ meats |
| *Selenium rich foods: brazil nuts, skip jack tuna, organ meats, mushrooms, halibut, beef, sunflower seeds. |
| *Zinc rich foods: oysters, sardines, beef, lamb, turkey, split peas, pumpkin seeds, almonds, ginger root |
| *Magnesium rich foods: dark green veggies, almonds, seeds, legumes, soaked brown rice and millet |
| *Vitamin D: sun exposure without sunscreen at midday in spring, summer and fall; and egg yolks, butter, liver, sun-dried shiitaki mushrooms, fermented cod liver oil, wild cold water fish (especially salmon, sardines, cod, and mackerel) |
| Iron: clams, oysters, organ meats, white beans, lentils, spinach |
| *B-Complex rich foods: Nutritional yeast, organ meats, egg yolks, fish, beans, almonds, walnuts |
| *Cultured foods/take probiotics |
| Green tea or green tea extract (EGCG) |
| *The herbs/supplements: Ashwaghandha, coleus forskohlii, guggol gum, phosphatidylserine and blue flag all support the thyroid. |
| Activities to boost hypothyroid: Avoid heavy metals, toxins, and anti-bacterials. Perform liver detoxification; singing, exercise, rebounding, yoga shoulder stands, stress management; and sleeping 7-9 hours nightly, |
| Massage the thyroid with coconut oil; it helps to increase blood flow to the gland. |
| *Avoid soy and <u>raw</u> cruciferous vegetables-they deplete iodine. (Examples: kale, broccoli, cauliflower, collards, mustard greens, radishes etc.) Cook them very well to deactivate goitrogens. |
| *If Hashimoto's Thyroiditis: avoid gluten or all grains for one year. Also get tested for delayed food allergies, and leaky gut. |
| *Take an iodine loading test to determine iodine deficiency status and to get a baseline to establish how much iodine is needed. Find an Iodine literate practitioner for this purpose. Iodoral and Lugol's Solution iodine supplementation should then be started. |
| Supplementation: zinc, B-complex, Omega 3's, vitamin A retinol, vitamin D3, selenium, magnesium citrate, resveratrol, green tea extract, pine bark extract, and probiotics. iodine is often dieficient in hypothyroid patients. Also try thyroid support supplements with above nutrients, such as *Thyroid Synergy by Designs for Health*. |

## Toxicity and Weight Loss Resistance

Toxins are everywhere! Thousands of new chemicals are introduced every year. (In the air, in water, in food; offgassing in building and home materials; in plastics; in cleaning supplies and in personal care products etc.) These toxic substances often referred to as obesogens are absorbed into our blood and get stored in our fat cells, thus increasing our body's fat accumulation. The body, in its infinite wisdom perceives toxin buildup as a threat, and escorts these toxins out of our blood and into the safer fat cells to protect us. Our body will naturally resist reducing fat deposits to avoid dislodging the toxic chemicals. Obesogens often throw off our sex, thyroid, digestive and stress hormones; sending wrong signals that our body doesn't understand. These incorrect signals can send our fuel (food) into fat storage; instead of being used beneficially for energy.

Toxins are also anti-nutrients which decrease our body's temperature. Low body temperatures slow down our metabolism and calorie burning potential by as much as 30%. A high toxic load frustrates our attempts at weight loss by impairing our liver, thyroid, and our cell mitochondria. With a poor functioning liver our body has difficulty neutralizing these toxic substances.

Fortunately, reducing our toxin exposure, and implementing a liver detoxification program will aid in improving our fat metabolism and weight loss. Reducing our toxic load, combined with an elimination diet can be an effective weight loss approach for those inividuals who have high toxic loads and impaired liver detoxificatiion.

**Tips to support detoxification**: (See also Total Load/Liver chapter)

- Assess your total toxic burden and eliminate what you can. Toxins are contained in refined sugar, artificial sweeteners, microwaved food, processed foods, hormone laden conventional animal proteins, excess alcohol, excess caffeine, teflon cookware, dry cleaned clothes, house-hold products with chemicals, pesticides; commercial personal care and beauty products, and plastic derivatives. Eliminate toxic products to reduce toxic load. (See oxidative stress section for other toxins)
- Consume onions, garlic, cruciferous vegetables, citrus, berries, beets, dandelion leaf, whey protein powder, lemon and water, ginger, turmeric, cinnamon, oregano, rosemary, dill, and spirulina to detoxify and diminish fat storage from xenoestrogens.
- Herbs/supplements for detox: green tea, dandelion tea, milk thistle extract, buffered vitamin C extract with bioflavonoids, and chlorella.
- If toxin levels are extremely high, it is recommended to work with a nutrition professional who can guide you on a liver detoxification program and provide you

with a pharmeucutical grade detoxification support formula. **Designs for Health Paleo Cleanse** is an easy to use kit that can accelerate the elimination of toxins.

*Exercise 7c: Determine which metabolic factors are causing your weight gain: carb sensitivity, insulin resistance, metabolic syndrome, food hypersensitivity, hormone imbalances, and/or toxicity? Determine from symptom list and/or lab testing. Follow nutritional support plan for dysfunctional metabolism issues from above.*

---

 Impaired Metabolism Plan of attack

If you have several metabolic factors that may be causing your weight gain, it is recommended to work on them sequentially so as to not become overwhelmed. It is more effective to focus on only one metabolic area at a time. However, it's beneficial to journal about your emotional eating triggers on a regular basis. The best strategy when applying this metabolic support protocol is to focus on one type of a dysfuncional metabolism for 60 days before adding the next area of need for 60 days. (Cooper, 2007)

### Order of Progression: focus on one issue at a time

1. Emotional eating (Continue to focus throughout your life.)
2. Carbohyrate sensitivity, insulin resistance or metabolic syndrome
3. Food hypersensitivities
4. Hormonal Imbalances:
   o Leptin Resistance support
   o Stress support
   o Thyroid support
   o Estrogen dominance support
5. Impaired liver detoxification support (Do not attempt to detox when you feel fatigued or weak)

Note: You may follow these metabolic protocols while implementing the weight-loss plan outlined on the next page.

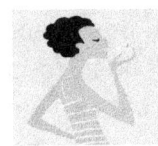

# A Healthy Weight Loss Plan

It is vital to be mindful that the <u>most important goal</u> of any weight-loss plan is overall health improvement. The following weight loss plan will aid in achieving this goal. The plan is characterized by moderate amounts of healthy proteins; heart-healthy fats; large quantities of vegetables; and fruits that are low in sugar. This is a low-glycemic food plan which will limit blood sugar and insulin surges. The less insulin is triggered, the less fat will be stored on the body. Research has found that it is excess starchy carbohydrates and high-glycemic carbs that cause undue weight gain, rather than fats, as previously thought. Therefore, it is fine to eat healthful fats in moderation on this plan.

When endeavoring to lose weight, think of yourself as being on a "healthy food plan," as opposed to being on a "diet." A consistant food intake of whole, natural, organic foods, coupled with an abundance of veggies will help expedite weight loss without needing to go on a "diet;" which we eventually go off of anyway. Generally, most people gain the weight back after being on a "diet" because they never really internalize healthy eating habits.

When we balance nourishing eating with consistant vigorous exercise, stress reduction, and good sleep; our body will maintain a healthy metabolism, and fat burning hormones will be activated. We then will reap the rewards of a healthy and slim body.

Note: It is not advised to eat an inordinately <u>high quantity of protein</u> combined with a very low amount of carbohyrates, such as in the currently popularized <u>High Protein/Low Carbohydrate</u> diets. This type of dieting leads to high-acid conditions, immune suppression, metabolic imbalances, and possibly kidney failure. It also doesn't effectively provide the brain and the body with the glucose (sugar) it needs for thinking and energy; often causing brain fog and fatigue, as well as insomnia. Another side effect of a super high protein diet is bad breath and constipation. What's more, it's also very difficult to sustain this way of restricted eating; and the majority of people gain the weight back. Therefore, eating <u>one small serving of a starchy savory complex carbohydrate</u> (whole grain, winter squash, cooked root veggies, yams) one to three times daily, with a few low-glycemic fruit servings daily is a viable plan that will support weight loss and energy.

**The following page** has a step-by-step list of measures to take to start internalizing good eating and lifestyle habits; and sequential steps to help you reduce high carb foods for easy and successful weight loss. See carb swap chart for alternate carb ideas. If you feel highly motivated; you can skip some of the early steps in this plan.

It is always a good idea to start with the easiest, most encouraging strategies when implementing a weight loss plan. In this plan, you will be introducing healthy eating habits into your daily routine, and won't feel like your are going into deprivation mode right away- as you won't be required to restrict any food or serving sizes the first week. After one week of continued healthy eating routines, your next step is to start restricting carbs. You will need to follow the other suggestions concerning proteins and fats that I have summarized in other areas of this book, as they are not included in this weight-loss plan.

## First Week: Cultivating Healthy Habits

Practice the following first nine steps for one week to acquire a healthy eating and lifestyle routine. You will not be required to eliminate any foods at this stage or worry about serving sizes. This will facilitate the next level of steps.

1. **Upon rising drink the juice of ½ lemon in filtered water.** Supports alkalinity and liver cleansing. You can drink lemon water throughout the day also.
2. **Have a protein packed breakfast every day** within an hour of waking to jump start your metabolism. If you skip breakfast, your body goes into starvation mode, which slows your metabolism and makes it harder to lose weight. <u>Option One</u>: A whey protein powder smoothie* (undenatured and grass-fed), or Well Bet X meal replacement protein powder* or yellow pea protein powder (1 scoop) with 1/2 cup berries, 1 cup almond milk, cinnamon, spirulina, nutritional yeast and 2 Tbsp. flax meal. Old fashioned oatmeal can be an additional side dish if you are still hungry. (lightly sweetened)

    <u>Option Two</u>: 3 eggs scrambled with garlic, onion, basil, spinach, and tomato with buttered whole grain sprouted toast, or on a bed of unsweetened oatmeal. Oatmeal is a great toast substitute when prepared in a savory manner with salt and pepper, and topped with scrambled or poached eggs.

    * <u>Natural Factors Well Bet X PGX-Meal Replacement</u> protein powder (for those with insulin resistance, and metabolic syndrome) or Undenatured grass-fed whey protein powder or yellow pea protein powder (for general weight loss.)
3. **Have two protein-rich healthy snacks between meals. Make sure that you eat every 3-4 hours:** This maintains blood sugar balance, activates our metabolism, and avoids uncontrollable hunger surges. Example: a handful of nuts with raisins; bean dip with celery sticks; 1-2 Tbsp. almond butter split on 2-4 *"Mary's Gone Crackers"* crackers; a small apple with a small chunk of cheese; seaweed topped with avocado, cucumber and tamari; or a meal replacement protein powder shake. etc.
4. **Stay hydrated** 75% of Americans are chronically dehydrated. Drinking adequate water has been shown in studies to shut down midnight hunger pains. Many individuals confuse hunger for thirst. It 's advised to drink at least half your weight in liquids: filtered or mineral water, fresh diluted vegetable juices, broths and herbal

teas. Drink every ½ hour. Green tea is a good hydrator, as it has also been shown to be thermagenic (fat burning.)

5. **Add extra leafy and crunchy vegetables to your meals**. They are very high in fat burning fiber, detoxifying and very low in carbohydrates. Make sure you load up on these vegetables at each meal to fill yourself up. Eat a large salad at lunch. At dinner eat a pound of leafy and crunchy vegetables: have a big salad with at least 5 leafy and crunchy vegetables before your main dish at dinner. Then fill half of your dinner plate with cooked vegetables
6. **Eat a sensible lunch and dinner** with 15-20 + g. protein per meal (depending on your weight) and add healthy fats: 1-2 Tbsp./per meal. (olive oil, olives, butter, dried coconut, coconut oil, avocado, flax meal or oil etc.) Eat a serving of fish 3-4 times a week to restore insulin sensitivity. Add a starch serving of: winter squash, cooked root vegetables, sweet potato, basmati brown rice, quinoa or bread. Etc
7. **Begin to do some form of exercise** at least 3 times a week to burn calories, increase energy levels and build muscle (which supports weight loss) Walking is always a good start. (See exercise chapter on a walking program)
8. **Take a deep calming breath** before eating. Have gratitude for your meal, and chew your food slowly and thoroughly (until soupy consistency.) Consider putting your fork down between bites to slow down the eating process. Take a half hour to calmly eat your meals.
9. **Stay mindful of your fullness cues.** Avoid absent-mind eating in front of T.V. etc.

## 2nd Week: Elimination Phase- Keep up with the suggestions from above

1. You may start to use **meal replacement protein powders** in shakes to substitute for one or two meals a day, but this is optional. (morning, lunch or snack) One scoop *Paleo Meal, or Natural Factors Well Bet X PGX*, or any other undenatured grass-fed whey protein powder. Add 1 cup almond milk or coconut milk- diluted with 1 cup water or green tea, ½ cup berries, cinnamon, 2 Tbsp. flax meal, 1 Tbsp. dried coconut, nutritional yeast and spirulina (1/4 tsp to 2 tsp.)
2. Eliminate the most carbohydrate-dense foods in your diet first. These are **sugary drinks, and refined snack foods (soda, sweet drinks, candy, chips, french fries etc.)** These foods rapidly get turned into sugar, and are absorbed into the blood quickly; causing high insulin surges; an inability to limit intake; and ensuing weight gain. Eliminate one can of soda or sweet drink per day until none are consumed.

## 3rd Week

1. **Eliminate refined white flour and processed grain products** (bakery items, white bread, tortillas, white rice, and semolina white pasta etc.) These foods also exert a high insulin rise, and promote over-eating. Eliminate white bread and substitute with gluten-free brown rice bread (*Food For Life* brand) or sprouted whole grain

bread such as *Food for Life Ezekiel 4:9 bread, Berlin Natural Bakery,* or *Alvarado Street Bakery Etc.*

## 4th week

1. **Reduce/eliminate whole grain "flours" in baked goods, breads and pastas**: (wheat, brown rice, buckwheat, corn, quinoa etc.) All flours, even whole grain flours cause a rise in insulin, and encourage over-consumption. Use 1 less piece of bread at lunch (ex. ½ sandwhich) Eat one less cup of pasta at your meal (ex.1/2-1 cup instead of 2+ cups) Substitute with low-glycemic bean and nut flours- now found in breads.

2. **Substitute certain varieties of whole grains for other low glycemic counterparts**: Long grain brown rice, especially brown basmati rice has a lower gycemic load than short grain varieties. Instant oatmeal has less fiber than old fashioned oatmeal, and therefore has a higher glycemic load. Steel cut oats are also a good oatmeal substitute. When trying to lose weight, it's best not to eat a high quantity of grains, as they promote overeating by stimulating an exaggerated blood sugar response. Eat ½-3/4 cup of cooked grains instead of 1+ cups.

## 5th Week and thereafter

1. **Substitute high-fiber starch alternatives for some or all of the higher glycemic starches (potatoes, corn, and whole grains.)** This is especially important for high insulin secretors. The following foods will provide enegy, and help you to feel full: sweet potatoes, garnet yams, peas, baked carrots, beets, and turnips; winter squash (pumpkins, butternut squash, kabocha squash, spaghetti squash, acorn squash etc.) and other cooked tubers and root veggies etc. They have a lower glycemic load, and a higher nutrient profile; and will provide satiety. Pumpkins, kabocha and spaghetti squash have very low glycemic loads, and can be eaten freely. Always choose several small potatoes or yams instead of one large one to increase fiber content, and lessen glycemic load- as there is more fiber rich skin on several smaller potatoes.

2. **Reduce dairy**. Dairy contains carbohydrates due to its lactose content. (a form of sugar) Milk and cream contain the highest amounts of carbohydrates. Cheese has lower carbohydrate amounts. Goat cheese, cheddar cheese, and parmesan cheese have the lowest carb levels. (0.5 grams or less per oz.) Mozerella, gouda, blue cheese, and swiss cheese contain only a gram or less of carbohydrates per oz. Choose low carb options in moderation. Cheese servings are the size of 3 dice. Cultured lactose-free yogurt with "live and active cultures," has lower carb levels than standard yogurt. Eat a ½ to 3/4 cup yogurt serving.

3. **Reduce/eliminate high carb fruits**: Eat mostly low carb fruits such as berries, green sour apples, whole cranberries, acai, and grapefruit. Limit to 3 servings a day.

Lemons and limes diluted in water can be eaten or sipped in drinks in abundance. See glycemic load chart.

4. **Consume legumes daily** (beans and lentils) They contain high fiber and protein. Important for lowering blood sugar and insulin response to meals. Be sure to soak 12 hours. Cannelini beans are especially weight-loss friendly because they stop carbs from breaking down into sugar, and thus prevent fat storage. Eating the cannelinni beans whole in salad and soup before eating starchy carbs is an Italian custom.

5. **Eat high fiber foods**: Fiber forces us to chew longer; which slows down our eating. It also supports lowered glucose and insulin release. Try for 35-50 grams daily. Start slowly, as an abrupt increase can cause gas and bloating: avocado, kale, broccoli, collard greens, almonds, green beans, blueberries, carrots, seeds, shredded coconut. 2-4 Tbs. flax seed meal throughout the day. Put flax in smoothies, oatmeal etc. (grind seeds in coffee grinder.)

6. **Eat moderate amounts of beneficial monounsaturated and omega-3 fats**: They improve insulin sensitivity: olives, olive oil, macadamia nuts, avocado, almonds, flax seed meal, chia, pumpkin seed, salmon, sardines, anchovy etc.

7. **Increase probiotic rich foods/supplements**: These support weight loss. Fermented vegetables and refrigerated saurkraut, beet kvass, yogurt, and kefir with "Live and Active" bacteria on label.

8. **Increase thermogenic (fat burning) foods**: Proteins, mushrooms, celery, broccoli, cauliflower, cabbage, leafy greens, asparagus, chili peppers, berries, apples, turmeric, ginger, cayenne pepper, maca, cardamom, black pepper, and green tea.

9. **Thermogenic Botanicals**: Green tea and Green tea EGCG supplements.

10. **Weight Loss Supplements**:
    - White kidney bean extract-stops carbs from breaking down into sugar, and thus prevents fat storage. Eating the cannelinni beans whole in salad and soup before eating starchy carbs has the same effect.
    - African yam (irvingia gabonensis) activates fat burning potential (thermogenic); improves response to insulin
    - Garcinia cambogia- Asian fruit estract that suppresses appetite, and helps you feel full with smaller amounts of food.
    - Fucoxanthin-Japanese brown seaweed extract that reduces appetite and switches on fat burning genes
    - *Carbxzyme and Thermo EFx by Designs for Health*. Helps boost fat burning.
    - 7- Keto- Suppots fat burning. Thermogenic.

11. **Brisk exercise** 5-7 days a week/brisk walking etc. Start out with 15 min. a day-3 times a week. Work up to 45-60 min 5+ days a week. Wear a pedometer to measure

walking progress throughout the day: ultimate goal-10,000 steps daily, or cross train w/burst, strength, and flexibility routines.

12. **Manage stress-**. The stress hormone, cortisol if activated too often can promote weight-gain. Deep breathing is helpful.

## Metabolism Boosting Eating Tips

| Drink 1-2 meals a day using whey protein powder or yellow pea protein meal replacement smoothie | Proteins: Eat 3-4 oz. animal protein or 6-12 oz. vegetable protein at each meal | Fats: 1-2 Tbsp. per meal omega-3 and monounsat. (olive oil, coconut oil, avocado, seeds, nuts, olives) | Non-starchy carbs- 1 Lb. at supper: (Crunchy/leafy veggies- raw and cooked). A large salad and ½ plate of veggies | Starchy veggies: ½-3/4 cup 1-3 x/day (sweet potatoes, yams, winter squash, cooked carrots and beets) |
|---|---|---|---|---|
| Gluten-free grains: ½ cup 1-2x/day (quinoa, oats, buckwheat, millet, amaranth, wild rice, basmati rice) | Fresh low glycemic fruit: 1-3 pieces or 1-3 cups/day of: berries, green apple, ½ grapefruit acai, cranberries. Unlimited Lemon/lime juice | Beverages: ½ cup everyhour; ½ your weight in oz.daily; Water, tea, broth, or fresh diluted veggie juice (50% diluted) | Increase thermogenisis (fat burning)w/ turmeric, cardamom, ginger, cayenne pepper, green tea, apples, green beans, chili peppers, cabbage, brocolli etc. | *Fermented Foods: veggies, kefir, yogurt *High fiber foods-flax seed, green beans, carrots, almonds, kale, broccoli, blueberries, avocado |

*Exercise 7d: Print out the Healthy Weight Loss plan, and the metabolism boosting meal Plan. Follow the plan for as long as you need to. Refer to the carb food swap chart for healthy carb suggestions.*

Note: Many individuals have also been very successful with weight loss by following the Paleo Diet, outlined in the next chapter.

*Affirmation: Everyday my relationship with food becomes healthier. My metabolism is healing. I can achieve my healthy body composition.*

Chapter 8

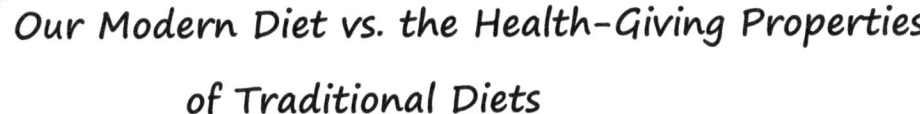

# Our Modern Diet vs. the Health-Giving Properties of Traditional Diets

We have deemphasized the importance of food and mealtimes in our modern culture. According to Dr. Mark Hyman, author of the *Blood Sugar Solution*, our diets have been "turned upside down since the advent of agriculture and industrialization." He, and other health advocates contend that our early ancestors would not have recognized 60% of our food calories today; mostly coming from factory made processed foods.

However, that wasn't always the case. In our not too far past humans had a reverence for their food and paid a lot of attention to food preparation and meal times. Eating was a pleasurable experience and one in which the diners took time to eat in a relaxed manner. Today our food is often of poor quality, nutrient depleted, and hastily eaten.

Many individuals today are looking to the past to restore more healthful ways of eating into their lives. It makes sense to look at what our earlier ancestors in traditional cultures have eaten and thrived on for thousands of years. A growing body of research has now associated traditional diets of the past with a lower incidence of disease, and greater longevity. Many medical professionals in the early 20$^{th}$ century including Dr. Westin Price of the U.S.; Albert Schweitzer of Africa; and Sir Robert Mc Carrison of India, noted that isolated primitive races had little or no evidence of modern "western" diseases.

Dr. Weston Price, the Author of the book, *Nutrition and Physical Regeneration*, and a dentist in the early 20$^{th}$ century, carried out groundbreaking research on the value of traditional diets of primitive cultures around the world. Price followed traditional cultures from remote villages in Switzerland, Africa, the South Pacific, the Hebrides, and the Inuit cultures etc. for twenty to forty years; and documented the advent of crooked teeth, cavities and degenerative diseases as their traditional dietary practices changed to a more industrialized "civilized" western diet. He also made expeditions to warmer parts of the world to determine if there were tribes who could obtain all their requirements for good health and a high state of physical efficiency by subsisting on plants and vegetables alone. The conclusion of his studies revealed that all indigenous tribes put great value on animal foods, especially organ meats. He found that even the agricultural tribes in Africa consumed insects and small fish; however, they were not as robust as tribes that hunted, fished or kept herds. Dr. Price's extensive global search could not locate any group that was building and maintaining good health exclusively on plant foods.

Additional experts subsequently began studying the diets of traditional cultures. Drs. Burkitt, and Trowell; scientists and authors of the book; *Western Diseases: Their Emergence and Prevention*, published in 1981, noted that when primitive cultures abandoned their traditional diet of unprocessed whole foods in favor of processed western foods there was a sharp increase in chronic diseases such as obesity, heart disease, diabetes, cancer, arthritis and gout,

Dr. Price's work is now being carried on by the Weston A. Price Foundation, founded in 1999 by Sally Fallon and Dr. Mary Enig. They have authored the highly recommended classic cookbook entitled *Nourishing Traditions*. Sally Fallon summarizes Dr. Price's research by identifying the:

### Ten Underlying Characteristics of Healthy Traditional Diets.

You can improve or maintain your own health by incorporating some or all of these characteristics of traditional diets.

1. No refined or denatured foods
2. Traditional diets all contained some animal proteins, especially valued were organ meats. At the minimum, traditional cultures ate dairy and insects that happened to fall in their rice. (East Indians) Dr. Price found that the healthiest cultures always ate fish and seafood. Critical nutrients such as the vitamins: retinol A, D, B12 and cholesterol are only found in animal foods. (Some individuals may have difficulty making the conversion from plant sourced vitamin A-beta-carotene to animal sourced vitamin A.) Butter, liver, fish eggs, cream, and animal fats were the sacred foods of traditional cultures. Dr. Price analyzed native diets and found that they consumed 10x more animal sourced vitamin A and D than Western diets.
3. Extremely nutrient dense. Everything they did maximized nutrients. They ate organ meats preferentially over muscle meats. They ate animal fats over vegetable oils. They ate pastured animals, and raw or fermented dairy products. Super nutritious fish eggs and fish liver oil was widely sought after.
4. Raw foods: raw dairy, raw marinated fish, and raw meats for enzyme and high vitamin B6 content.
5. Fermented or lacto-fermented dairy, animal proteins and enzyme-rich vegetables (sauerkraut, kefir etc.) with every meal for digestive efficiency and probiotic content.
6. They soaked, sprouted, soured, or fermented their seeds, nuts, legumes, and grains to support digestion.

7. No polyunsaturated oils. All used animal fats.
8. Equal amounts of omega-3 to omega 6 oils. Omega-6 sources from nuts and seeds. Omega-3 sources from fermented fish, cod liver oil, fish eggs, egg yolk, organ meats, seaweed, algae etc.
9. All contained unrefined salt for protein digestion, adrenal gland health, and brain development.
10. They all made use of bones- usually in bone broths. Very high in easily absorbable minerals like calcium, magnesium and phosphorous. Rich in digestive and liver supportive gelatin. Helpful also for leaky gut, youthful skin, allergies, and fatigue.

## Traditional Diet Components

| No refined or denatured foods | Animal proteins in the diet | High nutrient density: animal fats, organ meats, cod liver oil, eggs, sea veggies, algae | Raw foods: Dairy, fish, meats (must freeze meats before eating to avoid pathogens) | Fermented/lacto-fermented vegetables, fish, drinks, and dairy |
|---|---|---|---|---|
| Soaked, sprouted, or soured grains, nuts, seeds, and legumes | No polyunsaturated refined oils Only animal fats, coconut oils, palm oils and extra virgin olive oils | Balanced 0-3 to 0-6 oils: nuts and seeds w/ pastured animals, eggs, wild fish etc. | Colored sea salt: not pure white refined salt. Can be gray or pink. | Homemade bone broths. They also ate small bones in fish (sardines, salmon etc.) |

## Homemade Bone Stocks

Homemade bone stocks have been a dietary mainstay for millennia. Not only does bone stock impart delicious flavor to any soup or dish- It is a nutrient packed "super food." it strengthens our immune system and is full of absorbable minerals such as calcium, magnesium, potassium, phosphorous, and sulfur. Bone broths also provide an excellent source of the protein- collagen which nourishes our joints, tendons, ligaments, skin and mucous membranes. The amino acids glycine and proline contained in collagen have many therapeutic applications as they are instrumental in repairing thinning and damaged intestinal linings (leaky gut): a common occurrence as we age. A thinning lining can also be the contributing factor to autoimmune diseases, food allergies, ulcers, Chrone's disease, and ulcerative colitis. The glycine protein in bone stock has also been found to be calming and to improve gastric acidity secretions, (HCL) thus benefiting our protein digestion. Additionally, the gelatin and glucosamine and chondroitin sulfate derived from bone stock are preventative/restorative for osteoarthritis and bone loss. Lastly, bone broth has youth enhancing qualities due to its hyaluronic acid and collagen content; which aids in moisturizing and building smooth and strong skin.

Bone stock is easy to make. Simply put bones, and skin (necks/backs/feet etc.) from any animal in a large pot of filtered water with 2 Tbsp. of apple cider vinegar to draw out the minerals. You can add onions, garlic, carrots and celery; and herbs such as parsley, thyme, rosemary, and bay leaf. Bring it to a boil then skim off the layer of scum that forms on top. You can simmer it from 1-3 days. Refrigerate the broth or freeze the broth in ice cube trays to add to sauces later. And of course it is invaluable in soups.

Note: Chicken feet are especially collagen-rich.

---

## *Modern Traditional Diets*

There are still some surviving cultures today that are exhibiting high level health and longevity. Studies have shown that the healthiest and longest lived current cultures in the world continue to have a wide and varied traditional diet. The dietary practices of these cultures have been shifting towards western patterns recently, but many elders still adhere to their traditional diets. These vigorous cultures still eat predominantly unprocessed natural whole foods, often similar to the traditional diets of their early ancestors. Two of the most well studied cultural diets are the Mediterranean diet and the Okinawa diet. These specific dietary patterns are being adopted by non-native people today with the aim of helping to alter their eating habits to more resemble those of these healthier cultures.

**The heart healthy authentic Mediterranean diet** has been studied extensively. Demographic data has shown that until the recent adoption of the American diet, people in the Mediterranean region lived longer, and had far less diabetes, heart disease and obesity than Americans. The *Lyon Heart Study* revealed that adhering to the Mediterranean diet is far more heart- healthy than the American Heart Association Diet. A study published in the *New England Journal of Medicine* followed 7,400 people at risk for heart disease for five years. The study showed that those adhering to the Mediterranean diet had a 30% reduced risk for heart disease and stroke compared to those participants on a low fat diet. Another recent study published in the medical journal, *Neurology*, followed over 17,000 participants over the age of 45 for four years, and found that those who closely adhered to the Mediterranean diet were 19% less likely to suffer from cognitive decline and Alzheimer's disease. Other benefits of the Mediterranean diet include cancer and osteoporosis prevention.

The Mediterranean diet is a widely enjoyed and sustainable plan because it is not a strict deprivation diet. There are many Mediterranean diet cookbooks that give a framework to work with- which can be easily suited to individual needs.

### Benefits of the Mediterranean Diet/Decreased Risk Factors for

| Heart disease, stroke | Cancer | Alzheimer's disease | Type 2 diabetes |
|---|---|---|---|
| Lower oxidized cholesterol and blood pressure | Weight loss | Increased vitality and energy | Osteoporosis prevention |

The Mediterranean diet features almost entirely homemade food, often coming from the garden. It's characterized by generally fresh, seasonal, local and organic minimally processed foods; with an abundance of fare from plant sources, plus plentiful herbs and spices. The diet consists of between 7 to 10 servings of fruits and vegetables daily, with large quantities of tomato based sauces. Whole grains, olives, beans, nuts, and seeds are featured, and the principal fat consumed in abundance is extra virgin olive oil. A wide use of citrus juice is used in cooking. Fish and poultry are eaten more commonly than red meat of which is consumed approximately one time a week or less. Seafood and fish are enjoyed several times a week. Sugar intake is low, with fruits predominating for dessert. One to two 1 oz. servings of raw nuts are eaten daily. Small amounts of cheese, bread and pasta are also enjoyed. A daily glass of red wine is imbibed with meals. Cannellini beans are eaten often in soups and salads

***Tomatoes, tomato sauce, and tomato paste*** are regularly enjoyed in abundance in the Mediterranean countries. Tomatoes, especially cooked tomatoes are rich sources of the antioxidant lycopene. It is lycopene that is identified in many studies as the compound responsible for the prevention of oxidized "bad" LDL cholesterol caused by free radicals. This oxidation contributes to arterial plaque, and heart attacks. In a lycopene study performed on human subjects, tomato products were served one-to-two times a day for one week. The participants were shown to have a reduced quantity of oxidized cholesterol after the end of the week.

Research has found that lycopene is better absorbed with cooked tomato dishes and with meals that include fat or oil. Raw tomatoes can be served with olive oil to increase its nutrient absorption.

**Tomato meal ideas**: Eat cooked vegetables and quinoa with tomato sauce. Make meatballs with tomato sauce; add tomato slices to your sprouted grain sandwiches. Use canned organic tomatoes to make soups and sauces. Add tomatoes to your egg dishes. Put sun-dried tomatoes (without sulfur) in your salads and eat alone as snacks. Drizzle tomatoes with a little olive oil, and serve with basil and mozzarella cheese. Buy the freshest tomatoes at your local farmers' market, CSA, or grow your own!

## Mediterranean Meal Plan

- A typical breakfast might include: poached eggs with asparagus on tomato slices; sprouted whole grain toast with drizzle of olive oil/ or oatmeal, and grapefruit segments.
- A typical lunch might include lentil soup, mixed green salad with arugula, tomatoes, olives and almonds, with a homemade Italian dressing, and an apple.
- A typical dinner might include a small mixed green salad with olives, cannellini beans, tomato and Italian dressing; sautéed shrimp with thyme; whole grain risotto with tomatoes; and baked Brussels sprouts
- Snacks/Desserts might include dates with walnuts, or hummus and carrots, or fresh fruit.

## Other Tips to Shift to a Mediterranean Diet

- <u>Pair each meal and snack</u> with a colorful vegetable or fruit. (Especially tomatoes)
- Swap out animal proteins at lunch or dinner for legume dishes, and soups instead: using lentils, fava beans, cannellini beans, peas, garbanzo beans, hummus, and black-eyed peas.
- Have bean dips as snacks with vegetables.
- Stir frozen peas into casseroles.
- Serve fish/seafood instead of meat several times a week.
- Add walnuts, almonds or seeds to salads, granolas or fruit desserts.
- Prepare nut and seed pesto, which can be served with whole grains, or veggie sticks
- Eat olives and olive oil abundantly!

---

## The Okinawa Diet

The Okinawa island of Japan boasts the highest percentage of people in the world that live past 100.(they have the longest documented life expectancy) Over 25 years of research has proven that the elders have one of the healthiest diets in the world, which contributes to their lower heart disease, cancer, dementia, osteoporosis, and other age-related disease rates. Women also suffer from less menopausal problems. In 1975, the *Okinawa*

*Centenarian Study* headed by Dr. Suzuki found an unusual number of centenarians to be lean, energetic, and youthful looking and enjoying low rates of disease.

## The Okinawa Diet lowers risk factors for:

| Breast and prostate cancer | Menopausal problems (don't need estrogen replacement due to soy) | Osteoporosis | Dementia |
|---|---|---|---|
| Heart disease | Autoimmune diseases | Inflammation | Diabetes |

The traditional dietary habit practiced by the Okinawa elders is caloric restriction, with the practice of eating until 80% full. *The Journal of the American College of Nutrition* reports that the elders typically consume 500 fewer calories per day than people following western diets. This type of restriction has been shown in studies to slow down the aging process.

The traditional Okinawa diet has an antioxidant rich, low glycemic load, nutrient-dense dietary pattern. It is predominantly plant based with high complex carbohydrates, mostly from vegetables, with few grains or sugars. The major component of the diet is green and yellow vegetables with the Asian sweet potato being the staple in lieu of rice. The diet is high in fiber, vitamins, minerals, and antioxidants with an average of nine fruits and vegetable servings a day. It is high in anti-inflammatory mono-unsaturated fats and omega-3 fats. A little red meat is consumed, with raw goat and pig eaten several times a month. Miso soup with tofu cubes, legumes, and fish are the primary proteins. A minimum amount of dairy is consumed, and alcohol is limited to an occasional drink. Desserts are few.

Other common foods in the Okinawa diet are immune enhancing shiitake mushrooms; trace mineral-rich sea vegetables such as kombu and hijiki; burdock root; blood-sugar stabilizing bitter melon (a cucumber-like gourd); konjac starch, asparagus, bok choy, fennel bulb, cultured vegetables, citrus: and an array of herbs and spices such as fennel seeds, peppers, mugwort and anti-inflammatory cold turmeric tea.

---

**Sea Vegetables:** (aka seaweeds) are "super foods" that offer the broadest range of minerals compared to any other food; with the widest variety of trace minerals as well. Seaweeds contain all the nutrients found in the ocean, which are the same minerals found in our blood. They are also an excellent source of B-vitamins, and the antioxidants vitamin A and C. Seaweed is most prized for its rich source of iodine; a vital component of breast, uterine, prostate and thyroid tissue. Many women as they age develop low thyroid or thyroiditis; and seaweed can balance this condition. Seaweed also offers benefits for menopausal women and supports osteoporosis prevention as well. The sea vegetable Wakame is especially high in bone-building calcium and magnesium. Seaweed also supports cardiovascular and blood pressure health and heart attack prevention due to its high magnesium profile. Sea vegetables are excellent detoxifiers, and even can mitigate radiation exposure. Finally, sea weed contains high quantities of cancer-protective lignans, which are especially beneficial for combating breast cancer. Choose organic wakame, arame, dulse, nori, sea lettuce, kombu, and sea palm etc. Nori is the commonest form of sea weed in America- often sold in large and small sheets, or wrapped around sushi.

### Okinawa Meal Plan

- A typical Okinawa breakfast might include miso soup, with eggs and mustard greens; a pear and jasmine tea.
- A typical lunch might include stir fried fish and bok choy; some raw veggies with a small Okinawa sweet potato and jasmine tea.
- A typical dinner might include a bowl of miso soup flavored with sea weed; sea vegetable salad; stir fried shrimp with bitter melon, shiitake mushrooms, and other vegetables; a purple sweet potato; and jasmine tea.
- Snacks might include fresh fruit or vegetable sticks

---

### The Traditional Paleolithic Diet

*The Paleolithic Diet*, also known as the Paleo or caveman diet, is our most ancient traditional diet. It is now experiencing a resurgence due to recent scientific findings. The diet is based on research which examined the types of foods our hunter-gatherer ancestors ate in the Stone Age. Our early ancestors hunted, scavenged, and foraged until the advent of agriculture and animal domestication (about 10,000 years ago) at the start of the Neolithic era. However, it is important to note that many cultures and ethnicities ate traditional hunter-gatherer diets until fairly recently.

Dr. Loren Cordain, the author of the book, *the Paleo Diet* is a leading expert on Paleolithic nutrition. He asserts that over ten thousand years ago during the Paleolithic period, humans did not consume grains, sugar, vegetable oils or dairy; the products of the agricultural era. He acknowledges that they primarily ate vegetables, fruits, tubers, roots, nuts, seeds, eggs, fish, fowl and game meat. Scientific findings of these Paleolithic societies have shown that these ancient people were muscular, energetic and healthy and had an absence of modern chronic diseases such as heart disease, cancer, obesity and diabetes. Dr. Cordain and other Paleo experts assert that our bodies have not evolved to eat the evolutionarily newer foods developed during the rise of the agrarian, and industrial period. He believes that our genes have not had time to catch up with these changes; and that there have been major declines in our health since agriculture has taken hold. (*Note*: Paleo critics contend that there is evidence that humans have evolved significantly since the stone-age and continue to do so.)

Dr. Cordain and other advocates of the Paleo diet feel that returning to a diet that mimics our ancestors' diet is a logical way to increase our health, strength and energy levels. There are many benefits of eating a Paleo diet. One of the most prominent benefits is that it keeps blood sugar levels steady, and has shown usefulness with individuals who are pre-diabetic or diabetic. According to the scientific literature, it is also beneficial for:

| Poor digestion | Leaky gut | Food sensitivities | Autoimmune conditions | Weight loss/optimal body composition |
|---|---|---|---|---|
| Blood sugar stability, diabetics, pre-diabetic, insulin resistance | Joint pain and inflammation | Gaining muscle mass/athletic performance | Rashes, acne, eczema, psoriasis, dermatitis | Fatigue |

The Paleo diet advocates abstaining from <u>all grain containing foods</u>, refined sugars and soft drinks, and dairy. Some Paleo proponents feel that legumes should also not be consumed. However, in 2013 researcher Dr. Stephen Guyenet posted that legumes were indeed a part of our ancient diet, as there is evidence of fava beans and peas being found in ancient Paleolithic sites. Additionally, it was discovered that current hunter-gather cultures such as the Kalahari Bushmen and the Australian Aborigines consume legumes in the form of the tsin bean and the acacia legume. Kriss Kresser, author of the book, *Your Personal Paleo Code,* believes that legumes in small quantities are fine, but not to displace the more highly nutrient-concentrated animal proteins in the diet. The paleo diet can be practiced short or long term.

## A Typical "Paleo" Diet Features:

1. Meats in the form of grass-fed or organic beef, buffalo, ostrich, chicken, game meats, lamb, goat; organ meats and bone marrow, pork, turkey, goose, and duck etc.
2. Wild fish, shellfish, and fish eggs
3. Nuts and seeds (soaked and dried), plus their flours and butters.
4. All vegetables
5. Sea vegetables
6. Low glycemic fruits. (Berries etc.)
7. Unrefined fats/oils: coconut oils, extra virgin olive oil, lard, avocado oil, coconut milk, macadamia oil, red palm oil
8. Legumes in small quantities.

## Paleo Meal Plan

- o  A typical breakfast might include: 3 egg omelet made of roasted pepper and kale with ½-3/4 cup sweet potato hash, and fresh cranberries
- o  A typical lunch might include: Cilantro turkey burger with guacamole (without the bun) a fermented veggie; 2 cups of a raw leafy and crunchy veggie salad, and 1 cup mixed berries
- o  A typical snack might include 2 oz. beef jerky or 1 oz. almonds with 1/2 cup strawberries.
- o  A typical dinner may include wild salmon, 2 cups cauliflower and broccoli sauté, a fermented veggie, a yam, and a colorful salad.

---

## Cultured and Fermented Foods

Fermented foods that possess beneficial bacteria have been a major staple of traditional diets for thousands of years. Fermentation was a necessity in order to preserve foods, and it also enabled these cultures to have vegetables for the long winter months. Our early ancestors also knew that this would enhance their digestion. Every tradition was known to ferment and culture their foods and many still do.

Native Americans fermented their meats, fish and vegetables. Germans consumed sauerkraut and kvass. Russians drank milk kefir. The Chinese ate, and still eat fermented cabbage and soy sauce. Indonesians also currently consume tempeh. Japanese ferment natto. Bulgarians consume yogurt. Latin Americans consume cortido and Koreans dine on Kimchi.

In America, our once healthy fermented foods: cheese, yogurt, soy sauce, pickles, and sauerkraut are now pasteurized, but this high heat destroys the beneficial enzymes and health-giving probiotics. Refined vinegar is now added instead; depleting our mineral stores.

Fermented foods are the missing piece in our modern diets, and have acquired a super-food status due to their superior health-promoting qualities. They contain essential beneficial bacteria that nourish and strengthen our gastrointestinal tract, improve digestion and protect our gut lining; which often becomes weakened as we age. Probiotic rich foods are vital for helping our immune system stay in good working order by keeping pathogens out of our gut. Fermented foods also manufacture B vitamins, a necessary component of mood and brain health; and they also synthesize vitamin K2, which is linked to cardiovascular and bone health. Cultured foods also help us to absorb minerals in our foods by increasing absorption rates; and they can also assist in controlling sugar cravings. Last, but not least, fermented foods are detoxifiers; as beneficial bacteria ingest pesticides, mercury, and other toxins and remove them in the stool. It is interesting to note that 70% of our stool is comprised of bacteria.

Alternately, when pathogenic bacteria dominate our digestive system we can suffer from absorption issues, poor elimination, and inadequate detoxification. A whole host of problems can arise due to bad bacteria overload or a leaky-gut caused by harmful bacteria. Here is a list of some of the prominent conditions caused by a microflora imbalance.

| OCD, Bipolar disorder, schizophrenia, depression, anxiety | Acne |
|---|---|
| Arthritis | IBS, leaky gut, food allergies |
| Candida | Vaginal infections |
| Cancer | Decreased immunity |
| Inflammation | Autoimmune diseases |

## Prebiotics

Beneficial bacteria need to eat to thrive, and prefer to eat "prebiotics;" which provide nourishment for them. Prebiotics are found in fiber-rich foods. Excellent prebiotic foods are: berries, garlic, leeks, onions, flaxseeds, dandelion, spinach, kale, tomatoes, lentils, chickpeas, and black beans. It is a good idea to emphasize these foods when endeavoring to increase a healthy microflora population.

## Homemade Lacto-Fermented Vegetables

Culturing or fermenting vegetables is an ancient tradition in which raw and shredded vegetables have been left to ferment with sea salt for 3 days or more. This fermentation process allows the naturally present beneficial bacteria to multiply which produces an enzyme, vitamin, and mineral-rich super-food that is the perfect food for individuals who want to achieve high level health. The beneficial bacteria contained in cultured vegetables such as lactobacillus bacteria strains and bifido bacteria strains help to repair the damaged gut mucous lining that is associated with irritable bowel syndrome, leaky gut syndrome and many other diseases. It is very simple to make your own fermented veggies, and several companies sell starter cultures with vitamin K2 synthesizing bacteria for this purpose including: *Body Ecology, Cultures for Health, and Dr. Mercola.* Fermented veggies are also sold in the refrigerated section in health food stores. See fermented vegetable recipe on page 275.

*Exercise 8: Input in your plan some aspects of the four traditional diets that you would like to incorporate into your own life. Make sure to incorporate fermented and cultured foods. Traditional diet cookbooks are listed in the back.*

*Chapter Nine*

# Common Nutrient Insufficiencies in Midlife
## (Plus Herbal/Dietary Supplement Usage)

Our body's nutrient status has a strong impact on our daily life; it effects how we feel, our energy levels, our moods, thinking processes, our aging, and even our sleep. If our body has sub-optimal levels of essential vitamins, minerals, and nutrients- we are likely to be robbed of our vitality, health and quality of life. Many conditions and diseases are tied to nutritional shortfalls. However, longstanding insufficiencies can be overcome by making choices that improve our diet, and lifestyle, and by using nutritional supplements if necessary.

Many individuals in midlife suffer from inadequate levels of nutrients. Years of eating a poor high-sugar diet, compounded by chronic stress, toxin exposure, and waning digestive function can cause accumulated nutrient shortfalls. There are several very common nutrient insufficiencies that afflict middle-aged people, especially prevalent are: vitamin D, vitamin B, vitamin K2, zinc, magnesium, iodine, and omega-3 fatty-acids.

The following chart lists the most universal nutrient inadequacies that a middle-aged person may experience. Look over the chart to discern if you may have symptoms of suboptimal levels. It may be beneficial to use targeted dietary supplements for several months to gain back healthy nutrient stores. The optimal and most absorbable supplements and dosages are listed when applicable. The dosage given is the optimal daily allowance; (ODA) which is a value that allows the body to thrive, not just survive. Always take in divided doses throughout the day when taking larger doses. For some nutrients it is better to obtain from food sources alone. Read the symptom list; then check-off the nutrient box that you may have a possible shortfall in. Follow the supplement dosage directions on the label- if no dosage is noted on the chart.

Note: Always take supplements under the guidance of a medical professional. If you are not taking medications, only take targeted dietary supplements for three months without direct supervision from a nutritional/medical professional. If you are taking meds, do so under the guidance of a physician; as there are many drug-vitamin-herb interactions. Refer to the book: <u>A-Z Guide to Drug-Herb-Vitamin Interaction: 2<sup>nd</sup> Edition</u> by A. Gaby.

See charts on next three pages. Soak all grains, legumes, nuts and seeds for mineral uptake.

## Common Nutrient Insufficiencies

| NUTRIENT/SUPPLEMENT | FOUND IN: FOOD & FOOD-LIKE HERBS | SYMPTOMS/CONDITIONS |
|---|---|---|
| **Zinc-most common** Vital mineral. Depleted by stress, and sugar. Zinc orotate, glycinate or aspartate or Zinc Supreme: 15-30 mg (Causes nausea on empty stomach.) | Oysters, red meat, lamb, poultry, liver, egg yolks, pumpkin seeds, ginger root, oats, sesame butter, sea veggies, sage, nettles, dulse, skullcap, chickweed | Sugar/carb cravings, poor immunity, poor digestion, brittle nails, poor wound healing, insomnia, low stomach acid, mental lethargy, anxiety, racing thoughts, hormone imbalances, Alzheimer's, Parkinson's, eye diseases |
| **Vitamin D3-most common** *Depleted by insufficient sun exposure in the midday (sun screen blocks vitamin D) Vitamin D3- 2,000+ IU. Take with vitamin K2 to avoid calcification of arteries | Sunlight, egg yolks, cold water fish (salmon, sardines, and herring) cod liver oil, butter, sun-dried mushrooms. * Vit D3 supplements should be taken in winter (Oct.-Feb.) - if you live in northern latitudes. | Poor immunity, Osteoporosis, auto immunity, depression, breast and colon cancers, pre-diabetes, muscle pain, inflammation, fibromyalgia, Alzheimer's. Vitamin D Impacts every part of our biology and DNA. Optimal range: 50-70ng/ml on labs |
| **N-Acetyl Cysteine (NAC)** common: 600 mg. *Depleted by stress, poor sleep, medication and toxins | Poultry, yogurt, ricotta, oats, garlic, onions, broccoli, Brussels sprouts, red peppers, all fruits and veggies | Free radical overload, poor toxin elimination, poor immune function, cancer risk, cataracts, low glutathione, high homocysteine |
| **Vitamin K2-most common:** 85% of Americans deficient if not eating grass fed animal protein or natto. * Essential for bone health Mk-7:150-200 mcg (take with fat/oil) | *Only from grass-fed animal protein: Pastured eggs, grass-fed butter, organ meats, grass fed dairy (especially in brie, edam, gouda, goat, gruyere, swiss) *And in fermented foods such as fermented vegetables and natto. | Tarter build up, osteoporosis, arterial calcification, inappropriate calcification as heel spurs and kidney stones, heart disease, stroke, cancer |
| **Iron-** Depleted by poor stomach acids *You should not take in a supplement after menopause *Iron overload can cause cognitive decline | *Heme-iron best absorbed: meat, poultry, fish, organ meats *Non-heme iron- less absorption: leafy greens, molasses, horsetail, nettles, dandelion leaf/root, plantain leaf, peppermint. | Anemia, brittle and spoon shaped nails, impaired immune function, fatigue, heart palpitations, headaches |
| **Magnesium-Very common** *Depleted by stress, sugar, poor HCL levels, coffee, alcohol, excess synthetic vitamin D2 *Magnesium Citrate, aspartate, glycinate: 320-1,000 mg. Take w/Vit. B-6/ 25 mg. Epson salt baths | *Leafy greens (spinach, swiss chard), nuts, seeds, beans, peas, sea weed, figs, mineral water, sage, dandelion greens, parsley leaf, oat straw, nettles, burdock root, horsetail, red clover, carrot tops, dulse, chickweed. | Constipation, IBS, High blood sugar, heart attack, irregular heartbeat, insomnia, nervousness, anxiety, depression, constipation, eye twitching, muscle cramps, noise sensitivity, PMS, restless legs, irritability, asthma |
| **Vitamin E** Very common Depleted by refined grains/ refined oils, free-radicals *Mixed tocopherols- 400-800 IU. w/tocotrienols | Cold pressed vegetable oils, eggs, seeds, nuts, whole grains, avocado, spinach, asparagus, kale, sweet potatoes; uncooked peas and green beans; liver, alfalfa, nettles dandelion leaf, and seaweeds. | Wrinkles, age spots, hot flashes, dry skin and hair, PMS, eczema, psoriasis, cataracts, poor reflexes, autoimmune conditions, fibrocystic breasts, blood vessel damage, lung and heart problems, oxidative stress |

| NUTRIENT/SUPPLEMENT | FOUND IN | SYMPTOMS/ CONDITIONS |
|---|---|---|
| Probiotics: most common depleted by sugar, refined foods, antibiotics, steroids, stress, birth control pills, and antibacterial products *Designs for Health Probiophage DF* or Probiotic Synergy or Innate Response-Flora 20 or 50. | Cultured vegetables, uncooked miso, tempeh, natto, beet kvaas, kefir and yogurt with "live and active cultures." <br><br>*Kombucha: fermented tea has been known to cause sensitivities in some individuals due to wild fermentation. | Vaginal infections, fungus on toe-nails, jock itch, headaches, digestive problems, constipation, GI diseases, auto-immune conditions, poor immunity, skin conditions, rashes, food/ environmental allergies, asthma, sick often., low mineral status. |
| Vitamin B6: common *Depleted by stress, and a lack of leafy greens. Individuals with an anxiety condition known as Pyroluria may be deficient. *P5P (coenzyme active form) 50 -100 mg | Leafy greens, lightly cooked liver, organ meats, fish, poultry, egg yolk, beans, lentils, broccoli, prunes, banana, walnuts, cauliflower, cabbage, avocado, nutritional yeast | Depression, anxiety, sleep and cognitive problems, decreased lymphocytes, homocysteine overload, PMS, swollen stiff fingers in the morning, carpal tunnel syndrome, poor dream recall, prefer not to eat breakfast, motion sickness, morning nausea |
| Vitamin B12 very common *if low HCL levels- than low B12. Vegans require it. Birth control pills deplete. Sublingual methyl cobalamin: 500 mcg | Fish, meat, organ meats, oysters, yogurt, egg yolk, crab, cheese | Dementia, poor memory, fatigue, constipation, anemia, constipation, digestive problems, numbness and tingling in hands and feet, nervousness, depression. Chrone's disease |
| Folate-very common Folate 5-MTHF: 400 mcg <br><br>Birth control pills deplete | Leafy green vegetables, black-eyed peas, lentils, garbanzo beans, turkey, asparagus, nettles, parsley , sage, alfalfa, peppermint | CVD risk, fatigue, insomnia, premature hair loss, impaired immune function, anemia, depression, hearing loss |
| Vitamin C: very common Not stored/keep a daily supply. *Depleted by stress. Ester-C-1,000-3,000 mg/day or liposomal vitamin C in divided doses. | Strawberries, kiwi, red bell peppers, citrus, snow peas, tomatoes, celery, potatoes, guava, broccoli, Brussels sprouts, red chili pepper, camu camu, acerola cherry, raspberry leaf, red clover, dandelion, paprika, plantain, pine needles, watercress | Bleeding gums, loose teeth, easy bruising, impaired wound healing, tiredness, low immunity, wrinkles, sick often, chronic stress, homocysteine overload |
| Vitamin A: common retinol comes from animal sources; carotenes come from plant sources and convert to vitamin A using zinc/vit. C *Fermented Cod Liver Oil: 1-2 tsp. or retinol: 5,000 IU | Fermented cod liver oil, eggs, liver, kidney, butter, cream, grass-fed whole milk; orange, yellow and red veggies and fruits, spirulina, dark leafy greens *Potential toxicity with long-term high dosages of retinol supplement | Poor night vision, wrinkles, dry bumpy skin on back of arms; asthma, infection prone; taking a long time for eyes to adjust to a darkened room; hypothyroid; fat malabsorption, diabetes, psoriasis |

| NUTRIENT/SUPPLEMENT | FOUND IN | SYMPTOMS/CONDITIONS |
|---|---|---|
| **\*Iodine: most common** Iodized salt is an insignificant source of iodine. \*Depleted by soil depletion; goitrogens in unfermented soy, and raw cruciferous vegetables; chlorine, bromine, and fluoride<br><br>Supplement: Iodoral iodine | Sea weed- especially dulse, kelp, and bladder wrack; seafood, and dairy products. (secondary source) Dr. David Brownstein, author of the book, *Iodine, Why You Need It, Why You Can't Live Without It*, believes that Iodine deficiency is an under-recognized epidemic across the U.S. | Hypo-thyroid, thyroiditis, poor hormone production, impaired breast and ovarian health, breast cancer, fibrocystic breasts and uterine fibroids, prostate enlargement, prostate cancer, hearing loss, fibromyalgia, brain fog, poor brain function, lung problems, sinus issues, atherosclerosis, headaches, toxic metal poisoning |
| **Omega -3 fatty acids: very common**: conversion of plant sourced (ALA) into DHA/EPA is not efficient. Fermented Cod liver oil: 1-2 tsp. or *Designs for Health OmegAvail Line* or its *XanthOmega krill oil* (2 soft gel capsules)<br><u>Vegans</u>: algae w/DHA | Wild pacific salmon, mackerel, herring, sardines, anchovies<br><br>Flax seed meal, hemp seed, chia seed, walnuts, pumpkin seeds (not always efficient) | Poor mood and brain function, depression, heart disease, high blood pressure, inflammation and pain, diabetes |
| **Calcium-very common** Calcium Citrate or glycinate- Don't take calcium without magnesium. The ratio of calcium to magnesium must be in balance or the body will create calcium deposits. Ratios of Ca to Mg should be 600 mg Ca/400 mg Mag. Age 50+:1200 mg calcium 1:1 ratio of Ca/Mg after menopause | Dairy, cheese, yogurt, broccoli, dark leafy greens, cabbage, hazelnuts, oysters, canned salmon and sardines with bones, fermented soy, soaked almonds, sesame seeds, tahini, whey, seaweeds, sweet potatoes, parsley, nettle, horsetail sage, peppermint, yellow dock, chickweed, oat straw, raspberry leaf, red clover, lambs quarters. | Osteoporosis, osteoarthritis, muscle cramps, acute anxiety, irritability, insomnia, tooth decay, colon cancer risk, leaky gut |
| **Vitamin B1, and B2: very common** Depleted by stress, refined foods *Co- enzyme B-Complex 50-100 mg | Organ meats, brown/wild rice, nutritional yeast, whole grains, spinach, avocado, cauliflower, almonds, sunflower seeds, peas, beans, asparagus, mushrooms, eggs, collard greens, almonds, shellfish, nettles, peppermint, alfalfa, rose hips, fenugreek seed, yellow dock | Age related cognitive decline, Alzheimer's disease, fatigue, decreased heart function, poor thyroid function, anemia, cataracts, stress conditions. |

➡ Home <u>Zinc Challenge</u> Test: Taste test for zinc deficiency by <u>Designs for Health</u>
Take 1 Tbsp. and swish in mouth for 10 sec. No or mild taste= zinc deficiency.

## Common Nutrient Deficiencies in Vegans

**Abstaining from animal protein altogether can lead to deficiencies and health complications.**

| Protein/carnitine/sulfur | Vitamin D | Vitamin K2 | Calcium |
|---|---|---|---|
| Iron | B12 | Zinc | Omega-3 |

## Mineral Excess and Toxicity

There are two common mineral excesses that can cause oxidation and free radical damage in the body. These excesses are copper and iron.

- Many women and men experience <u>high copper levels</u> in America. Stress, adrenal exhaustion, copper pipes, high carb diets, vegetarian diets, synthetic estrogen and birth control pills can all create toxic copper levels in the body.
- Anxiety, panic attacks, depression, PMS, mind racing, acne, allergies, headaches, brain fog, candida overgrowth, hypothyroid and osteoarthritis are linked to high copper levels.

Usually, it is found that if an individual has low zinc levels they will also have high copper levels; therefore it is recommended to eat a diet that is high in protein and zinc to manage high copper levels. (Red meat, ginger root, oysters, soaked nuts, and seeds, and seafood) Supplement with zinc: 30mg; N-Acetyl Cysteine: 1000-2000 mg, Manganese: 5-20 mg, and vitamin C: 3 to 6 g/day to rid the body of excess copper. To assess copper levels it is advised to get a hair mineral analysis, and to work with a medical professional if high copper is indicated.

- <u>Excess iron levels</u> in the body can promote disorders such as heart disease and diabetes. Toxic iron levels can also cause or aggravate arthritis. Use supplemental N-Acetyl Cysteine: 1,000 mg/day; Manganese: 5-20 mg/day; or donate blood to lower high iron levels. To assess iron levels- have hematocrit, and serum ferritin blood levels checked.

**Exercise 9a:** Assess your possible nutritional insufficiencies or excesses with symptom/lifestyle list. Input these and food and nutrient dosage suggestions into your wellness plan.

## Nutritional Dietary Supplements

Using nutritional supplements to fill nutrient gaps in our diet or to target specific health challenges can be an effective tool to get our health back in balance. Although there has been past controversy about dietary supplements, it has been reported by the *Orthomolecular Organization* that according to the *American Association of Poison Control*, vitamins haven't caused a single death in 27 years. One of the safest track records on the market! Prescription drugs however, kill over 100,000 people every year, even when properly prescribed. In 2002, after 30 years of research in relation to chronic illness, *The Journal of the American Medical Association* (JAMA) reversed its longstanding anti-vitamin position, and recommends daily multi-vitamin/mineral supplements for all adults.

Taking a high quality food-based multi-vitamin/mineral can be your insurance against deficiencies in your diet; unless you have food allergies-then lab made is better. It can be a way of making sure that your body is supplied with all of the essential nutrients; especially if you have eaten a poor diet for many years. Many studies have found that daily multivitamin use predicted a moderate reduction in overall cancer risk. Dr. Alan Gaby, author of the book *Nutritional Medicine*, also has claimed that double blind trials have found positive effects from multivitamins intake for reducing cognitive decline.

When you do shop for multi-vitamin/mineral supplements, ensure that you choose ones with natural organic "whole food concentrates." These are the closest to natural whole foods, having synergistic effects. Check that there is at least 1,000 IU of vitamin D3, and at least 400-800 mg of folate (not folic acid). Also the vitamin E form should contain the four mixed tocopherols. (Even better- with the added four tocotrienols) You also may need to take extra magnesium; as many Multi's don't supply enough. The ratio of calcium to magnesium should be 1:1 or even additional magnesium than calcium if you are post-menopausal. **Innate Response's Women Over 40, and Men Over 40** are excellent choices.

When choosing minerals, always look for chelated forms; these minerals are bound with other compounds that enhance their absorption. Examples are minerals that have citrate, glycinate or aspartate after their name. Avoid any mineral labeled oxide, as it is poorly absorbed.

If choosing other supplements to target specific imbalances, you do need to be savvy about assessing the quality of the products- as some are ineffective, or contain known toxins. As with food, it is important to read product labels. There can be many ingredients used in the manufacturing process that can lead to health problems. These ingredients are known as excipients. A long list of excipients on the label, just as in foods, is an indication of a poor quality product.

In addition, several categories of dietary supplements have a reputation for spiking their products with pharmaceutical drugs, or synthetic ingredients. This is common with diet, muscle building, and high energy products. The FDA is responsible for taking action against any proven unsafe dietary supplement; hence these products are often flagged by the FDA, and removed from the shelves.

Many manufacturers however do add additives, dyes, binders, fillers, flow agents, and sometimes even heavy metals to their products. Supplements that are sold in drug stores almost universally contain unhealthy excipients; but health food stores are not immune to carrying questionable excipients either.

There are some excipients that are considered safe however, such as: micro-crystalline cellulose, vegetable cellulose, rice flour, silica, glycerin, and potassium sorbate (in liquids.) Gelatin capsules are made of animal proteins, and are hard to digest for people who have low stomach acids. Vegetable capsules, (HPMC) are easier to digest. Try to buy supplements in capsule form, as there are less binders in them. Liquid supplements are more absorbable, and are recommended for vitamin D3.

The following chart shows **harmful excipients** to look for on the labels.

| Talc: carcinogenic | Dyes-Tartrazine etc.: linked to asthma, brain toxicity | Artificial flavors: asthma, GI problems, headaches | Parabens: hormonal impairment, cancer causing |
|---|---|---|---|
| Titanium dioxide: carcinogenic | Maltodextrin | MSG | Magnesium Stearate, calcium stearate, stearic acid: suppresses immunity, and absorption |

There are some vitamin store or natural food store products that have high quality- pure nutrients, and follow good manufacturing processes (GMP.) Such brands are: Solgar, Now, Natrol, Pioneer, Rainbow light, New Chapter, Garden of Life, Mega Food, Natural Factors, and Source Naturals.

Companies that sell high quality excipient-free brands are: Enzymedica Enzymes, Pure Encapsulation, Thorne Research, New Chapter Organics, Pure Synergy, and Healthforce Nutritionals.

The <u>premier</u> quality supplements are <u>"professional" health care practitioner brands</u>. These are pharmaceutical grade and have been used clinically with proven therapeutic effects. You can obtain these from health care and nutrition professionals. These include: Standard Process, Innate Response, New Mark, Metagenics, Thorne Research, Apex Energetics, and Designs for Health etc. Contact the author for more information on purchasing these products.

## A Note on Supplements for Osteoporosis Prevention

Our bones need a blend of supportive nutrients to prevent bone loss and osteoporosis. Many women mistakenly take an excessive amount of calcium to confer some bone protection. According to bone experts taking calcium supplements without the co-factor support of other vitamins and minerals is dangerous because it does not support its absorption and metabolism. Instead it is deposited in soft tissue, heart tissue, and arteries causing blockages and calcification. The following is a list of the vitamins and minerals needed for bone-loss prevention. Remember, don't just supplement with calcium; you will do more damage than good. Look for these nutrients in bone-support supplements also.

- Vitamin K2 (Mk-7): 200 mcg/ Pastured eggs, pastured dairy, yogurt, kefir and cheeses, organ meats, fermented veggies, natto and natto capsules.
- Vitamin D3: Daily midday sun exposure for 15 min. to one-half hour (10-2pm) spring through fall- All people in northern latitudes should take Vitamin D3 in winter. Fermented cod liver oil (contains vitamin D) or 2000+ IU Vitamin D3 (under Dr. supervision-up to 10,000 IU, if test levels are below 50 ng/ml)
- Magnesium Citrate or Glycinate: 1000 mg/ green leafy vegetables, beans, sunflower seeds, nuts, sea weed, (nori, dulse, kelp) bone broth.
- Calcium citrate: 1000 mg/dark leafy greens, dandelion, sesame seeds, sardine and salmon bones, bone broth, dairy
- Strontium citrate: 680 mg (elemental strontium) Stimulates bone formation-whole milk/dairy-especially cheddar cheese, shell fish, sea weed (caution: don't take strontium supplement at the same time as calcium supplement-don't take if have kidney disease or blood clotting issues)
- Boron: 3 mg/apples, dried fruit
- Manganese: winter squash, sweet potatoes, nuts
- Silicon: Horsetail grass herbal tea/infusion, cucumber, avocado, onions, strawberries
- **Women's Health Network's Better Bones Builder** supplement supplies the above nutrients.

---

**Remember that supplements** are just that. They are meant only to **supplement** a healthy diet. They never can take the place of one. Additionally, it has been found that taking an excess of supplements can lead to insomnia from overstimulation. If you want to optimize your health, it is wise to consume a wide variety of whole natural organic foods with plenty of vegetables and sprouts. Nutrient powerhouses such as: bone stock, sea vegetables, nutritional yeast, green algae powders, and fermented vegetables can also stand-in for supplements. Food-like herbs and "super foods" or booster foods can additionally substitute for them.

It is important to take note that medications can additionally cause nutrient depletion. The website **pilladvised.com** can give you information on what nutrients are being depleted from your body when you take certain medications. These depleted nutrients will need to be supplemented in your diet or with dietary supplements for as long as you take the meds.

*Additionally, you should always consult with a medical professional when you begin using supplements, especially if you are on medications. If you are taking supplements to target a specific health challenge, do so for three months; and then check in with yourself to examine if the supplement has been effective and if conditions have improved. If they have improved, stop usage of the supplement and continue emphasizing foods/herbs rich in the particular nutrient. Then monitor if symptoms return. You may resume usage for another three months if there is little improvement in your symptoms. (Only under a medical professional's guidance) Even if you take supplements long term, it is always advised to take a break from them from time to time.

Caution: A variety of supplements may infrequently cause a bad reaction in sensitive individuals. Supplements may also interact negatively with an array of medications. When you first try a new supplement, take a small quantity of it to observe how it affects your body. If a bad reaction is experienced, simply take 500 mg. of vitamin C (detoxifier) every 15 minutes or so until you find relief.

## *Herbals/Botanicals*

Susan Weed, prominent herbalist and author of numerous books on botanicals, acknowledges that herbs are exceptionally nourishing and therapeutic, but need to be used with care. She divides herbs into four categories:

- **Food-like nourishing herbs** with high-level nutrients: Alfalfa, borage, chamomile, chickweed, comfrey, fennel, fenugreek, nettles, oat straw, plantain, raspberry, red clover, rose hips, and slippery elm are featured in this book. These can be used on an ongoing basis; as they are the safest herbs. (Caution red clover may increase the size/bleeding of fibroids)
- **Tonifying Herbs** (tonics) Act slowly, and are used in small quantities for extended periods of time- which have a cumulative effect (slight chance of side-affects): Milk thistle, black cohosh, chaste berry, dandelion root, don quai, Echinacea, ginseng, hawthorne, horsetail, motherwort, wild yam and yellow dock are featured in this book.
- **Sedating/Stimulating herbs** cause rapid-reactions and need to be used in moderate doses for fairly short periods of time: Catnip, hops, kava kava, licorice, passion flower, sage, skullcap, uva ursi, and valerian are examples featured in this book.

- **Potentially poisonous herbs** are best taken in tiny amounts for a very short period of time: cayenne and goldenseal are featured in this book.

There are several forms of herbal remedies. Some are considered more effective than others. Dr. Andrew Weil suggests using standardized extracts; as the compounds have been evaluated for quality and accuracy. He also recommends using long-lasting tinctures and freeze dried capsules. Additionally, Susan Weed proposes using longer brewed herbal "infusions" over the shorter steeped herbal teas to extract more nutrient and medicinal substances from the botanical. She advises preparing infusions in pint or quart jars by pouring boiling water over an ounce of jarred herbs and infusing them for a certain duration. Afterword, strain the herbs from the herbal liquid and place in the refrigerator. Can be sipped hot, warm or cold:

| |
|---|
| Roots/barks in a pint container for 8 hours (minimum) |
| Seeds/berries in a pint container for 30 min. (maximum) |
| Leaves in a quart container for 4 hours (minimum) |
| Flowers in a quart container for 2 hours (maximum) |

(Weed, 2002)

Caution: Herbs may interact negatively with a variety of medications.

Note: Herbal supplements if not from reputable suppliers can be contaminated with metals and pesticides. Always buy organic herbs from reputable companies. Herb Pharm, Gaia Herbs, Avena Botanicals, Blessed Herbs, Catskill Mountain Herbal, Frontier Herbal Coop, Green terrestrial, Red Moon Herbs and the Standard Process-*MediHerb* line are highly regarded herbal suppliers. (Non-food-like herbs should not be taken daily for a long duration-stop usage periodically) Herbal usage also should be under the guidance of a medical professional; as herbs can be very powerful and can cause occasional side effects.

*Exercise 9b: Input any information on dietary supplements that you would like to remember, including osteoporosis prevention.*

*Chapter Ten*

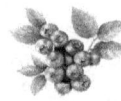 ## Free Radicals, Antioxidants and Aging

According to our current aging theory, the major factor that promotes premature aging is **Free-Radical** overload. (An accumulation of unpaired electrons in our body.) Free-radicals have been the subject of hundreds of scientific studies over several decades. This research supports the fact that in order to forestall premature aging, it is necessary to neutralize these destructive free radicals.

Unfortunately, free radicals are everywhere: in the air we breathe; the products we use; the food we eat; and even from the process of absorbing oxygen to make energy in our body. Free radicals cause a progressive damage to our cells and organs, known as "**oxidative stress.**" If our body has an insufficiency of antioxidants to neutralize these ever-present free radicals; oxidative stress (cell damage) will take place.

In much the same way that metals rust, oxidation happens in our bodies. Another illustration of free radical damage is when we cut an apple in-half and leave it out for a while; the interior will turn brown due to oxidation. This will hasten the deterioration of the fruit. This is much the same way that free radicals and oxidative stress affect our body. Virtually all degenerative diseases have been shown to be the result of oxidative stress. It has particularly been found to be the causative factor in a weakened immune system; excessive fatigue, hormone imbalances, heart disease, inflammation and pain; poor memory, mood disorders, damaged DNA, wrinkled and aged skin; premature cell death and cancer.

Dr. Bruce Ames, a professor at U.C. Berkeley estimates that the average person experiences 10,000 DNA free radical assaults every day. Even one free radical is capable of destroying an entire cell or strand of DNA. However, our body can neutralize many of these hits; but as we age this ability weakens. These assaults take a toll on our vitality, and can age a person by 10 years or more.

See free radical chart on next page.

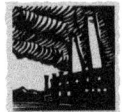 Here is a list of some of the worst "Free Radical" offenders:

| Refined and processed foods | Vitamin and mineral deficient diets | Low fiber diets | Dehydration (less than 7-8 glasses of water or tea) | Excessive refined salt (sea salt/Himalayan salt is okay) |
|---|---|---|---|---|
| Sugar/high fructose corn syrup, artificial sweeteners | Pesticide containing foods (non-organic) | GMO containing foods (non-organic soy, corn) | Hormone and antibiotic laden factory farmed nonorganic meats and fish | Inadequate sleep |
| Food additives and preservatives artificial food colorings and flavorings | Pesticides, herbicides exposure from sprays | Vegetable oils (corn, safflower, canola, peanut, sunflower, soy) (except unrefined olive oil which is very beneficial) | Oils/meats heated to high temperatures (fried or over 250 degrees) causes oxidized fat | Excess alcohol |
| Stress factors: chronic stress, worry, anxiety, trauma, disease | Excess anger | Chemicals in personal care products: especially parabens (See list on E.W.G. skindeep.com) | infections in the body (fungal overgrowth, parasites, bacteria) | Sedentary lifestyle |
| Hydrogenated oils (trans fats) partially hydrogenated fats | Air pollution, cigarette smoke, smog, soot, air fresheners, deodorizers | Chemical and heavy metal toxins, chemical laden household cleaning products, | Chlorinated/fluoridated tap water | Food and water in plastic containers |
| Indoor mold | Fluoride (in toothpaste and water) | Bromine (often in baked goods and bread) | Medications/ drugs | Toxic waste |
| Auto exhaust | Ionizing radiation from x-rays, cat scans, EMF's, cell phones | Excessive UV light from the sun (a small amount is beneficial) eyes are the most vulnerable-wear a hat & protective clothing | Excessive exercise (more than 2 hour of strenuous exercise a day) | Our bodies produce free-radicals as a by-product of metabolism (when it burns nutrients for energy!) |

**Exercise 10a:** Make a short list of some free radical offenders that you can limit or eliminate from your life in the next few months. Input them in your Personal Wellness Program.

*I know the free radical list is overwhelming ....but here is where* <u>Antioxidants</u> *come in to save the day!*

Antioxidants destroy free-radicals! Yes, antioxidants boost our body's defense system by preventing or reducing cell damage caused by free-radicals. They do this by donating an electron to an unpaired free-radical electron; which then makes it stable. This can be equated to leaving a sandwich out on the counter. The air will make the bread go stale and the meat go bad; but if we put it in a container in the refrigerator it will be preserved. Similarly, if we take the sliced apple mentioned earlier and squeeze lemon juice on it, it will be preserved due to the abundance of antioxidants found in the lemon juice.

The same antioxidants can preserve and repair our cells from oxidative damage and our cells last longer. The most significant strategy to slow down the aging process and neutralize damaging free radicals is to saturate our tissues with as many antioxidant-rich foods as possible. We can accomplish this by fortifying our body with antioxidants every time we sit down to eat. Antioxidants are supplied in our diet from vitamins, minerals, amino acids and phytonutrients.

Antioxidants are classified as <u>water soluble or fat soluble</u>. Water soluble antioxidants patrol and target the liquid interior (cytoplasm) of the cell, and the watery areas outside and between cells. Water soluble antioxidants include vitamin C, glutathione, alpha lipoic acid and the flavonoids: resveratrol, anthocyanin, and catechin.

Fat soluble antioxidants target the external, fatty area of the cells (Cell membranes.) Fat soluble antioxidants like vitamin E, vitamin A, beta carotene, astaxanthin, CoQ10, and alpha lipoic acid protect fats from oxidation and cell membranes from lipid (fat) peroxidation. (Oxidative damage to cell membranes.)

*Note that <u>alpha lipoic</u> acid is a very powerful antioxidant in that it is both water and fat soluble; therefore it can access all regions of the body. It also regenerates other antioxidants such as vitamin C, vitamin E, CoQ10 and glutathione after they have done their work. Alpha lipoic acid is derived from organ meats, green leafy vegetables, and nutritional yeast, and can also be found in supplement form; which according to the Linus Pauling Institute is more bio-available to the body. CoQ10 is synthesized from organ meats and fish.

## <u>The ACESZ</u>

There is also a <u>vitamin/mineral antioxidant</u> defense system of the body known as the **"ACESZ."** The "ACESZ" include **vitamin A, vitamin C, vitamin E, selenium and zinc.** When we eat plenty of foods with the "ACESZ," we will be able to quench excess free-radicals and slow down our aging process.

**Vitamin A Rich Foods (retinol and beta-carotenes):** Important for immune, skin and eye health. Animal sourced preformed vitamin A (retinol) found in fish, shellfish, meats, poultry, milk, cream, cheese, butter, organ meats and fermented cod liver oil is the most readily absorbed, and the <u>most usable form</u> of vitamin A. Plant-sourced beta-carotenes derived from fruits and vegetables are a secondary source and can be converted to true vitamin A (retinol). Some individuals may have conversion issues, especially individuals who are on a low fat diet and people with low thyroid functioning. Therefore it is best in these cases to get a portion of vitamin A from animal products.

Fermented Cod liver oil is an excellent source of vitamin A and has been a sacred food and vitality tonic for many traditional cultures. The powerful Roman soldier was given a daily ration of it, as well as the Scandinavian Viking- who kept a drum of fermenting cod livers outside of his home.

Highest plant sources of pro-vitamin A: dark leafy green vegetables; and orange, red and yellow colored fruits and veggies. High levels are in spinach, kale, carrots, and collard greens. Other sources are Swiss chard, mustard greens, dandelion greens, parsley, broccoli, beet greens, mangoes, tomatoes, carrots, sweet potatoes, winter squash, and apricot. Try to have a serving at each meal. Put spinach leaves in a shake. Lightly scramble eggs with kale, onions and tomatoes. Melt butter on veggies with a squeeze of lemon.

**Vitamin C Rich Foods:** First line of defense against free radicals- which lowers the risk for many chronic diseases; immune-boosting; protective against cancer and early aging. A high stress lifestyle uses up Vitamin C. Highest sources: sprouts, kiwi, feijoa, strawberries, citrus, red bell peppers, broccoli, Brussels sprouts, kale, cauliflower, tomatoes, spinach, leafy greens, and papaya. Have several servings at each meal. Cooking lowers Vitamin C levels in foods. Try to eat a daily salad. Lightly steam or sauté vegetables to reduce vitamin C depletion.

**Vitamin E Rich Foods:** Lowers the risk of heart disease; slows down brain aging, supports menopause, and protects against the oxidation of fats. Highest sources: soaked raw nuts and seeds, (especially almonds and sunflower seeds) avocados, extra virgin cold pressed olive oil, olives, leafy greens, organ meats, whole grains, sea weed, sea foods, and wheat germ. Have several Vitamin E servings at each meal. Put nuts on your hot cereal in the morning. Have nuts and seeds for a snack. Soak them for at least 12 hours- then dry them in a dehydrator or in the oven- just under the lowest setting. Have organ meats once or more a week. Eat sea weed daily. Make your own salad dressing using 2 parts olive oil to one part raw apple cider vinegar or lemon juice; a raw garlic clove; and Italian herbs.

**Selenium Rich Foods:** Anti-cancer/immune boosting properties: enhances skin elasticity and thyroid function. Highest sources: Brazil nuts, crimini mushrooms, eggs, garlic, meat, and organ meats, nutritional yeast, seafood (cod, salmon, sardines, and halibut), oats, barley, brown rice, and un-denatured grass fed whey protein powder. Eat one serving of Brazil nuts daily (2 nuts only), Put whey protein powder in shakes or sprinkle on cereals, Eat up to 2 Tbsp. of nutritional yeast daily (put in shakes or sprinkle on vegetables). Eat up to 12 organic whole eggs per week. Eat wild cold-water oily fish 3 to 4 times per week. Have 2 to 3 servings a day of selenium rich foods.

**Zinc Rich Foods:** Promotes mental alertness; immune, mood and eye health, and wound healing. A high stress lifestyle depletes zinc. Highest sources: oysters, eggs, ginger root, pumpkin seeds, mushrooms, nutritional yeast, sea foods, turkey, meats and wheat germ. Eat 2-3 servings daily. Supplement when undergoing surgery or to heal injuries.

## High "ACESZ" Foods (more above)

| Vitamin A<br>1-2 ea. meal | Vitamin C<br>1-2 ea. meal | Vitamin E<br>1-2 ea. Meal | Selenium<br>2-3 daily | Zinc<br>2-3 daily |
|---|---|---|---|---|
| Dark leafy greens/broccoli | Sprouts/spinach/ leafy greens | Raw almonds/ sunflower seeds | Brazil nuts | Oysters |
| Eggs/beef/fish and chicken liver | Rose hips/camu camu/acerola | Whole grains | Crimini mushrooms | Eggs |
| Yams/sweet potatoes/carrots Winter squash/pumpkin | Strawberries Kiwi Citrus (and pith) Watermelon | Avocados | Eggs | Ginger root |
| Fermented cod liver oil | Cauliflower, cabbage | Organ meats | Organ meats | Pumpkin seeds |
| Butter, dairy, cheese, | Red bell peppers | Olives, and cold pressed Extra Virgin Olive Oil | Seafood | Turkey and other meats |
| Parsley/chili pepper/dandelion root | Tomatoes Broccoli | Dark leafy greens, spinach | Raw garlic | Sea foods |
| Mango, apricot | Feijoa | Sea weed/ sea food | Nutritional yeast | Nutritional yeast |

**Exercise 10b: Make a list of several ACESZ foods for each vitamin and mineral** to input in your health plan; and 1 or 2 vitamin supplements if desired: if you are on a low fat diet you may be deficient in the fat soluble vitamins: A, D, E and K.

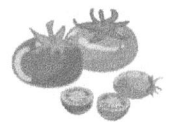

## Additional Categories of Antioxidants:

### Carotenoid and Flavonoid Phytonutrients

**Phytonutrients** (aka phytochemicals) are non-vitamin health promoting compounds that defend the body against oxidation and disease. They are found in the <u>deeply colored</u> pigments of plants and sometimes in animals. Phytonutrients are contained in the **deep blue, green, orange, yellow, red, and purple fruits; vegetables, beans, grains and micro-algae.** These pigments offer the plant itself protection from insects, fungus, and UV light etc., and they also confer antioxidant protection for humans who eat them. Therefore it is wise to eat a diverse array of various colored plant foods. "Eat from the rainbow," the adage goes. When shopping for produce, grains and beans- selecting the deeper colored varieties will supply you with the greatest antioxidants. (Example: black rice, red quinoa, dark brown flax seeds, little red beans, kidney beans, purple potatoes etc.)

**Carotenoids:** There are more than 600 naturally occurring pigments known as carotenoids. Carotenoids are the <u>yellow, orange, and red pigments</u> synthesized in plants. They can be classified into two classes of Carotenes: <u>*(alpha and beta)* and *lycopene*</u>. The second class is <u>*Xanthophylls. (beta-crytoxanthin, lutein, zeaxanthin, and astaxanthin.*</u>) The deeper the intensity of color it is, the higher the level of carotenes will be in the food. Studies suggest that a large intake of carotenes are cancer, heart disease, cataract, and macular degeneration protective. The carotenes known as lutein, zeaxanthin, astaxanthin, and lycopene have very high antioxidant activity.

Carotenoids are <u>best absorbed by eating fats with a meal</u>; cooking in oil or fat increases their bioavailability. Pouring olive oil on raw carotenes will also support carotenoid absorption. Individuals on low fat diets and smokers may be deficient in carotenoids. It's best to eat carotenoids as food instead of supplements.

*<u>Individuals who have conditions that reduce the body's ability to absorb fat</u> such as: pancreatic insufficiency, Chrone's disease, celiac, cystic fibrosis, surgical removal of the stomach; gall bladder and liver disease may need to take small amounts of a retinol vitamin A/carotenoid supplement to avoid deficiency.

### Eat From the Rainbow!

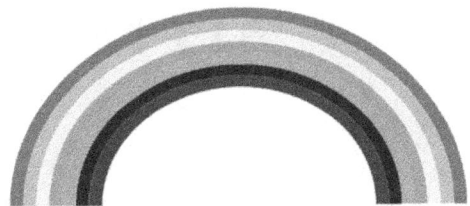

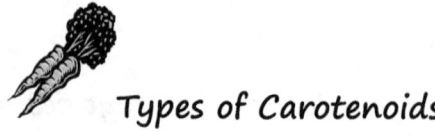

# Types of Carotenoids

- **Alpha and Beta-Carotenes**- The body converts these carotenes into vitamin A, also known as retinol A. Immune-boosting, cancer, eye and heart disease protective. Present in orange, yellow and dark green vegetables and fruits. Highest sources: canned pumpkin, carrots (juice and cooked), winter squash, spinach, sweet potatoes, collard greens, kale, turnips mango; and all dark green leafy vegetables.
- **Beta Cryptoxanthin**- Eye, arthritis, CVD, asthma, infertility, cancer (cervical, colon, skin) protective. Highest sources in cooked pumpkin, papaya, sweet red peppers, oranges, tangerines, and peaches.
- **Lycopene**- Cancer, cardiovascular disease, stroke, macular degeneration, and prostate protective: Present in red and pink vegetables and fruits. Highest sources in red tomatoes; (unsulfured sundried tomatoes, tomato paste, cooked tomatoes, raw tomatoes): red peppers, paprika, strawberry, pink guavas, watermelon, pink grapefruit, persimmons, chili peppers, and red cabbage. (Cooked tomatoes contain more lycopenes than raw.)
- **Lutein and Zeaxanthin**- Cataract, macular degeneration, CVD, stroke and cancer protective. Additionally protective of skin from UV light-generated free-radicals- as lutein can penetrate the deeper epidermis skin layers that sunscreens can't penetrate. Present in yellow and dark green vegetables and fruits. Highest sources in egg yolk (most bio-available), corn, orange peppers, parsley, spirulina, celery, cooked spinach, kiwis, grapes, zucchini, and squash family, and other cooked dark leafy greens.
- ***Astaxanthin**- The most powerful carotenoid free-radical scavenger and one of the strongest antioxidants. It is eye, heart, blood sugar, dementia, Alzheimer's, inflammation, cancer, tendon and joint protective. It is also useful as a natural sunscreen and immune booster. It enhances athletic performance and decreases sore muscles after workouts. Astaxanthin is sourced from red microalgae called- Haematococcus pluvialis and from the sea animals that eat it. Present in red or pink colored animals. Highest sources are in wild salmon, krill, shrimp, lobster, crab and other crustaceans. It is difficult to get high amounts of astaxanthin from food. In addition, it is unwise to eat a large amount of seafood- due to its high toxic metal content. An alternative is taking astaxanthin supplements. Dosage: 2 mg daily.

## Carotenoid Rich Foods

| Alpha/Beta Carotenes | Lycopene | Lutein/Zeaxanthin | Astaxanthin |
|---|---|---|---|
| Canned/fresh pumpkin | Canned/dried/fresh/cooked tomatoes | Egg yolk (most bio-available) | Red/pink seafood |
| Carrot | Red peppers | Corn | Wild salmon |
| Winter squash | Paprika | bell peppers (all colors) | Krill oil |
| Spinach | Pink grapefruit | Cooked spinach | Shrimp |
| Sweet potato/yam | Strawberries | Kiwis | Lobster |
| Tangerines/oranges/papaya | Red cabbage | Zucchini/winter squashes | Astaxanthin-from Haematoccus pluvialis Supplement |
| | | Parsley, celery | |
| Leafy greens | Rose hips | Dark leafy greens | Crab |

➡ Try to have 3 different colored fruits/vegetables at lunch and dinner. (Orange, yellow, red, purple, green) Try to eat carotenoid sources three times or more a day. (Beta-carotene, lycopene, and lutein/zeaxanthin) Raw, steamed or sautéed dark leafy greens are recommended daily. Make sure you use oil or fat to facilitate carotenoid absorption. Example: steamed greens with a drizzle of olive oil and lemon or apple cider vinegar; or greens sautéed in butter or coconut oil with garlic.

➡ **Paleo Greens Organic Powder** from *Designs for Health* is chock full of carotene-rich vegetables in an easy to drink powder form. Great for those who have trouble eating their veggies.

*Exercise 10c: Make a list of several foods, and any supplements if you desire, from each carotene group. Input them in your wellness plan: Alpha-Beta carotenes, lycopene, lutein/zeaxanthin, and astaxanthin or Paleo Greens.*

_____

# Flavonoids

A large number of powerful phytonutrients fall into the flavonoid category. Flavonoids have a long history of use in traditional medicines, and are involved in giving plants colorful pigmentation. Flavonoids block the damaging oxidation of fats that cause atherosclerosis and other conditions. Some Flavonoid classes are: **catechin, hesperidin, flavonols, ellagic acid, resveratrol, glucosinolates, anthocyanin, and pycnogenol.** Consuming coffee, refined sugar, artificial sweeteners, preservatives, additives, and pesticides deplete flavonoids in the body.

- **Catechins-** Cancer, brain, and heart protective. A very powerful catechin is green tea. It has the top flavonoid content and is more powerful than vitamin C and E. It also activates the body's own antioxidant system. Its most active compound is known as (EGCG). Green tea effectively blocks the formation of carcinogens, and is most effective for estrogen related cancers such as breast, ovarian and uterine cancer; and cancers of the gastrointestinal tract. Green tea has also been demonstrated to regulate cholesterol levels, reduce high blood pressure, protect against cognitive impairment, support autoimmune conditions and fight bacteria and viruses. The traditional Matcha green tea powder (sipped ritually) also has increased antioxidant value. There are two ways to enjoy its benefits: as an infusion with a tea bag/ tea leaves or from EGCG extracts or capsules. Some experts suggest up to 4 glasses daily. (can be iced) To naturally decaffeinate: pour a small amount of hot water over the tea bag; wait 10 seconds and then spill out the tea; next refill with fresh hot water onto the leached tea bag. This tea bag can be used several times, as it will still have potency. (Don't drink with milk)
  Other top catechin sources are mangosteen, unsweetened 70%+ dark chocolate or 100% cocoa powder. Make hot cocoa with almond milk, raw milk, or coconut milk, and add natural stevia sweetener to it.
- **Hesperidin-** Inflammation supportive. Found in rosehips, and citrus fruits- especially their pith and skins. After squeezing a lemon for your morning lemon juice- eat the inner pith.
- **Rutin-** Helps body utilize vitamin C and produces the skin building-block called collagen. Skin, hemorrhoid, varicose vein, bruising, hypertension, cholesterol, stroke, and senility protective. Rutin has been found to slow down the aging process. Highest sources in buckwheat, citrus fruit (pith and rinds) and in apple skins.

- **Luteolin-** Blocks brain inflammation; boosts memory; cancer protective. High sources in celery hearts, hot pepper, rutabaga, artichoke leaves, kohlrabi, celeriac, Brussels sprouts, beets, Chinese kale, lettuce, cauliflower, spinach, lemons, parsley, thyme, peppermint, basil, rosemary, sage, chamomile tea.
- **Flavonols-** The most well studied type is **Quercetin.** Asthma, allergy, cancer (inhibits tumor growth) and coronary heart disease protective. Quercetin prevents the release of histamines and can reduce watery eyes, runny nose, hives, and swelling. Highest sources in apples, onions, berries, and grapes.
- **Resveratrol-** Inflammation, heart disease, and cancer protective. Longevity increasing. Resveratrol activates a gene called sirtuin 1; which is known to slow down the effects of aging by activating cells to behave youthfully. Produces the same longevity benefits as exercise and calorie restriction. Highest sources in red grapes, (especially Muscatine grapes) red grape juice, and red wine. (Pinot Noir.) Seeing that these are high in sugar, limit the amounts ingested. The following lower glycemic foods contain smaller amounts of resveratrol: raspberries, cranberries, blueberries, mulberries, lingon berries, grape skin and seeds, and peanuts. Higher dosage resveratrol supplements are also available.
- **Ellagic Acid-** Promotes cancer cell death. Facilitates the liver in neutralizing cancer causing chemicals. Highest sources in raspberries, pomegranates, strawberries walnuts, and pecans.
- **Glucosinolates-** Powerful cancer preventatives. Highest sources in Brussels sprouts, cabbage, kale, broccoli, and all cruciferous vegetables. All must be cooked well to de-activate the harmful goitrogens. (goiter causing anti-nutrients.)
- **Anthocyanin- Very powerful antioxidant.** Vision, inflammation, circulatory, vein, Parkinson's disease, and cancer protective. Present in red, purple, and blue fruits, vegetables and grains. Highest sources in black raspberries, billberries, blackberries, blueberries, strawberries, black currents, cherries, cranberries, pomegranates, hawthorne berries, goji berries, acai fruit, and purple grapes. Also in red cabbage, eggplant, red onions, black beans and red beans.
- **Pycnogenol-**Vitamin C protective; capillary and circulation strengthening. Prevents allergies, restless legs, varicose veins, bleeding gums, glaucoma, strokes, and Alzheimer's disease. In addition, it blocks red blood cell seepage causing bruising and age related red spots on skin. Highest sources in pine bark extract and grape seed extract. Pycnogenol's flavonoids and acids are also found in parsley, spinach, onions, grapes, rhubarb, beets, chives, and green tea.

## Flavonoid Rich Foods

| Catechins | Hesperidin | Rutin | Quercetin | Resveratrol |
|---|---|---|---|---|
| Green tea, matcha green tea powder, or EGCG extract | Citrus | Buckwheat | Apples | Purple/red grapes, red wine, purple grape juice |
| Dark chocolate, hot cocoa | Citrus pith/rind | Apple skins | Red onions | Raspberries, grape skin and seeds |
| Mangosteen-Also contains xanthones | Rose hips | Citrus-pith/rind, Rose hips | Berries, Grapes | Peanuts, Cranberries, Blueberries |
| **Pycnogenol** | **Ellagic Acid** | **Anthocyanin** | **Glucosinolates** | **Luteolin** |
| Parsley, Spinach | Raspberries | Blue/blackberries Pomegranates | Cooked Brussels sprouts | Rutabaga, celery hearts |
| Onions, chives | Pomegranates | Strawberries | Kale | Kohlrabi |
| Pinebark extract | Strawberries | Cherries, Cranberries | Broccoli, cabbage, cauliflower, collard | Chamomile, Peppermint |
| Grape seed extract | Pecans | Bilberry/hawthorne | Mustard greens | Rosemary, sage, |
| Beets | Walnuts | Goji berries, acai Fruit, elderberries | Cruciferous veggies | Thyme, basil, parsley |

➡ Try for one serving a day of most of the listed flavonoids. Upon rising, drink the juice of one-half lemon in a full glass of water daily. This will gently cleanse the liver, and lymph system; increase alkalinity; and support a morning bowel movement. Drink with a straw, or rinse mouth out after drinking if you are concerned about tooth enamel damage. Have one to four servings of decaffeinated green tea daily. Include berries (fresh or frozen) in your daily diet. Do not eat more than 3 medium sized or ½ cup servings of fruits daily.

**Innate Response** makes an anti-aging drink powder formula named **Resveratrol Reds** that contains many of these flavonoids. **Apex Energetics** also sells flavonoid-rich **Nourish Greens**

**The Phytonutrients known as Terpenes** exert very powerful anti-cancer effects in both prevention and possibly cancer treatment. Terpenes also are great at cleansing the lymphatic system (circulates immune boosting white blood cells) which becomes sluggish as we age. **D-limonene** is a widely tested terpene. It is found in citrus fruit zest and rinds. Other terpenes are found in volatile oils such as: peppermint, thyme, and rosemary. Use these herbs liberally in your cooking.

*Exercise 10d: Make a list of one or two foods from each group of flavonoids, and any supplements if desired. Try to get one serving a day of most of these flavonoids. Add these to your wellness plan. Add several terpene-rich foods to your wellness plan also.*

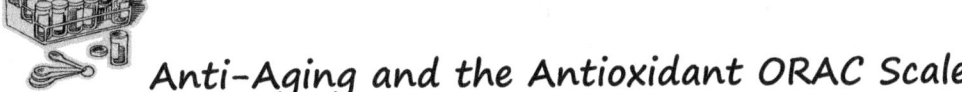

# Anti-Aging and the Antioxidant ORAC Scale

The ORAC scale (oxygen absorptive capacity) is a standardized test that rates the antioxidant capacity of different foods. It was developed by *The National Institute of Aging* in the *National Institute of Health* and was then adopted by the USDA. The test combines a measure of both the time an antioxidant takes to respond to a free radical and also its antioxidant capacity in a test sample. Foods with a high ORAC value, in theory, have a high free-radical destroying potential, and provide many times more capacity to neutralize free-radicals than low ORAC foods. High ORAC foods are packed with beneficial phytonutrients, minerals, vitamins, and amino acids, and are known as "Super-Foods" in some health circles.

➡ Interestingly **herbs and spices** have the highest ORAC value for their weight of any foods. They are at the very top of the rating scale. Try to add spices and herbs liberally to each meal.

- **Spices/Herbs** highest on the ORAC scale are: cloves, oregano, dill, rosemary, thyme, Ceylon cinnamon,* turmeric, sage, parsley, nutmeg, basil, chili powder, cumin, mustard seed, savory, paprika, tarragon, raw ginger root, peppermint, cilantro, garlic/organic garlic powder, curry powder, and black pepper. Dried and fresh herbs are both high in ORAC values. *Note: all cinnamons are antioxidant-rich because they are all in the same family; however Ceylon has the highest ORAC value.
  *Cinnamon is a highly esteemed therapeutic spice in many cultures due to its antioxidant and digestion boosting effects, and for its ability to lower blood sugar and reduce insulin resistance. Additionally, it aids in reducing bone breakdown which can help prevent osteoporotic bone loss. Try apples sprinkled with cinnamon; or put it in your morning smoothie; or on your hot cereals and granolas; add it to fried rice, or as a topping on a frozen banana. 1 tsp. a day is recommended.
- **Fruits** Highest on the ORAC scale are: black raspberries, cranberries, wild blueberries, elderberries, blueberries, pomegranates, raspberries, strawberries, lemons, blackberries, purple plums, red delicious and granny smith apples, red cherries, figs, oranges, purple grapes, rosehips, acai fruit, mangosteen, and gogi berries. (However, juices from these fruits in clear containers have lost much of their antioxidant power. It is suggested to get antioxidants from fresh or frozen produce and juice.)
- **Vegetables** Highest on the ORAC scale are: red cabbage, broccoli raab, red leaf lettuce, asparagus, red onion, artichoke, eggplant, purple cauliflower, sprouted radish seeds, broccoli, sweet potato w/ skin, savoy cabbage, beet greens, avocado, arugula, beets, radishes, spinach and kale.

- o **Legumes** highest on the ORAC scale are: small red beans, kidney beans, black beans, pinto beans, lentils, and aduki beans.
- o **Nuts** highest on the ORAC scale are: pecans, walnuts, hazelnuts, pistachios, and almonds. Have a ¼ cup serving daily or more.
- o **Fresh vegetable juices** greatly multiply antioxidant values. Try to have a fresh juice several times a week; or better-a daily juice. You will notice how well vegetable juice replenishes your energy. You can lower the glycemic load by including spinach and celery; and using root veggies in moderation.

➡ Misc. items very high on the ORAC scale are: green tea, unsweetened dark chocolate or cocoa, red wine, olives, and cold pressed extra virgin olive oil.

## High ORAC Foods

| Spices/Herbs | Fruits | Vegetables | Legumes | Nuts/Seeds |
|---|---|---|---|---|
| Oregano/Thyme | Fresh cranberries or frozen concentrate | Red cabbage | Kidney beans | Pecans/ Walnut |
| Rosemary | Blueberries | Broccoli raab/broccoli | Black beans | Almonds |
| Cinnamon/cloves Nutmeg | Pomegranates or Frozen concentrate | Red leaf lettuce/spinach | Pinto beans | Hazelnuts |
| Turmeric/cumin/curry powder | Black raspberries, Red raspberries, | Asparagus | Lentils | Pistachios |
| Parsley | Strawberries | Sweet potato w/skin | Aduki beans | Flax/chia seed |
| Onion/garlic/garlic powder | Blackberries, Elderberries | Avocado | Lima beans | Misc. High ORAC foods ⇓ |
| Chili powder/paprika black pepper | Lemons/oranges | Eggplant | Small red beans | Red wine |
| Dill/sage | Apples | Purple cauliflower | | Green tea, |
| Peppermint | Cherries | Kale | | Cocoa, dark chocolate |
| Mustard seed | Figs | Artichoke | | Olives |
| Cilantro | Acai/mangosteen | Savoy cabbage | | Olive oil |
| Arugula | Gogi berry | Radishes/radish sprouts | | Spirulina |
| Basil | Purple plums | Beets/ beet greens | | Chlorella |

**Exercise 10e: Make a list of several high ORAC foods**, and input them into your personal wellness plan. Try to have one from each group daily. Don't forget to add some spices and herbs! Use spices liberally in all of your meals. Remember to fill half of your plate or more with raw or lightly cooked vegetables. Try to eat a large salad with leafy and crunchy vegetables daily. Don't forget to eat from the rainbow! Have at least 5 colors a day.

**The brighter and deeper the color of the vegetable, fruit, seed, grain or bean- the higher the antioxidant values.**

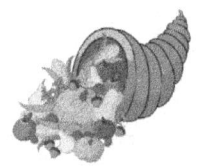

Chapter 11

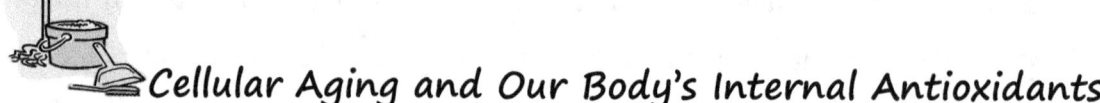

# Cellular Aging and Our Body's Internal Antioxidants

In the last several years, researchers have learned that the process we normally think of as aging is really not true aging, but the process of disease-states taking over our body. Typical age-associated diseases such as cancer, diabetes, heart disease, and arthritis are really a result of free-radical damage; which induces cellular aging. Research has found that our own body makes two of the most powerful antioxidants known. They are called Glutathione Peroxidase/Reductase and Super Oxide Dismutase.

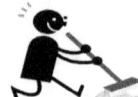

## Glutathione: Our Own Internal Master Antioxidant

Glutathione is a molecule that is vitally important to our overall health. It is the principle antioxidant in every cell of our body, and also exists in the liver. It is made from or synthesized by three protein building blocks: cysteine, glutamine and glycine. Glutathione, known as the "mother antioxidant" is a master at repairing any free-radical damage instantly. Glutathione also powerfully cleanses and protects our body from heavy metals, pesticides and other toxins; and the damage they cause. It does this by essentially "handcuffing" these free-radicals by donating its own electron to them; which can then be subsequently eliminated.

Glutathione is also essential for proper functioning of the immune system, and it keeps all other antioxidants performing at high levels. Glutathione can also recycle itself; although aging, toxins, poor food choices, excess alcohol, smoking, poor sleep, food intolerances, bad bacterial overload and stress decrease the body's production of it. Glutathione is one of the most important anti-aging, anti-cancer, and cardio-protective compounds in our cells. The depletion of glutathione stimulates people to age more quickly; and puts them at risk for lipid peroxidation, inflammation and immune and toxin-induced diseases including: cancer, cardiovascular disease, autoimmune and other degenerative diseases. However, encouraging experiments performed on animals demonstrated that increased glutathione-generating food intake boosted their longevity by about 40%.

Fortunately there are many glutathione-boosting foods. All foods that contain sulfur will synthesize glutathione. Sulfur-rich glutathione acts like fly paper; free-radicals stick to it, and then are neutralized. Regular moderate exercise also boosts glutathione. Additionally, eating an array of fresh organic produce will increase its levels. Lastly, soaking in one cup of sulfur-rich Epson salts will enhance its production and recycling.

## Glutathione Boosting Foods

- **Vegetables**: asparagus, crimini mushrooms, avocado, red peppers, tomatoes, squash, red beets, okra, spinach, cruciferous vegetables: broccoli, cabbage, kale, Brussels sprouts, bok choy, watercress, mustard greens, collard greens, turnip greens, napa cabbage, cauliflower, rutabaga, kohlrabi.
- **Herbs/Spices**: garlic, onions, parsley, turmeric, cinnamon, cardamom, and rosemary. Consider eating one or more raw garlic cloves daily or take aged garlic extract in supplement form.
- **Nuts**: raw brazil nuts (eat only 2-3) and walnuts (eat ¼ cup serving of nuts daily)
- **Legumes**: black eyed peas and pinto beans
- **Grains**: whole oats, wheat germ, rice bran
- **Animal Proteins**: unprocessed organic duck and other poultry; organic organ meats, wild fish (especially wild salmon), raw pastured egg yolks, plain organic yogurt or kefir with-"live and active cultures," raw organic cow and goat milk, un-denatured organic/grass fed whey protein powder. (for raw milk sources: go to realmilk.com)

## Glutathione Boosting Foods

| Veggies | Herbs/Spices | Nuts | Legumes | Grains | Proteins |
|---|---|---|---|---|---|
| *Asparagus | Garlic | Brazil nuts | Black-eyed peas | Oats | Poultry/duck |
| Crimini mushrooms | Onions | *Walnuts | Pinto beans | Wheat germ | Organ meats |
| *Avocado | Parsley | | | Rice bran | Wild fish/salmon |
| Red peppers | Turmeric | | | | Raw pastured egg yolks |
| Tomatoes | Cinnamon | | | | Plain yogurt/kefir |
| Okra | Cardamom | | | | Raw cow/goat milk |
| Cruciferous veggies & all raw veggies | Rosemary | | | | Undenatured organic whey protein powder |

*Note: Fresh organic raw foods support more glutathione production then cooked foods.

➡ Moderate sun exposure also boosts glutathione antioxidant levels. Try to get 20-30 minutes of midday sun exposure daily (10-2pm) in spring, summer, and early autumn. (Without sunscreen.) If you are sun-sensitive you can sit out for 5-10 minutes at a time- several times a day.

*Glutathione Synthesizing/Recycling Supplements/Herbs:*

| ** N-Acetyl Cysteine (NAC) | *Alpha lipoic Acid | *Milk thistle | Methylation vitamins: vitamin B6, B12 and folate | Selenium |
|---|---|---|---|---|
| *Vitamin C w/ bioflavonoids | Vitamin E (mixed tocopherols with tocotrienols) | Aloe Vera | * Melatonin (hormone that is a powerful anti-aging antioxidant) | Grape seed extract |
| L-glutamine | Cordyceps mushroom | Gotu Kola | Apex Energetics- *Glutathione Recycler* or *Oxicell* | Moderate sun exposure w/o sunscreen 20-30 min. daily |

**Exercise 11 a: Make a list of Glutathione Boosting Foods and supplements** if desired and input in your personal wellness plan. Try to get 3 or more servings a day.

_____

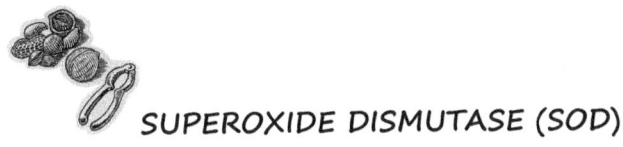

# SUPEROXIDE DISMUTASE (SOD)

*Our body's top anti-aging antioxidant*

The SOD enzyme was discovered in 1968, and is the key enzyme in the body created by our SOD1 gene. SOD's main function is in preventing the highly damaging and abundant internal free-radical known as "superoxide" from destroying our cells. Superoxide is a waste product from cell metabolism; a process which creates energy for our body, but also creates damaging free-radicals. Our life-saving SOD enzyme essentially transforms this "superoxide" free radical into hydrogen peroxide; which is then neutralized by the catalase enzyme into water and oxygen.

If our cells become overwhelmed by dangerous "superoxide," and we don't have enough SOD enzymes to neutralize them, our cells will be damaged and start to age, often causing cancer. Researchers believe that as we get older, our body's production of SOD diminishes. Fortunately we are able to enhance our SOD levels, even as we age; as it has been proven that humans who have more SOD in their cells live longer. Boosting SOD levels through optimal nutrition, exercise, and staying away from toxins may help guard against disease and keep our cells younger for a longer period of time.

*SOD plays a critical role in preventing/healing*

| Aging | Stroke |
|---|---|
| Heart attack | Arthritis |
| Lung disorders | Neurological disorders |
| Cancer/cancer therapy support | Collagen and Skin aging (wrinkles, sagging) by increasing skin elasticity; and reducing hyper-pigmentation and redness. Protects against UV rays |
| Wounds/burns | Inflammation (IBD, fibrosis, psoriasis) |

*Here are some SOD boosting foods and supplements*

- **Minerals:** foods rich in copper, zinc, and manganese boost SOD production. Calves liver, oysters, crimini mushrooms, pecans, brazil nuts, almonds, walnuts, sesame seed, pumpkin seeds, peanuts, buckwheat, split peas, barley, rye, oats, pineapple, spinach, chard, asparagus, green beans, green peas, spirulina, ginger root, lima beans, turnips. (Be sure to soak nuts, seeds, grains, and legumes 7-12 hours before eating to reduce phytates)

- **Green Vegetables**: barley and wheat grass, broccoli, Brussels sprouts, cabbage contain natural SOD
- **Fruits**: honeydew melon and cantaloupe contain natural SOD. Blueberries, guava, goji berries, citrus, and strawberries help the body make SOD in tandem with copper.
- **Gliadin**: If you eat a little wheat, rye, or barley (that contain gliadin protein) with your fruit or vegetables, it can help protect the SOD content of them from stomach acid. Note: many people have gliadin/gluten sensitivities, and should avoid eating these foods. Or use GliSODin supplement.
- **Vitamin E** (supplement-mixed tocopherols) has been shown to boost SOD by 30% Vitamin E foods: sunflower seeds, wheat germ and oil, almonds, spinach)
- **Oils**: flax oil/seeds have been shown to boost SOD levels significantly
- **Herbs/Fruit Extracts**: *Pterostibene, Juar tea, and extract of Andrographis paniculata,

### Copper, Zinc, Manganese-Rich SOD Boosting Foods

| Spirulina | Oats/rice | Calves liver | Oysters | Crimini mushrooms |
|---|---|---|---|---|
| Ginger root | Turnips | Green beans | Asparagus | Spinach/swiss chard |
| Pineapple | Pecans | Brazil nuts | Almonds | Walnuts |
| Strawberries | Pumpkin/sesame seeds | Buckwheat | Lima beans | Green peas |

### Other SOD Boosting Foods/Herbs/Supplements

| Veggies | Fruits | Vit. E | Oils |
|---|---|---|---|
| Wheat grass | Honeydew melon, Cantaloupe | Sunflower seeds | Flax oil/seed |
| Broccoli | Blueberries/strawberries | Wheat germ/oil | **Herbs/Supplements** |
| Brussels sprouts | Citrus | Spinach | Juar tea |
| Cabbage | Guava | Almonds | Andrographis paniculata extract |
| Barley grass | Goji berries | Avocado | *Pterostilbene |
| | | | GliSODin |

## The Catalase Enzyme

The catalase enzyme works together with glutathione and SOD to help neutralize free-radicals and to break down residual toxic hydrogen peroxide chemicals left behind from the detoxification processes. However, as we age the production of our catalase enzyme also starts to dwindle; which can result in the build-up of hydrogen peroxide. Interestingly, recent research has discovered that a build-up of hydrogen peroxide has been found to be the culprit for prematurely graying hair. Hydrogen peroxide essentially bleaches hair follicles from the inside out. There are foods that can stimulate the production of the catalase enzyme in our body, and some experts believe may hinder the loss of hair pigment and premature graying.

*Foods that stimulate production of the catalase enzyme*

| *Beef liver: very high source | Alliums: leaks, garlic, onion | Cruciferous veggies: kale, broccoli, cauliflower etc. | Avocado | Potatoes and sweet potato |
|---|---|---|---|---|
| | | | | |

**Exercise 11b: Make a list of at least 5 SOD and catalase boosting foods** to input in your personal wellness plan. If your SOD levels are kept high, you can keep your cells much younger for a longer period of time.

*Chapter 12*

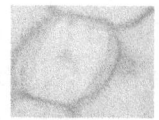 *Mitochondria: our "Cellular Batteries"*

A great way to slow or reverse aging is to boost our cells' mitochondrial function; as low energy output in our mitochondria is a major component of poor health as we get older. Mitochondria, if you remember from your high school biology class, are like mini power plants that generate power in our cells. They do this by taking food and converting it into usable energy for us. Children have the greatest quantity of mitochondria, (about 1,000 mitochondria per cell) and is why they are so lively and energetic. However, as we age, we can experience mitochondrial decay. By the time we reach age 50, we may have only half the amount we had as children; and as a result our body will produce less energy.

High energy organs that burn-up a lot of energy quickly such as our brain, heart, liver, kidneys, eyes, ears, nerves, and muscles particularly need a great deal of energy to do their job, and will suffer if mitochondria energy output declines. Mitochondria, for example take up 40% of the space inside our heart cells. Therefore, problems can occur especially with our heart, if we have poor functioning mitochondria. Other problems that can arise from mitochondria decay are: fatigue, slow metabolism, weight gain, memory loss, hearing and vison problems, psychological problems, immune dysfunction and pain.

Our mitochondria are sensitive to damage from excess sugar, nutrient-poor foods, and a sedentary lifestyle. Mitochondria are also affected by environmental toxins and infections. Additionally, if we have an excess amount of free radical damage and oxidative stress; our mitochondria can lose their power-generating capacity. This will result in energy loss, and added free-radical damage.

*Mitochondria–Related Symptoms and Dysfunctions*

| Cardiac problems | Stroke | Dementia |
|---|---|---|
| Migraine | Seizures | Fatigue |
| Weakness | Hearing loss (inner ear dysfunction) | Liver dysfunction |
| Eye disorders | Neuropathies | Insulin resistance/diabetes Pancreatic dysfunction |
| Kidney dysfunctions | Premature aging and pain | Obesity |

A nutrient deficiency can also lead to reduced mitochondrial energy production in our cells, but by implementing a nutritional support program we can help restore our mitochondrial health. Several key nutrient co-factors and antioxidants are needed to support mitochondrial function; thus helping our surviving mitochondria make more energy. These antioxidants include **Coenzyme Q10, lipoic acid, and carnitine.** They can be found in foods or purchased as supplements.

## Mitochondrial Supportive Antioxidant-Rich Foods

| CoQ10-increases ATP | Lipoic Acid | Carnitine increases ATP | Other |
|---|---|---|---|
| *Organ meats: liver, kidney heart | *Organ meats: liver, kidney, heart | *Red meats: lamb and beef | eggs |
| Fish-sardines, mackerel | *Brewer's yeast/nutritional yeast | Dairy products | nuts |
| Grass-fed beef | Dark leafy vegetables/broccoli | Legumes | *blueberry |

Other co-factors that restore mitochondrial function are glutathione, cysteine, vitamin E, vitamin C, carotenoids-(lutein/zeaxanthin), flavonoids, pterostilbene, and the minerals zinc, copper, selenium, and manganese. Co-factors needed for the cellular mitochondria-boosting Krebs cycle are vitamins B1, B2, B3, B5, and vitamin K; and the minerals, magnesium, phosphorous and sulfur. Examples are as follows:

- Nutritional yeast is very effective for improved mitochondrial function, due to its high vitamin B complex content.
- Dark leafy greens, nuts, and beans boost mitochondrial-boosting magnesium and vitamin K levels.
- Eggs, beans, and poultry are high in supportive sulfur; and eggs are very high in lutein/zeaxanthin.
- Activities that have been found to improve mitochondrial function are calorie restriction, reducing insulin production with low glycemic-load foods, and regular exercise.

Note: According to the Linus Pauling Institute, the lipoic acid in food is not as available as in supplemental lipoic acid. There are some side effects of long term use of supplemental lipoic acid however, such as a decrease in blood sugar and thyroid hormones.

## Additional Mitochondrial-Boosting Foods/Lifestyle

| Nutritional yeast | Dark leafy greens, | Nuts |
|---|---|---|
| Beans | Eggs | Poultry, |
| Calorie restriction | Low glycemic-load foods | Regular exercise. |

## Mitochondrial Supportive Supplements

*(Neutralize oxidative stress/glycation(o/g) and increase ATP)*

| *Alpha lipoic Acid:(o/g) 240-480 mg daily | *Pterostilbene: 250 mg (Sears, 2015)  *Branched chain amino acids (BCAA) | *B-vitamins: Benfotiamine: (Vit B-1) (o/g) Vitamin B2 (riboflavin), Vitamin B3 (niacin), Vit B6-P5P-50 mg. | Carnosine: (o/g) 500 mg 2 times daily |
|---|---|---|---|
| *Resveratrol (reverses mitochondrial aging process) 10-20 mg, Pomegranate extract: (o/g) | *CoQ10-hydrosoluble ubiquinone: Increases ATP/ if under 60: 50-100 mg if over 60/or on statin drugs: 100-200mg (Dr. Sinatra, 2015) | *L-Carnitine: Increases ATP/ 500-1500 mg daily | D-ribose-increases ATP (chronic fatigue support) 5 grams daily |

➡ Mitochondria lab testing: "Organic Acids" urine test. (Assesses metabolism steps)

### Mitochondria Multiplier: PQQ

Not only do mitochondria lose their power, they also become damaged and decrease in numbers as we age. Our heart and brain have the most mitochondria- as many as 2,500 mitochondria in every cell. In 2010, researchers discovered a powerful nutrient that can actually generate new mitochondria. It is known as *pyrroloquinoline (PQQ,)* and it is *referred to as* the *"mitochondria multiplier."* PQQ actually can *restore* the mitochondria that have been lost due to aging. You can purchase this as a supplement or in selected foods.

**PQQ supplement** Dosage: 10-20 mg/day

### Foods Rich in the Mitochondria Multiplier Nutrient PQQ

| Parsley | Green tea | Green pepper | Oolong tea | Kiwi fruit |
|---|---|---|---|---|
| Natto | Papaya | Spinach | Fermented cod liver oil | Tempeh/miso |
| Broad bean | Carrot | Cabbage | Sweet potato | Red potato |

**EXERCISE 12: Input several mitochondrial boosting and mitochondria multiplying foods/supplements** into you're your personal wellness plan. Try to have several each day.

*Chapter Thirteen*

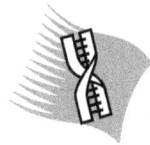

## *Telomeres and Our Anti-Aging Enzyme*

In 2009, Dr. Elizabeth Blackburn won a Nobel Prize in medicine for discovering an enzyme that actually reverses aging by stimulating our cells to grow younger. Her work focused on telomeres and the telomerase enzyme.

Telomeres cap the end of each strand of our DNA and protect them from unraveling when cells divide. This is much like how the plastic tips that cap shoe-laces protect them from fraying. Cells normally can divide about 50-70 times, but every time our cells divide our telomeres get shorter; and after many divisions, our telomeres become very short and frayed. Shortening telomeres are also likened to a bomb with a fuse; the shorter our telomeres get, the faster we grow old and experience age-related declines such as cancer.

Dr. Blackburn found through her research that the telomerase enzyme, known as telomerase, keeps our telomeres from wearing down excessively, and even can boost our telomere length. Recent scientific literature has revealed that there are substances and activities that <u>increase</u> telomerase action; as well as some that <u>decrease</u> the telomerase activity. "Oxidative Stress" (the inability to neutralize free radicals, as explained previously) lowers the activity of the telomerase enzyme; and as a consequence shortens our telomeres.

*Other behaviors and conditions that accelerate telomere shortening*

| Stress, pessimism and worrying | Smoking | Obesity, | Sedentary lifestyle (lack of activity) |
|---|---|---|---|
| Nutritional deficiencies | Dysbiosis/yeast overgrowth, parasites | Chronic disease | *Inflammation |

*Inflammation comes from an inflammatory diet of refined carbs, processed food, artificial additives and sweeteners, sugar, high fructose corn sweetener, transfats/hydrogenated fats, and processed meat consumption. Drinking soda has been shown in the latest research by Dr. Blackburn to dramatically decrease telomere length.

*Fortunately*, making healthy lifestyle choices; having good eating habits; and minimizing free radical exposure has a profound effect on the health of our telomeres and therefore on how well we age. A *University of California San Francisco* telomere *study* revealed that men who optimized their diets; got regular exercise; and calmed their stress through meditation, were able to increase the enzyme telomerase in their immune cells.

*Exer. 13a: Input foods/activities that trigger telomere shortening that you can reduce or eliminate.*

_____

There is also a commercially available telomerase activator that is a highly concentrated extract from the ancient Chinese herb astragalus, called TA-65. A person may pay up to several thousand dollars a year for this product.

*The following are budget conscious options to activate the telomerase enzyme:*

- Resveratrol containing foods: red wines from Burgundy or Argentina (Drink moderately and only if you presently drink alcohol), raisins, purple grape juice, cranberries, blueberries, mulberries, peanuts or resveratrol supplements such as <u>*Innate Response's Resveratrol Reds*</u>
- Green tea or green tea extract. (EGCG) Also combats skin aging
- N-Acetyl-Cysteine. (NAC) Also combats hearing loss.
- Vitamin E containing foods: raw nuts, seeds, avocados, olives, olive oils, spinach. Heart disease and cancer protective.
- L-Carnosine containing foods: Grass fed pasture raised red meat, chicken, fish. L-Carnosine optimizes organ function: cell regenerative, cataract preventative and kidney strengthener.
- Vitamin C containing foods: citrus, strawberries, kiwi, sprouts, broccoli, rosehips, and camu camu. Firm-skin promoting. Slows down telomere shortening by 62 %
- Vitamin D3 containing foods: fermented cod liver oil, sardines, mackerel, salmon, and midday sun exposure. Vitamin D3 prevents osteoporosis, cancers, and mood disorders; plus increased telomere activity by 19.2%
- Milk Thistle herb- Detoxifying properties, and liver protective. Researchers concluded that milk thistle increased telomerase activity 3-fold.
- B-complex vitamin rich foods: nutritional yeast, whey protein powder, and spirulina. Reduces excess damaging homocysteine levels- which build up in your blood stream when antioxidant levels drop
- Acetyl L-Carnitine rich foods: Grass fed pasture raised red meat (beef and pork) Brain booster
- Citrulline or watermelon concentrate
- Rhodiola Rosea

## Telomere Lengthening Supplements/Herbs

| Resveratrol | Milk Thistle | Green tea Extract | Omega 3-cod liver oil | N-Acetyl Cysteine | Acetyl L-Carnitine |
|---|---|---|---|---|---|
| L-Carnosine | Buffered vitamin C with bioflavonoids | Vitamin E mixed tocopherols/tocotrienols | Vitamin B Complex or nutritional yeast | Citrulline | Fiber: Flax seed meal, legumes |
| Vitamin D3 | Melatonin | Rhodiola Rosea | Spirulina | Chlorella | Grass-fed Whey protein powder |

### In addition, studies have linked a longer telomere length with:

- A varied, and large quantity of antioxidants (reduces oxidative stress)
- Consumption of ten servings a day of fresh and relatively uncooked or lightly cooked vegetables and fruits
- Mixed fiber (flax meal, beans, rice bran)
- Monounsaturated fats (avocado, almonds, olives, olive oil)
- Omega-3 fatty acids from cold water fish 3 times per week (salmon, sardines, halibut) or an omega-3, krill oil or fermented cod liver oil supplement
- High quality vegetable proteins (soaked beans, fermented miso, tempeh)
- A high quality multi-vitamin/mineral supplement
- Optimizing hormone levels with herbs or natural bioidentical hormone replacement
- Optimizing exercise with 1 hour per day of aerobic/burst, and resistance exercise
- Optimizing sleep to 8 hours per night
- Achieving ideal body weight with low body fat: 22% for women and 16 % for men
- Stress management/reduction
- Calorie reduction-reduce daily calorie intake by reducing starches and grains.
- Intermittent fasting for 12 hours each night at least 4 days a week. (easily done at night)

## Telomere Lengthening Foods/Activities

| Selenium-rich foods: Brazil nuts, sea food, garlic, liver, mushrooms | Green tea<br><br>Red wine (1 small glass only 1-3x wk.) | Balance hormones with herbs/bio-identical hormones | Free range/pastured Red meat, poultry, duck | Mono-unsaturated fats: olives/oil, avocado, almonds | Sardines, salmon etc. 3x wk. or fermented cod liver oil or krill oil |
|---|---|---|---|---|---|
| 10 serv. fruit/veg. daily Citrus, strawberries, kiwi, rosehips Kale, broccoli | Nutritional yeast, spirulina, undenatured whey protein powder | Daily midday sun exposure (10-2pm) in spring, summer, fall | Stress management/ 8 hours of sleep each night | Exercise one hour daily | Calorie reduction/fasting<br><br>Weight management |

➡ **Telomere Lab Testing:** If you would like to find out the length of your telomeres, and how well you are aging, telomere lab testing can be performed at Spectra Cell Laboratory. You can also retest to see if your lifestyle changes have improved the length of your telomeres.

*Exercise 13b: Make a list of 1-5 telomere lengthening foods/activities/supplements* that you can commit to for the next few months. Input them into your personal wellness plan.

Chapter 14

## Alkalinity/Mineral Reserves and pH

### (Oxygenation, Rejuvenation and Bone/Joint Health)

The pH of our body (the fluid in and around our cells) is one of the most important measurements of our health. Our blood pH effects how our body uses vitamins, minerals, and enzymes; it also regulates digestion, and our cellular activity. Our blood needs to stay within a narrow pH range; and if the blood pH becomes too acidic, calcium and other minerals will be leached out of our bones in order to alkalinize our blood. Our bones and other cells then can become depleted of necessary minerals. If a high acid environment (acidosis) is chronic; all the alkaline buffering mineral reserves such as calcium, magnesium, sodium and potassium, will be depleted- leading to chronic fatigue, osteoporosis and other chronic diseases.

Minerals are our acid neutralizers and maintain alkalinity for us. One of their jobs is to sustain pH homeostasis or balance. Our blood pH should be slightly alkaline; at 7.35-7.45. Our urine pH should be between 6.8 -7.2. (Close to neutral.) It is very common as we age however to experience mineral deficiencies and pH imbalances, primarily due to mineral depletion in our soil; commercial agriculture; poor food choices; a high-stress lifestyle; and compromised stomach acid production.

Yet, minerals are the most important nutrient in our diet due to the fact that they are co-factors in all the body's metabolic enzymatic reactions. Essentially, they are needed for all bodily functions. Additionally, they give structural support to our bones, connective tissue, and the vascular system. They are also hormone regulators, and cancer protectors. Minerals (zinc and selenium) are antioxidants, and give anti-inflammatory support. Most importantly, viruses, bacteria, fungi, cancers and diseases all thrive in a low mineral/acidic environment. As you can see, an inadequate mineral status can negatively affect your quality of life as you age.

Certain food choices also contribute to acidosis, such as eating refined/packaged foods, pasteurized dairy and sugars. Grains, breads, and pasta also lower pH, as grains are acidic; especially when grain is milled into flour. Also, consuming excessive portions of meat and other animal protein and fats at one meal without balancing them with mineral-rich acid-neutralizing vegetables will also contribute to acidosis. Vegetable proteins, such as beans and soy also promote acidity, but not to the extent that animal proteins do. It is not suggested that you eliminate animal proteins however from your diet; as they offer excellent nutritional density, and are important for the growth and repair of our cells. Just ensure that you eat only between 3-4 oz. at a meal; and balance the protein with 3 servings of vegetables. A good rule to follow to keep your mineral stores and your pH balanced is to consume more alkaline producing foods than acid producing foods: 80% alkaline forming mineral-rich foods (vegetables/fruits) to 20% acid forming foods. (Proteins/grains etc.)

*Symptoms/Conditions Related to Mineral Depletion and/or Acidosis*

| Joint pain/arthritis | Aching muscles | Chronic fatigue | Wrinkles |
|---|---|---|---|
| Nausea/stomachaches Gastritis | Kidney stones | Diabetes | Osteoporosis and osteopenia |
| Gout | Circulatory and cardiovascular weakness | Constriction of blood vessels | Cancer |
| PMS | Insomnia | Anxiety | Depression |

## Mineral-Rich Foods

*Emphasize these in your daily diet*

| Sea Veggies | Vegetable juices | Mineral broth, bone broth | Dark leafy greens | *Algae: spirulina, and chlorella |
|---|---|---|---|---|
| *Nutritional yeast | Organic soaked and/or sprouted seeds and nuts (7-24 hours) | Organic herb teas/infusions: nettles, horsetail, oat straw, comfrey, alfalfa | Nutritional mixed green powders with barley grass, chlorophyll etc. | Mineral water, glacial milk, sparkling mineral water |

## How to Build Mineral Reserves and Alkalinize the Body.

| | |
|---|---|
| Eat 3 servings of vegetables with each serving of animal protein in a meal- for pH balance. Parsley, kale, fennel and spinach have an alkalinizing effect on the body. | Fruit/vegetable goal: 10+ servings of vegetables and fruits daily. (2-3 servings of fruits only) |
| Eat sea weeds/add them to soups | Eat leafy greens daily |
| Drink fresh vegetable juices daily or weekly | Eat sprouted seeds and sprouted grains |
| Eat home-made vegetable broths | Take spirulina/chlorella powder daily |
| Drink barley grass/wheat grass juice | Drink beet juice |
| Blend in mixed alkalinizing green powders to smoothies. Spirulina and chlorella are often part of the ingredients, along with wheat grass or barley grass. **Paleo Greens** is a good formula. Alfalfa is the richest source of chlorophyll | Replace acidic forming grains with alkaline forming root vegetables (carrots, yams, turnips, parsnips, red potatoes,) and gourds (winter squash) at least 3-7 times a week |
| Eat grain in its whole form over the more acidic flour grain foods. (Pasta, baked goods, bread etc.) Replace flour products with unrefined whole quinoa, brown rice, millet, buckwheat, wild rice, and amaranth. | Squeeze alkaline forming fresh lemon or lime into your drinks throughout the day/squeeze some on your meals. Although citrus are acidic, they have an alkaline ash. |
| Drink sparkling mineral water (Gerolsteiner is high in minerals) | Add cinnamon, ginger, and other spices to your meals |
| Eat high alkaline forming extra virgin olive oil | Use raw apple cider vinegar (with the mother) and olive oil salad dressing on salads. |
| Take a high quality chelated mineral supplement (with calcium/magnesium/potassium citrate or glycinate) | Take the supplement- potassium bicarbonate with mixed minerals if high acid conditions persist |
| Sweeten foods with stevia or Lo han guo. Add one Tbsp. black strap molasses to water for high minerals | Dairy foods-Eat low acid producing dairy foods: "Live and active" cultured kefir and yogurt. Un-denatured organic whey protein powder is also low in acidity. |
| Eat/drink alkalinizing, mineral rich foods/herbs: kelp, dulse, kale, collard greens, parsley, apricots, dandelion greens, almonds, sesame seeds, nettles, oat straw, comfrey leaf, and red clover | Deep breathing increases alkalinity |

➡ **Home pH Assessment:** Monitor your morning urinary pH using a **pH test kit** which is intended to show pH values, and whether your body has a healthy store of minerals. The thin strip of pH paper changes color when it comes in contact with moist/wet substances. Track your first morning urine pH. (after at least 6 hours of sleep- without getting up to urinate) If your first morning urine is below 6.5 (acidic range) or if your first morning saliva is below 7.0; your bone alkali mineral reserves are probably low. This indicates that your bones are being depleted of minerals in order to buffer metabolic acids. A low morning saliva test, according to some practitioners also reveals whether chronic emotional issues are affecting your mineral status. To offset this excess acid condition, quickly drink some lemon water, lime water or apple cider vinegar in water. **<u>Microessentials- Hydrion pH paper</u>** is a very accurate pH test paper.

---

### Energy Boosters

*Nutritional yeast is a great energy booster, as it is packed with B-vitamins and minerals. Nutritional yeast does not contribute to candida albicans, as some people fear; as the yeast is no longer living. Start with 1/2 tsp. in a smoothie and work up to 2 Tbsp. per day. (But no more, as an excess can cause elevated phosphorous levels.) Nutritional yeast has a cheesy flavor, and can be substituted for parmesan cheese in foods such as pesto, grain and tomato sauce dishes. (Yeast tablets are also available.) Choose non-GMO yeast is possible.

***Spirulina and Chlorella** are also wonderful energy enhancers, and help detox the body. They are packed with chlorophyll, minerals, antioxidants and B-vitamins. They each have slightly different flavors and some people prefer one over the other. Start with 1/4 tsp. and work up to one Tbsp. (Tablets are also available.)

***Potassium rich fresh organic vegetable juices** combining celery, parsley, spinach, carrots, and beets with a clove of garlic or a slice of ginger can help raise flagging energy levels in the afternoon. Much better than coffee!

*Exercise 14: Monitor your morning urinary or salivary Ph. Make a list of 5-10 alkalinizing/energy boosting foods, activities and supplements that you can commit to within the next few months and input them in your personal wellness plan.*

Chapter 15

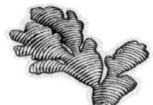 ## Hidden Inflammation and Immune Balance

Inflammation is a medical term that we've all been hearing about for several years now, but many people don't really understand what the condition is. We have all experienced inflammation at one time or another, particularly when we have gotten an infection, rash, allergy or a sprained ankle. This is a normal short term immune reaction our body mounts in order to bring blood and white blood cells to a damaged site in our body. After the threat is over and the condition is healed, the immune response is then turned off. Healthy inflammation is vital, as it is the body's mechanism for healing. Normal healthy responses of our immune defense system are needed to resolve infection and tissue injury, and to clear metabolic waste and environmental toxins.

The trouble arises when the defense system inside our body is not turned off, and runs out of control like a smoldering fire. This chronic slow burning inflammation creates free radicals that damage our organs and lead to rapid aging and illness. Hidden unrelenting inflammation limits the optimal functioning of our body, and experts believe is the root cause of joint pain and chronic diseases such as: heart disease, obesity, eczema, fibromyalgia, diabetes, dementia, cancer, depression, asthma, autoimmune disease, osteoporosis, rheumatoid arthritis and osteoarthritis. All of us, as we age, will have some inflammation; however by addressing the causes of inflammation, and living an anti-inflammatory lifestyle, we can limit inflammation and forestall or reverse disease.

The best way to prevent or control inflammation is to identify the triggers and causes of inflammation and then re-balance our immune system by giving it optimal conditions to cool its inflammatory fire.

### What Causes Inflammation?

**A Pro-inflammatory Diet:** Sugar, high fructose corn syrup, refined carbs, processed and packaged foods, trans-fats, refined vegetable oils, synthetic nitrates in meats, excessive commercial red meat consumption, excessive wheat usage, non-organic veggies and fruits, and particularly snack foods.

Potato chips, French fries, corn chips, and crackers contain **acrylamide**; formed from the heating (frying, baking, roasting) of proteins and sugars. Research from Poland revealed that people eating potato chips daily for a month had an increase in their

CRP (inflammation marker) levels. Other inflammation causing factors are listed in the following chart.

## Pro-Inflammatory Triggers

| Obesity/over eating | Sleep disorders | Periodontal disease | Smoking |
|---|---|---|---|
| Stress | Toxins: mercury and pesticides | Lactose/gluten intolerances and other hidden food allergies | Hidden or chronic infections with viruses, bacteria, yeast or parasites. |
| Indoor mold toxins and environmental allergens | Pro-inflammatory diet<br><br>Nutrient deficiencies | Oxidative stress with too few antioxidants | Medications: Antihistamines, NSAIDS (Motrin), Corticosteroids (Prednisone), Cox 2 Inhibitors (Viox, Celebrex) block immune function |
| High blood sugar | Lack of exercise or over-exercising: more than 15 hours a week | Hormone imbalances | Weak digestion |

It is important that you discover what contributes to your inflammatory condition. It could be lifestyle, environment or hidden infections that trigger a heightened immune response and cause cell damage. Food intolerances, candida overgrowth, leaky gut, parasites, heavy metals, and indoor mold toxins are often the source of inflammation when other risk factors have been ruled out. See Digestion and Detoxification pages for more info.

➡ Anti-inflammatory medications such as NSAIDS (Motrin, acetaminophen, aspirin) Steroids (prednisone) and Cox 2 inhibitors (Viox, Celebrex) block not just the inflammation causing the problem, but **all immune function**, and inhibit the body's natural mechanism for healing itself.

Exercise 15a: Determine if you may have high inflammation with self-assessment/chart. Then make a list of a few substances/activities that trigger inflammation that you can eliminate or limit. Input in your wellness plan.

## Anti-Inflammatory Foods/Supplements

An anti-inflammatory diet is one of the most effective ways to calm inflammation.

- *Eat a whole foods plant-based diet: Load up on veggies especially dark leafy greens and celery. (for brain inflammation) Eat fruit in moderation.
- *Omega- 3s: <u>very important.</u> Small cold water fish: sardines, herring, sable, halibut, wild salmon, mackerel, and anchovies. Eat 3-4 times a week. One of the most important factors in lowering inflammation.
- Eat adequate protein at every meal.
- Increase fiber intake: flax seed meal, beans/legumes and crunchy veggies. Put 1-2 Tbs. flax meal in morning protein smoothie. For freshness, grind seeds in a coffee grinder.
- Gamma Linolenic Acid (GLA): black currant seed oil, borage oil, evening primrose oil, spirulina, hemp seeds/oil.
- *Healthy Fats: cold pressed extra virgin olive oil, avocados, olives, and coconut oil
- Other vegetables: peppers, broccoli, eggplant, carrots, winter squash, fresh vegetable juices
- Fruits: citrus, berries, green apples, yellow and orange fruit (3 servings daily) only
- Nuts/seeds: raw walnuts, hazelnuts, sunflower seeds, omega-3 flax seed and meal; chia seed, hemp seed/oil
- Non-gluten grains
- Lentils (less starch than beans, thus have a lower inflammatory rating)
- Herbal Teas: green tea, holy basil (tulsi) tea, turmeric tea and ginger root tea (boil 1-2 inch piece of fresh ginger root for 15-30 min.)
- Herbs: ginger, oregano, turmeric (curcumin) Use these liberally on foods. Grate fresh ginger on salads. Put 1/2 tsp. of turmeric powder in protein smoothies.
- **Innate Response Formula's- Inflama-Complete** is a very effective anti-inflammatory herbal supplement.

## Anti-inflammatory Activities

- Release Stress: Chronic stress weakens immune function, and inhibits the body from repairing injured cells. Learn to actively relax to engage your vagus nerve; the powerful nerve that releases your entire body, and lowers inflammation. Practice yoga, deep breathing, meditation; and Epson salt baths (one cup)
- Exercise for 20 minutes to 1 hour at least three times a week
- Rebalance a weak digestion with daily probiotics: ("beneficial bacteria") 20 billion CFU of bifidobacteria and lactobacillus species. Or eat cultured foods. Use HCL and enzymes with meals to support digestion/assimilation.
- Sleep 7-9 hours per night.

- Take a high quality vitamin and mineral supplement.
- Determine if you have food allergies/sensitivities/intolerances. Many people are sensitive/intolerant to wheat and dairy. Assess reactive foods in your diet and stop eating them. Do an elimination diet with suspected foods for one month to observe health improvements. See dysfunctional metabolism chapter.
- Determine if you suffer from dysbiosis, candida yeast overgrowth, parasites, or a leaky gut. Many individuals have these conditions as they age, and it is a prominent reason for inflammation. Find a holistic practitioner that can help you resolve these issues.

➡ **There are two primary pro-inflammatory pathways** in the body, and are known as the COX and LOX inflammatory pathways. (COX-2 enzyme/5-LOX enzyme) Reducing levels of pro-inflammatory substances across both of the inflammatory pathways is the most effective way to resolve inflammation and pain. Note that curcumin, (sourced from turmeric) resveratrol, and Vitamin A and E are able to inhibit both inflammatory pathways.

*Anti-Inflammatory Botanicals and Supplements that inhibit both the LOX and COX pathways*

| COX-2 Enzyme inhibiters | 5-LOX Enzyme inhibiters |
|---|---|
| Cod liver oil/krill oil | Boswellia |
| *Curcumin | *Resveratrol |
| Bromelain (empty stomach) | *Curcumin |
| Quercetin | Marine lipid extract |
| Ginger | Selenium |
| *Resveratrol | Holy basil |
| Hops | Phosphatidylserine |
| *Vit. A & E | Vit. A, C, & E |

➡ **Lab testing for inflammation:**

- C-reactive protein test (under .55 mg/L for men -- under 1.50 mg/L for women)
- Fibrinogen test (under 300 mg)

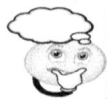

**Exercise 15b:** Make a list of 5-10 anti-inflammatory foods/activities/supplements that you can commit to for the next few months. Input them in your Personal Wellness Program. Input lab information

## Strengthening and Balancing our Immune System

**Our immune system** also defends us from harmful substances and organisms that we absorb from the environment, such as viruses, bacteria, fungi, and parasites. It in addition protects us from cancerous growths. When we have too little immune activity, we can come down with colds, the flu, or other infections. We can also develop a microbial overload or possibly cancer.

However some individuals suffer from excessive and imbalanced immune activity, which can lead to autoimmunity. This is where the body's defense system attacks its own tissues. However, the goal for achieving vibrant health is to have balanced immune functioning; not too overactive; yet not weak.

There are many factors that can weaken our immunity or cause it to become overactive. The following chart reveals some culprits.

### Factors that Weaken or Imbalance Our Immune System

| | | | |
|---|---|---|---|
| Excess sugar/refined carbs | Excessive alcohol, caffeine | Chemical exposures | Excessive exercise |
| Poor diet, nutrient deficiencies; low protein, damaged fats | Food hypersensitivity | Sleep deprivation | Lack of sun exposure (Vit. D) |
| Antibiotic overuse, microflora imbalance | Chronic stress, lack of R&R, depression, mood issues | Leptin resistance | Leaky gut (Increased intestinal permeability) |

➡ **Eating nourishing food**; maintaining stress reduction practices; and making sure to get adequate rest and downtime are the primary factors that maintain optimal immunity. Here are some additional immune enhancing aids.

### Immune Enhancers

| | | | |
|---|---|---|---|
| Organic whole plant-based diet w/ optimal protein, pastured red meat, wild sea food, leafy greens, berries, citrus and seeds. | *Chicken bone stocks/vegetable broths | Herbs/teas: green tea, Echinacea, astragalus, cats claw, licorice root, elderberry, holy basil, turmeric, ginger, olive leaf, oregano | *Fermented cod liver oil |
| *Garlic (raw) or aged garlic extract | Undenatured grass-fed whey protein | *Mushrooms-cooked or dried maitake, shiitake, reishi, cordyceps or AHCC (very powerful fermented mushroom extract) | *Stress reduction & management |
| Chlorella, spirulina aloe Vera | *Fermented foods: raw apple cider vinegar (with the mother) yogurt, kefir, veggies, kvass, miso etc. | Supplements: vitamin C, zinc, vitamin A, selenium, magnesium, vitamin D3, vitamin B. | Moderate exercise, R&R, good sleep, weight loss, sun, leaky gut repair. |

## Auto-immunity

If you suffer from auto-immune conditions, you will need to address your state of hyper-immunity and will need a protocol to balance immune function.

The following is a list of some autoimmune conditions: Rheumatoid arthritis, asthma, Hashimoto's thyroiditis, Grave's disease, vitiligo, Crohn's disease, I.B.D., Addison's disease, M.S., dermatitis, eczema, psoriasis, alopecia, type I diabetes, urticaria, pernicious anemia, celiac etc.

### Auto-Immunity/Hyper-Immunity Support Protocol

| | | | |
|---|---|---|---|
| Avoid gluten and possibly dairy. Paleo diets followed for one year are often successful. | Avoid commercial animal proteins. Choose lean organic proteins | Use extra virgin olive/ coconut oil as main oils | Sulfur-rich diet: garlic, onion, cruciferous veggies |
| Calorie restriction/fasting | Heavy metal chelation: cilantro, sea weed etc. | Nutritional yeast | Fermented cod liver oil (vit. A, D) |
| Probiotics/fermented foods | Vit's D3, E, and C, NAC, CoQ10, alpha Lipoic acid, EPA/DHA, GLA | *Green tea extract, turmeric, rosemary, oregano, ginger, grape seed extract, pycnogenol, resveratrol | Stress-reduction, self-loving thoughts, gentle exercise, Support leaky gut issues, sun exposure |

**Note:** Not to be used with Lupus or Ulcerative Colitis

**Exercise 15C**: *Make a list of some immune boosters and/or immune balancers, and input them in your plan to incorporate into your daily routine.*

_____

Chapter 16

# Nitric Oxide and Optimal Circulation

Nitric oxide, referred to as "the spark of life," is a vital "feel-good" gas molecule that is produced and released in the interior surface of our blood vessels. Nitric oxide's function is to widen our blood vessels in order to keep our blood moving smoothly. It is vital to our cell health and every biological system, as it facilitates delivery of nutrients and oxygen.

In 1998 three American pharmacologists were awarded the Nobel Prize for discovering this molecule, and studying how it aids in relaxing and expanding our blood vessels. Our body creates nitric oxide naturally out of the food that we eat. Nitric oxide is particularly important for our cardiovascular system as it keeps our arteries young and flexible; increases blood flow and circulation; and stops plaque buildup. Expanding arteries are critical to our optimal health as they are the means for bringing more oxygen to our heart, brain, and other organs.

Dr. Valentin Fuster, past president of the *American Heart Association* and head of cardiology at Mt. Sinai Hospital proclaimed that: "The discovery of nitric oxide and its function is one of the most Important in the history of cardiovascular medicine." Children and athletes have the most efficient nitric oxide system, but as we age free-radical damage; inflammation, a poor diet, smoking, worry, anxiety, and a sedentary lifestyle weaken our circulation, and deplete nitric oxide levels. After we reach age 40, there is a 50% decline in nitric oxide. Without sufficient nitric oxide levels we can feel tired and worn out. An "NO" deficiency is also linked to certain conditions such as: hypertension, heart disease, stroke, insulin resistance, diabetes, asthma, arthritis, Alzheimer's, erectile dysfunction, and osteoporosis.

## Nitric Oxide Benefits

| Energizes the brain and helps support memory by transporting information between cells | Strengthens the immune system at fighting bacteria and tumors | Reduces blood pressure/improves cardiovascular health/stroke prevention |
|---|---|---|
| Reduces inflammation | Improves sleep | Triggers positive emotions, Increases sense of smell |
| Supports good bowel function | Increases strength and endurance | Reverses erectile dysfunction and boosts libido in women by increasing blood flow |

## How to Boost Nitric Oxide (NO) Levels

Ongoing research has revealed that certain foods are able to boost NO levels in the body. An impressive nitric oxide MRI study was performed on subjects who drank beet juice in the morning. The MRIs amazingly showed that just hours after drinking beet juice, the subjects were flooded with a steady flow of blood to the brain. This blood flow indicates that an abundance of oxygen and nutrients nourished and energized the brain cells of these subjects. It is easy to see that NO promoting foods ought to be a part of our brain-boosting, as well as our cardiovascular strengthening arsenal.

We can also increase nitric oxide levels by eating foods rich in L-arginine; (nuts, fruits, pastured organic meats, and raw dairy) vitamin C, and vitamin E. Additional NO boosting foods are pastured eggs, wild cold-water fish, and brown rice. A high content of naturally occurring nitrates in certain vegetables additionally synthesizes nitric oxide in our blood. Mediterranean diets also have been found to produce NO. Nitric oxide only lasts a few seconds in the body, so the more we consume antioxidant rich foods throughout the day, the more stable and long lasting the NO levels will be.

Additionally, beneficial bacteria in our gut and mouth produce NO. When we do not have an adequate amount of friendly bacteria in our gut and mouth, we may not get the full benefits from an NO boosting diet. Now we have another reason to improve our gut bacteria status through probiotic-rich foods and supplements!

### Very high NO boosting foods (6,825-312 mg)

| Highest -Green leafy Vegetables-*kale, (cruciferous), *swiss chard, *arugula, *spinach, beet leaves, red leaf lettuce, bok choy, Chinese cabbage, cabbage, mustard greens | Chicory |
|---|---|
| Red beets and beet juice | Pomegranate juice (fresh/frozen) |

*highest sources

### High NO boosting foods (50-250 mg)

| | |
|---|---|
| celery | Endive |
| Fennel | Leek |
| Parsley | Radish |
| Garlic | Cauliflower |
| Carrot | Broccoli |
| lettuce | Asparagus |
| Artichoke | Kohlrabi |
| Mustard greens | |

**\*NOTE:** Spinach, parsley and beet leaves are very high in kidney stone forming oxalates, which can be a problem for some people (anti-nutrients which bind with calcium to synthesize calcium oxalate kidney stones) It is recommended to not eat these foods in high amounts or make them a staple of your diet if you have a family history of kidney stones. **Also** be careful with eating raw goiterogenic cruciferous vegetables (kale, bok choy, mustard green, cabbage, broccoli, cauliflower etc.) as they can block thyroid function if eaten in excess. Studies have shown that goiterogens are reduced by 1/3 when steamed, and reduced completely when boiled for a half hour.

*Activities that increase NO*

| Deep breathing | Exercise | Laughing, positive emotions |
|---|---|---|
| Taking naps | Taking hot baths/saunas | Acupuncture |

*Supplements that Increase NO*

Note: L-Arginine is not effective after age 40. (R. Williams, 2004)

| *Beet root powder | *CoQ10 | *Hawthorne extract or tea |
|---|---|---|
| B12 | Niacin | Magnesium Citrate or Glycinate |
| L-Citrulline | Vitamin C | Vitamin E |

*Best sources

- **Home Nitric Oxide Assessment-** Monitor your NO status with an **NO test kit** using your saliva and test strips. This is a simple way to observe if your NO boosting diet and lifestyle efforts are really working. **Neogenis Labs** sells high quality, precise test strips. First, test your baseline level of NO upon rising. Test again a week later to determine if food/supplements and lifestyle are improving your circulation status. (Brisk walking, greens or beet juice etc.) Then, test your saliva every other week.
- **Neogenis** offers a supplement: **Super Beets-** Organic Beet root crystals. Or try **Nox Synergy by Designs for Health**

*Exercise 16: Determine if you may have low nitric oxide levels with symptom assessment.* Make a list of 5-10 foods/activities/ supplements that can support your nitric oxide levels and heart/brain health for the next few months. Add them to your Personal Wellness Plan.

Chapter 17

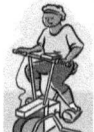 Exercise and the Anti-Aging Human Growth Hormone

Exercise is one of the best ways to maintain our health as we age. It has been found that people that exercise have a life expectancy that is 7 years longer than sedentary people. In fact, exercising just 30 minutes a day with vigorous exercise can cut our risk in half for many age-related diseases. Exercise offers us a plethora of health benefits. It supports blood sugar balance; healthy leptin levels and insulin sensitivity. It supports our heart and lung health. It is one of our best stress busters, as it lowers our stress hormones, and supports weight management. It has also been shown to trigger an increase in mitochondrial concentration in our cells.

According to Dr. William Kannel and Dr. Helen Hubert from the Boston School of Medicine; our lung strength tells us how long we will live. Our lungs begin to shrink if we are inactive as we age. The smaller our lungs, the less able our body will be in fighting off infections and pneumonia. Poor lung function increases our chances of dying from all diseases. Conversely, exercise maintains the size and strength of our lungs- increasing our chances for a longer life. In fact, practicing high intensity exercises that produce labored breathing have been shown to improve lung strength by 14%; although moderate and regular aerobic exercise can also benefit lung function.

Breaking a sweat with vigorous walking is really all that is needed to maintain or increase our lung strength. It's best however to avoid endurance exercises longer than 2 hours a day, as they tend to break down muscles, and can contribute to oxidative stress and inflammation. Practicing yoga also improves our lung capacity and facilitates oxygen delivery to our cells. It is an ideal exercise to do as we get older; as it maintains our balance and suppleness.

Some form of weight-bearing exercise or muscle strength training is also recommended 2-3 times per week, as it helps keep our bones strong and prevents muscle loss; which is a universal problem as we age. It also benefits the heart and boosts mood and weight loss, plus prevents chronic pain. One study showed that strength training in the elderly reversed oxidative stress and returned many of their genes back to youthful levels. Studies also show that strengthening quadricep muscles in our legs will aid stamina, stability and balance; extremely important for falling prevention as we get older. Simple squats or lunges are all is needed to increase quad strength.

If you are new to exercise, consider implementing a movement/walking program into your daily routine; as prolonged sitting can weaken our health due to the increased force of gravity on us. If you feel too weak to walk far; just standing every twenty minutes can counteract the force of gravity and support your health.

The best way to assess how much we move throughout the day is to use a pedometer, and it's best to wear the pedometer all day from morning 'till night. Pedometers are very inexpensive, and can be easily worn. If you would like to implement a walking program, a typical goal is to reach 10,000 steps per day by the end of six weeks.

## Pedometer Walking Program

| |
|---|
| **Week 1.** The first day of wearing the pedometer you will be checking how many steps you take in the course of your day, just doing normal routines. The rest of the week you will be adding an additional two thousand steps to your day. (about a mile more) You can break up the walking sessions in whatever way is easiest for you. (morning, afternoon, evening) |
| **Week 2.** Add to your daily walking by another one thousands steps. |
| **Week 3.** Increase your daily walking by another one thousand steps. (At least 7,000 daily steps) |
| **Weak 4.** Increase to eight thousand daily steps. Pick up the pace a bit. |
| **Week 5**. Increase to nine thousand daily steps. |
| **Week 6**. Increase to 10,000 steps. (about 5 miles) Congratulations! You should be feeling pretty good by now. You can increase your speed or duration if you feel strong enough. |

*Note this protocol can be modified to be made easier by adding only 250-500 steps per week with the goal of walking 5,000-7, 000 steps per day.

*A special bonus of exercise* is that it boosts our body's own natural production of our anti-aging hormone known as Human Growth Hormone. (HGH) HGH is a hormone secreted by our pituitary gland that helps us to feel young and energetic, and is responsible for our body's ability to withstand the aging process. HGH creates stronger and more powerful muscles and bones and protects them from atrophying. In addition, HGH has been shown to help promote healthy, taut skin; rapid hair and nail growth; increase our libido; and our cardiac output. Lastly, it is responsible for enhanced disease resistance, as it helps our internal organs heal faster.

Our natural production of HGH declines as we age, particularly around middle age; and by seventy years old we only produce 1/10 of the amount of HGH generated by a twenty year old. Additionally, certain lifestyle factors can blunt our HGH production. Several chief reasons for a deficiency of HGH are: having a sedentary lifestyle; eating a high glycemic-load diet; excess stress; and not getting enough sleep. Some deficiency symptoms may include: a reduction in lean body mass and bone mineral density; a worsened cardiovascular profile; erratic sleep, and increased body fat.

Fortunately there are many ways to naturally increase our HGH. It is important to work numerous major muscle groups to activate HGH. The most effective way to trigger its release is to perform high intensity short burst exercises. The goal is to get to the point where the body begins to pant and feel slightly winded. High Intensity Burst Training is an example. (HIBT) HIBT engages super-fast twitch muscle fibers, which efficiently stimulate the release of HGH. This is done by bursting one's heart rate above the anaerobic threshold for 20-60 second intervals- 5 or more times in a workout. Doing hill sprints is effective at releasing HGH also. Weight training with high repetitions is additionally an effective way to signal its release.

In addition, there are other non-exercise methods we can utilize to increase our HGH production. Given that HGH is released during the first few hours of sleep, it is advantageous to maintain normal sleep habits and to get adequate sleep. Eating a high protein/low carb snack before bed will help facilitate its production. (However, if you have sleep difficulties the opposite is advised.)

Our diet also has a lot to do with the quality of our HGH production. Eating a low glycemic-load diet, and high quality lean protein meals with cruciferous veggies (broccoli, kale, cabbage, and collards) can support optimal HGH levels. Zinc rich foods like oysters, lamb, ginger and pumpkin seeds also are HGH enhancers. Chlorella also contains a compound known as Chlorella Growth Factor, (CGF) which offers some of the same benefits found in natural human growth hormone. Lastly, reducing our belly fat can reverse the decline in our HGH production.

The goji berry, nicknamed the "longevity fruit" is also renowned for stimulating Human Growth Hormone production. It is one of the chief foods in the diet of the natives in the Ningxia Province of China, which boasts the greatest number of centenarians in all of the country. These inhabitants exhibit tremendous vigor and youthfulness. Eating a handful of goji berries (dried or fresh) daily can be a great addition to our HGH-boosting lifestyle. You can even grow it in your own backyard!

*Supplements to Boost HGH Production (take before bed)*

| Melatonin: .5-3 mg. | Vitamin D3: 2000+ IU. | Gaba: 1.5-3g. | L-arginine/L-lysine 3-5 g. |
| Glutamine: 2-10g. | Aged garlic extract | Chlorella | Pycnogenol |

*Don't forget the goji berry!*

## Athletic Injury Prevention and Management

As we age we can be prone to more sports/joint injuries, osteoarthritis; and pain due to nutrient shortfalls, over-exercising, overuse and muscle loss. We can lessen our chances of suffering from athletic and joint injuries, and osteoarthritis by emphasizing antioxidant-rich foods in our diet such as: vitamin C, vitamin E, cysteine (glutathione precursor), lipoic acid, selenium, carotenoids, lycopene, and bioflavonoids. Whey protein powder is also very useful as it promotes muscle development and repair.

| Vitamin C: red bell peppers, kiwi, citrus, Brussels sprouts, kale, broccoli, cauliflower, sprouts | Vitamin E: sunflower seeds, almonds, mustard greens, chard, turnip greens | Cysteine: eggs, garlic, onions, yogurt, poultry, oats, broccoli, red peppers, Brussels sprouts |
|---|---|---|
| Selenium: brazil nuts, crimini mushrooms, undenatured whey protein powder, fish | Lipoic Acid: organ meats, leafy greens | Carotenoids/Bioflavonoids/Lycopene: leafy greens, red, purple, yellow, and orange fruits and vegetables. |

## Remedies for Sport's/Joint Injuries

| |
|---|
| For all sports injuries: Increase protein, and add anti-inflammatory rich nutrients (vitamin E, C, carotenoids, bioflavonoid and lycopene-rich foods) Supplement with vitamin C: 3-8 g, zinc:30 mg, vitamin E: 800-1200 IU, MSM 1500+ mg. |
| Carpel tunnel syndrome: Vitamin B6 (P5P form) 50-150 mg (divided doses) |
| Plantar fasciitis: MSM- 1,500 mg to start, than 3g, (in divided doses) turmeric, nettle, ginger |
| Tendonitis: Buffered vitamin C: 3-8 g, (in divided doses) zinc, vitamin A, magnesium, MSM (500-1,500 mg), DMSO cream (applied to injury)  If chronic: SAMe -1200 mg (divided doses) |
| Tennis Elbow/bursitis: Omega-3s, vitamin B's, vitamin C, MSM, glucosamine/chondroitin, boswellia. White willow bark, ginger, bromelain or Wobenzyme. (on empty stomach) |
| Osteoarthritis: *Arthroben by Designs for Health*-Stimulates joint/cartilage repair/pain-relief. 1½ Tbsp. 1-2 times daily. Beneficial effects after 3 months of usage. |
| Cartilage problems/ joint popping/cracking/ pain between shoulder blades: Zinc deficiency |

## Natural Pain relief

It is suggested to avoid NSAID's (over the counter pain remedies) when suffering from athletic injuries, as they depress immunity; and are known to impair the health of the liver and GI tract. To manage acute or chronic pain, consider using the following strategies on the next page to avoid relying on regular doses of pain medication.

See next page.

## Nutrition for Sports Injury/Osteoarthritis Pain relief

| High protein for repair-Eliminate sugars and high carbs (increases inflammation/pain) | Sulfur rich foods: alliums, beans, cruciferous veggies Bathe in sulfur-rich Epson salts/MSM powder | High antioxidants: bright colored foods, lycopene, vitamin c | High mineral foods: sea veggies, leafy greens, chlorella | MSM: begin w/ 1500 mg then 3-10g |
|---|---|---|---|---|
| Curcumin: 400-600 mg (3x/day) on an empty stomach<br><br>Quercetin: 2-3 g with vitamin C | Ginger: 1 ginger capsule (4x daily) or 4 cups of fresh ginger root tea (one inch piece boiled in 2 cups of water for 20 minutes) | Omega 3 fish oil or krill oil<br><br>California Poppy tincture (for pain)<br><br>Black cumin seed oil (for Pain) | Wobenzym N or bromelain (between meals 3x a day) | For conditions with acute or long term pain: K-Laser Therapy, acupuncture or TENS (battery operated nerve stimulator) |

➡ *__Designs for Heallth- Arthroben__* has been found to decrease joint pain, inflammation and stiffness just as well as Aleve or Advil without the GI side-effects. 1½ Tbsp. 1-2 times daily.

Exercise 17: Input exercise and HGH info into your wellness plan, and any sports medicine info. Set a fitness goal for yourself by inputting how much exercise you are willing to do weekly.

Chapter 18

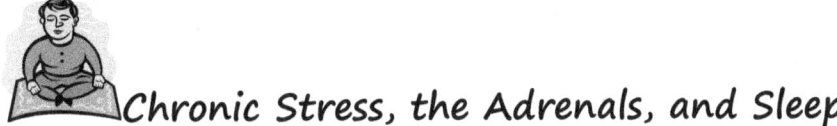

# Chronic Stress, the Adrenals, and Sleep

Stress is a common 21$^{st}$ century condition. Almost everyone suffers from it at one time or another. But what is it exactly? According to the Merriam–Webster dictionary, "Stress is a physical, chemical, or emotional factor that causes bodily or mental tension that alters an existent equilibrium, and may be a factor in disease causation."(Merriam-Webster, 2014)

We are seeing a silent epidemic of stress-related disorders in our society. In fact, it has been proposed that 95% of all illness is caused or worsened by stress. Research suggests that how effectively we handle stress is more important than any other risk factor in influencing whether we will live a healthy and long life. Aside from eating breakfast, some experts believe that the biggest predictor of longevity is mental and emotional resiliency. Due to our powerful mind/body connection, how well we handle our challenges has an immense impact on the wellbeing of our body. Our body just can't tell the difference between real stressors, such as life threatening situations (fleeing from an attacker) and harmless situations that cause psychological stress. (Being late for an appointment) They both create the same stress response and if chronically activated, will cause damage to our body.

Stress comes in many different forms. In addition to the more common psychological triggers of stress, there are other ways that our body can experience stress. Our body will react in the same manner no matter what produces the stress. Chronic stress weakens the "stress fighting gland" known as the adrenals, and uses up excessive amounts of nutritional reserves. Stress also overwhelms our nervous system. In addition, most people don't eat well when they are "stressed out;" which adds to the body's overload. It is vital to fortify ourselves with superior nutrition during periods of stress to give it the extra reinforcement it needs to keep up with the body's increased burdens.

### Emotional and Psychological Stressors

(Can contribute to accelerated aging and adrenal and nervous system dysfunctions)

| Anger, anxiety, sadness, guilt, shame | Tumultuous personal relationships | Divorce |
|---|---|---|
| Chronic worrying about relationships, children, finances, health problems | Job pressures | Chronic Pessimism |
| The perception of overwhelm: that there is not enough time to do everything. | Perfectionism | Death of a loved one |

### Physical stressors that overwork the adrenal glands

| Physical overwork | Constant rushing | Physical injury and illness | Surgery | Lack of Sleep |
|---|---|---|---|---|
| Lack of exercise | Excessive exercise | Yeast and parasite infections | Hormonal Imbalances | Food intolerances |

### Chemical Stressors

(Must be detoxified from the body; putting stress on the liver and adrenal glands)

| Poor diets high in refined and over-processed foods | Stimulants: coffee, alcohol, sugar and recreational drugs |
|---|---|
| Chemical substances: environmental pollutants, pesticides, GMO's etc. | Cortisol like medications |

The Hungarian/Canadian endocrinologist Hans Selye first popularized the term "Stress." He was the first to research the physiology of the stress response, which he called the "General Adaptation Syndrome." In this response the body responds to stress initially with an **alarm reaction**, also known as **"The fight or flight reaction."**

When a person experiences an initial stressor a two-part alarm system is set off. One activates the nervous system, (norepinephrine) and the other is hormonal (cortisol). The response begins in the hypothalamus with CRH (Corticotropin-releasing hormone) which stimulates both systems. The alarm is linked from the brain to the adrenal glands located on the upper pole of each kidney; which release norepinephrine, the neurotransmitter that triggers the sympathetic nervous system for the fight-or-flight response. This alarm also initiates the adrenal glands to produce epinephrine, also termed adrenalin, which makes us hyper-alert, and synthesizes glucose for energy supply. In addition CRH activates the HPA axis (hypothalamus-pituitary-adrenal axis), which discharges the major stress hormone-cortisol from the adrenal glands. The hormone DHEA is also released to boost the immune system.

These physiological responses cause a person to be extraordinarily alert, and ready to fight or flee from the "saber toothed tiger," or an invading enemy in our early history; or any other stressful event in our current day. The heart rate; breathing rate; blood pressure and metabolism speed up to boost the flow of oxygen to the fleeing or fighting muscles. Pupils dilate to heighten vision. The liver releases stored glucose to raise energy for the increased requirement. A person will begin to sweat to cool the body, and the immune system will be on full force to heal wounds, or to fend-off bacteria or viruses that might have come about during the crisis. Important regular physical processes that aren't needed to survive the emergency are curbed; as blood flow to the hands, feet, scalp, and intestines decreases. Additionally, this causes digestion to slow. Blood clotting is also heightened to control the possible loss of blood, and natural painkillers (endorphins) are released to alleviate pain which would aid an injured fleeing victim.

According to Selye's "General Adaption Syndrome," the **Second Stage** of the stress response is the **Adaption/Resistance Phase**. Historically and physiologically, the "fight or flight" response was meant for dealing with a short term crisis. After surviving a perilous experience, our ancestors would have had time to calm down and recuperate from the wounds or terror that they had undergone, thus allowing the adrenals to rest and recover.

Today, however, our stressors, often **_Psychological_**, as well as **_Environmental_**, and **_Physical_** are pervasive and ongoing; producing consistently and excessively high and damaging cortisol levels. According to Selye, if our stress is persistent, and our body produces an excess of cortisol; our body adjusts by switching into a hormone activity known as "pregnenolone steal."

Pregenenolone steal causes our "mother hormone" known as pregnenolone to be diverted into making cortisol at the expense of ("stolen from") our other vital hormones, such as estrogen, progesterone, testosterone, thyroid hormones and DHEA. (Immune/anti-aging hormone) The purpose for this process was to help us through the stressful period that typically only lasted a short time, but many people are in a constant state of pregnenolone steal in our modern age; which has led to a rise in hormone imbalances.

At this stress-response stage, the Hypothalamus-Pituitary-Adrenal Axis starts to be strained, and we can experience fatigue and insomnia. We will also suffer from lowered testosterone, progesterone, thyroid and DHEA hormone production. We additionally may experience estrogen depletion or dominance. Many people at this time resort to sugar, carbs, caffeine, and fat to stimulate and soothe themselves. But, these behaviors only worsen our health, and deplete our body.

Instead, it is imperative at this time to be diligent about increasing nutrient-rich foods into our diet. If we possess a strong constitution and maintain our nutritional reserves we may have the fortitude to withstand a large amount of stress. However, the best approach is having some sort of stress management/reduction practice in place to modulate the stress response.

If we haven't ensured proper nutrition or stress management during stressful times: Selye's **Third Stress Response: the Exhaustion Stage**, could take place. This is when the adrenals break down, and result in low cortisol, DHEA, and epinephrine levels; which contribute to what is known as "adrenal fatigue syndrome." This is a condition in which our adrenals are extremely debilitated and can't renew our energy. Our immune system, which is normally kept in check by balanced cortisol levels, becomes hyperactive; allowing inflammatory conditions to exist. This can cause allergies, asthma, or autoimmune disorders like Hashimoto's thyroiditis, arthritis, lupus, and M.S. (Simpson, 2011)

If the adrenal glands are weakened, these systems will also be compromised, and start to dysfunction:

- Energy levels will start to decline, and fatigue will set it.
- Blood sugar levels will initially increase producing weight gain in the abdomen, otherwise known as "central obesity." In more advanced adrenal dysfunction, low blood sugar will prevail.
- High stress hormones will cause high blood pressure. In advanced adrenal impairment, low blood pressure will be experienced.
- In addition, constant activation of the stress response system will produce muscle atrophy.

## Associated Conditions of Stress

Stress has sweeping effects on every facet of our health because our body systems are all interrelated; one aspect influences every other aspect. Additionally, certain conditions will come about according to our own genetic weaknesses.

| Low stomach acid (HCL) | Inflammatory Bowel Disease | Irritable Bowel Syndrome | Allergies | High Blood Pressure |
|---|---|---|---|---|
| Low Blood Pressure | Canker sores in the mouth | Chronic Fatigue Syndrome | Insulin Resistance and Type 2 Diabetes | Low Blood Sugar |
| Gall Bladder Dysfunction/ Gall Stones | Mania, Schizophrenia | Psoriasis | PMS | Progesterone Depletion/ Estrogen Dominance |
| Menopausal symptoms | Infertility | Impaired Brain Function and Memory/Dementia | Impaired Thyroid Functioning | Immune Dysfunction |
| Weakened Bones | Sleep Problems | Nutrient Deficiency | Acidosis | Accelerated aging |
| Leaky Gut | Dysbiosis | High stomach acid/GERD | Anxiety | Depression |

## Symptoms of Adrenal Hormone Overproduction (cortisol and adrenalin)

### First and Second Stage of Adrenal Dysfunction

These symptoms show that the stress response has been triggered often, thus shutting down many normal bodily processes to focus on the perceived threat. In this state our immune system is suppressed. Our organ functioning and cell reproduction also become sluggish. We are bothered by poor sleep and diminished brain and heart function. Cortisol, the fat promoting hormone will start to store fat around our middle. If stress is not managed at this juncture, sustained overproduction of adrenal hormones eventually leads to adrenal exhaustion; chronic underproduction of adrenal hormones; and hormone imbalances.

## Symptoms of Over-Production of Adrenal Hormones

| | | | | |
|---|---|---|---|---|
| Excessive agitation, irritable feelings | Worrying often, anxiousness, guilt often, panic attacks | Bruising easily, slow healing wounds | High cholesterol with high LDL and Low HDL | Fluid retention |
| Food/carb/sugar cravings, increased appetite | Trouble sleeping | Cold sores or mouth ulcers | Look older than your age | Memory or cognitive problems |
| Muscle weakness | Thin skin, non-pregnancy related stretch marks | Excessive hair growth on face (woman) | Light-headed and dizzy when stressed | Unusually fast heartbeat, fast breathing |
| Excessive sweat | Infection prone | Excessive caffeine and alcohol drinking | Disinterest in sex | Excessive urination |
| Heartburn, reflux | Headaches | Restlessness | Face or skin flushing | Trembling hands |
| Breathing trouble | Blurry vision | Thin extremities, round moon face | Excessive weight around belly, apple shape | Osteopenia or osteoporosis |

## Signs/Symptoms of Adrenal Fatigue & Underproduction of Adrenal Hormones

### Third and Fourth Stage of Adrenal Dysfunction

Adrenal exhaustion is caused by continual or extreme exposure to emotional or physical stress for a long duration, causing the adrenal gland to burn-out and atrophy.

| | | | | | |
|---|---|---|---|---|---|
| Chronic fatigue | Pale face, and lips | Cold sweats | Anxiousness, panic attacks | Muscle and joint pain | Heat sensitivity |
| Under eye circles | Excessive alcohol drinking | Swollen lymph glands | Internal shivering feeling | Moody and irritable | Tired in morning, even with adequate sleep |
| Perfume, chemical or pollution sensitivity | Long term respiratory infections | Scaly skin | Sick often | Sunken eyes or cheeks | Higher energy in the evening |
| Need for coffee to boost energy | Abdominal pain, gas or nausea | Socially isolated | Cold and clammy palms | Unable to take deep breaths | Eye sensitivity to light |
| Sweet, salty and carbohydrate. cravings | Sensitive to color, sound and smells | Hissing sounds in ears | Easily angered | Brain fog, and inability to concentrate | Cognitive decline |
| Signs of dehydration- sharp wrinkles | Weak, stiff muscles | Red palms or fingertips | Weight gain around middle | Thin muscles | Pain in mid- back area |
| Frequent urination in small amounts | Insomnia | Weak or slow pulse | Poor memory | Lack of sweat | Swollen fingers or ankles |
| Poor appetite | Easily defensive | Dizzy when standing | Chronic infections | Inability to handle stress/overreaction to small issues | Thin face |
| Hypoglycemic | Depression | Low blood pressure | Low thyroid | Difficulty in losing weight | Reduced sex drive |

**Exercise 18a: Input whether you may be suffering from a possible stress disorder/adrenal dysfunction** (gleaned from assessment/charts) If so, what stage is likely?

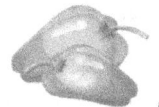

## Nutrition for Stress, Adrenal Regulation, and Repair

The ideal and most important approach to manage chronic stress is to try <u>to keep cortisol levels down</u>; this way we avoid overworking and weakening the adrenals, and prevent hormone imbalances. The following list details how to reduce cortisol levels or keep the cortisol hormone from being triggered.

- The most important factor to support adrenal health is to eat a protein-rich building diet using high quality animal and plant proteins. Eating at least 60 grams of protein a day is often recommended. Read food labels to determine protein intake.
- In addition, healthy fats and complex carbohydrates should be eaten at every meal. This will support optimal cortisol, serotonin, blood sugar, and insulin levels throughout the day.
- Eat smaller, more frequent meals, and don't skip meals. When the body goes too long without food, cortisol will be released. Eat breakfast within one hour of waking. It establishes the blood sugar foundation for the day. Our physiology is programmed to digest a high amount of calories in the morning.
- In addition, it is important to alkalinize the blood with fruits and vegetables, which will also add plenty of anti-oxidants to neutralize free radicals.
- Make sure you drink half your body weight in purified water to keep yourself hydrated.
- It is also essential to eliminate all sugars, and high sugar fruits to avoid insulin resistance.
- You will also need to avoid drinking caffeinated drinks, as these raise cortisol levels.

### Stress/Adrenal Support Target Foods

- *<u>**Drink stress supportive herbal teas**</u>: Very effective-Tulsi, passion flower, chamomile, catnip, kava kava, hops, valerian, skullcap, lemon balm. You can also take these in capsules. Drink oat straw tea for an overwhelmed nervous system. Make a blend of these herbs, and drink throughout the day. (hot or cold)
- <u>**Algae**</u>: Spirulina and Chlorella contain anti-stress components; methionine, calcium, and B-complex vitamins.
- <u>**Seaweed**</u>: contains high mineral content and B vitamins.
- <u>**Increase healthy fats**</u>: olive oil, avocado, olives, nuts, and coconut oils to sooth a stressed-out nervous system.
- <u>**Eat chlorophyll packed green vegetables**</u> to calm a stressed-out nervous system.

- ***Vitamin C rich foods:**  anti-stress effect/reduces cortisol levels: red chili peppers, guavas, kiwis, strawberries, red peppers, kale, parsley, collard greens, green peppers, broccoli, Brussels sprouts, mustard greens, watercress, cauliflower, persimmons, red cabbage, strawberries, papaya, spinach, oranges, lemon juice (and pith and rind) grapefruit, sprouts. Supplementation is recommended when chronically stressed. 3,000 mg of buffered Vitamin C with bioflavonoids.(In divided doses)
- ***Pantothenic Acid (Vitamin B5) rich foods**: "The anti-stress vitamin." Reduces adrenal insufficiency: Brewer's/nutritional yeast, liver, peanuts, mushrooms, soy, split peas, pecans, oatmeal, buckwheat, sunflower seeds, lentils, garbanzo beans, broccoli. Vitamin B5 Supplementation recommended: Dosage: 500 mg 1-3 x a day.
- **Whole Food B-complex** is recommended in addition to vitamin B5 for all stress conditions. Also add B-complex foods. High Sources are: rice bran, nutritional yeast, clams, eggs (raw or lightly cooked), spirulina, dried beans, various greens, and walnuts.
- ***Magnesium rich foods**: The "anti-stress mineral" has a calming effect on the nervous system and relaxes muscles. The substances alcohol, caffeine, and sugar all deplete magnesium. Rich in: sea vegetables, nuts, greens; and beans, kelp, dulse, almonds, cashews, N. yeast, buckwheat, brazil nuts, millet, pecans, rye, tempeh, dried coconut meat, brown rice, dried figs, apricots, bok choy, spinach, kale, collard greens, shrimp, avocado, cooked beans, brown rice, salmon. Therapeutic dosage recommended: 1,000 mg daily. Best forms of magnesium are Magnesium Citrate and Magnesium Glycinate.
- ***Zinc rich foods**: Levels are lost (excreted out through urine) during times of stress. Zinc is Important for immune function; to protect against immune compromising effects of stress. Food Sources: oysters, lamb, red meat, pumpkin seeds, ginger root, pecans, split peas, Brazil nuts. Dosage: Zinc aspartate 10-30 mg.

*Stress/Adrenal Support Target Supplements*

- ***Phosphatidylserine**: Decreases high cortisol levels. 300-800 mg per day.
- ***Melatonin**: Stress decreases melatonin levels significantly, causing insomnia. Take before bed. Spray/time-release supplements are most absorbable. Dosage: 1.5-3mg.
- ***Betaine HCL**: Stress decreases hydrochloric acid in the stomach. Take with each meal containing protein. Dosage: start with one 650 mg capsule, and work up until a slight burning sensation is felt in stomach; then reduce by one.
- **Desiccated Adrenal Cortical Extracts:** have been used to treat adrenal fatigue since the 1800's. Best sources are from pastured animals. 300mg 2 x a day
- **Fish oil and Omega-3 fats** has been shown to lower cortisol levels. Eat 3 cold water oily fish a week such as sardines, salmon, mackerel, and anchovies. Or take a fish oil

supplement made from whole bodies of fish from Alaska or New Zealand. Fermented Cod Liver Oil is also suggested. Dosage 1,000-4,000 mg a day

### Stress/Adrenal Support Target Adaptogenic Herbs

**Adaptogenic herbs** are an <u>essential aspect of adrenal support</u> as they help our body to adapt well to stressful conditions; in essence strengthening us against stress. Different adaptogens are used for the different stages of stress. Stage 1 and 2 would use the following herbs. Stage 3 and 4 would use the next section's list.

**Adaptogenic Herbs (for stage 1 and 2 adrenal dysfunction) Limit to 1 or 2.**

- *<u>Ashwagandha</u>, also called "Indian Ginseng" is used by Ayurvedic doctors in India. Studies show that it fortifies one's ability to cope with stressful situations by assisting it to process stress; thereby lessening the workload on the adrenals. In clinical trials ashwagandha has been shown to lower cortisol levels during times of stress by 26%. It also supports anxiety, mental acuity, and reaction time. Dosage 500 mg 3x a day. ( Life Extension Media, 2003) Especially useful for women.
- *<u>Rhodiola rosea</u>: A Russian adaptogen which controls excess cortisol release. It is effective in mitigating psychological and physical stress. Dosage 100-200 mg a day.
- <u>Asian Ginseng</u> (Panax Ginseng) and American Ginseng (P. quinquefolius) Improve adrenal function, and reduce the levels of cortisol. A study found that when menopausal women took 6 grams of Asian Ginseng root a day for 30 days, they experienced significant reduction in anxiety, insomnia, fatigue, and depression. Dosage: 500-600 mg/day. Take for 2-3 weeks, followed by a 1-2 week break, then repeat. (Life Extension Media, 2003) May increase facial hair if taken long term.
- <u>Green Tea</u> with the active ingredient, theanine. The amino acid theanine increases the production of Gaba, a calming brain chemical. Theanine also produces the brain chemical, Dopamine which improves mood. Green tea/theanine produces a tranquilizing effect without drowsiness or mental acuity impairment. Dosage: Green tea-3+ x day, (Make sure that you decaffeinate the tea naturally by steeping it for ten seconds in a small amount of hot water, drain that water, and then reinsert the tea bag in more hot water.) Theanine capsules-100mg 4x a day. Supports sleep also.
- <u>5HTP</u> for low serotonin and high cortisol levels at night- causing insomnia. Dosage 50-300 mg/45 min. before sleep.

### Cortisol Reducing Activities: For stage 1 and 2 adrenal dysfunction

- Exercise reduces cortisol levels, and metabolizes the excess blood sugar and insulin that stress produces.
- Love-making reduces cortisol levels and calms the nervous system.
- Meditation reduces cortisol levels.

- Yoga reduces cortisol levels, and increases GABA levels. (calming neurotransmitter)
- Forgiveness lowers cortisol levels.

## Nutrients/Activities that Lower Cortisol Levels

| Vitamin C | Magnesium | Vitamin B5 | Phosphatidyl Serine | Ashwagandha | Rhodiola |
|---|---|---|---|---|---|
| Panax Ginseng | Green tea/Theanine | 5HTP | Passion Flower | Holy Basil | Vitamin B5/ B-complex |
| Eliminate caffeine/sugar | Frequent protein-rich meals. Omega-3 fats. | Yoga, Love-making | Meditation, Forgiveness Stress-reduction. (see below) | Exercise | *Designs for Health-Adrenatone* or *Apex Ener.* pregeneolone |

### Stress Management Ideas:

- Let go of perfectionism and high self-expectations.
- Release catastrophizing and obsessing about bad experiences and comments. Emphasize the positives in your life.
- Practice gratitude and appreciation. Daily gratitude journals/prayers are effective.
- Meditate
- Practice deep breathing.
- Bathe in lavender and Epson salt baths. (1-2 cups) Rich in calming magnesium.
- Try the website "MeQuanimity" to start deconstructing your stress reactions.
- Try a meditation app. called "Heartmath, Inner Balance" You can use this app. on your i Phone, which guides you through a stress releasing and calming activity.
- The biofeedback computer game: *Journey to Wild Divine*: supports deep relaxation
- A small biofeedback device called *Resperate* helps with relaxation training
- *Stress Eraser* (heart rate variability monitor) activates the stress response.
- The Relaxation Company: Music and Relaxation C.D.'s

**Adaptogenic Herbs for Low Cortisol Conditions** (level 3 and 4 adrenal fatigue and exhaustion) Note: If you are suffering from serious adrenal failure, it is advised to seek professional help.

- **Licorice** helps sustain cortisol levels by slowing its break down in the body. Best Forms: Licorice tea - Drink tea 3 x a day for a short duration. Capsules are also available. Be mindful that long term use can lead to high blood pressure.
- **Eleuthero or Siberian Ginseng** has been used in China for 2000 years for invigorating the Qi (vital energy). It is an adaptogenic herb, which can restore fatigued adrenal function and prevent adrenal atrophy due to low cortisol. Ginseng boosts energy levels and DHEA and Testosterone. 20 drops of tincture 3x /day. Or 400-500mg capsules a day. (Life Extension Media, 2003)

## Insomnia and Sleep Disorders

Adequate sleep is vital for our physical health, as our body and brain use this time for rest, repair and detoxification. However, sleep disorders are a very common issue as we age, and chronic stress and high cortisol/adrenalin levels at night are often at the root of the problem. Other insomnia promoters are:

| Poor thyroid functioning | *Melatonin depletion-very common as we age | Poor sleep hygiene/disturbed rhythms |
|---|---|---|
| Low blood sugar | Liver problems | Low serotonin or GABA transmitters |
| No downtime before bed | Caffeine/alcohol/medications | Suboptimal B vitamin, zinc, magnesium, calcium levels |

### Insomnia Support

Follow the previous recommendations for stress and adrenal support and the following sleep promoters:

| Early to bed (by 10pm) and early to rise (stick to sleep schedule) | Regular exercise | Keep bedroom comfortable/no TV in bedroom |
|---|---|---|
| Wind down an hour before bed w/ low lighting/no screens | Bathe w/ Epson salts (1-2 cups) and lavender oil before bed | Meditation/yoga before bed |
| Have a high complex carb meal at supper (beans and quinoa/ potatoes etc.) Don't eat supper after 7pm | Herbal infusions: passion flower, oat straw, hops, scullcap, kava kava and valerian.(drink throughout day and before bed) | California poppy tincture (menopause support) |
| Supplements: Tryptophan: 1,000-1,500 mg or 5HTP 300 mg; or L-theanine: 100mg 4x a day; and/or melatonin 1-3 mg (all before bed) | B-Complex vitamins, Magnesium Calcium Zinc Vitamin D3 | Support low blood sugar with adequate protein throughout the day, and low glycemic foods. |
| Limit alcohol/caffeine Perform liver detoxification (see next chapter) | Practice Earthing (see Earthing chapter) | Manage Electrosensitivity issues (see chapter on Electrosensitivity |

**Exercise 18b: Stress Support.** Input target foods, adaptogenic herbs, supplements, and stress-reduction activities to support chronic stress conditions and adrenal dysfunctions. Input sleep suggestions if you suffer from insomnia.

Chapter 19

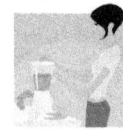 Reducing "Total Load,"

## Liver Cleansing and Detoxification for Vibrant Aging

Toxins have permeated our air, water, home, and food supply. Three billion kg of toxic chemicals are released every year into the environment. If we are in midlife, we are sure to have accumulated a great deal of unnecessary toxins, as research demonstrates that 70 different toxins can be measured in the average adult today. There is convincing evidence that even low-level toxin exposures contribute to the development of a variety of chronic health conditions including: fatigue, poor memory, headaches, hormonal disruptions, cancer, and chronic degenerative diseases.

For this reason cleansing and detoxification are a vital aspect of quality aging. Additionally, it is critical to reduce the overall number of toxic burdens that are stressing our body. "Total load" is the term used to refer to the total number of burdens that are contributing to an unhealthy body state, and involved in causing illness and disease. Many of these toxins are stored in our fat tissue. These stressors come from unhealthy foods, heavy metals, chemical toxins, microbe waste products, and lifestyle imbalances. Interestingly, our indoor environment in our homes has been found to be twice as polluted as our outdoor environment. (Out-gassing etc.). A high "total load" of pollutants is often at the core of mystery diseases. Most chronic diseases generally aren't caused by one single factor however, but multiple factors.

We may not be conscious of damaging toxins flooding our system, but our body will give us some warning signs of their disturbing presence; such as chronic fatigue, "foggy" thought processes, headaches, muscle aches, chemical sensitivity, allergic reactions, nausea, and just feeling "unwell" much of the time.

Single factors don't typically contribute to a disease state because the liver is designed to handle numerous toxins. However, problems arise from the "**_total cumulative effects_**" of many assaults to our system.

Lightening the total load that our body is under, and minimizing toxin exposure is one of the best things that we can do to support optimal aging. Our organs will begin to improve their capacity to endure stress, which will decrease our chances of developing chronic diseases.

## Factors That Increase Our "Total Load" & Substitutions to Lighten the Load

| | | | |
|---|---|---|---|
| Excess alcohol (more than 1 glass daily) Excess coffee: Drink only one coffee daily (Replace with green tea) | Excess sugar/high fructose corn syrup (replace with stevia, lo han guo, or fruit) | Toxic metals from industrial waste products in water supply, amalgams, hair dyes, aluminum pots (Use water filters, stainless steel pots, natural hair dyes) | Lack of essential nutrients (add or increase leafy/crunchy vegetables/ sea weed/algae nutritional yeast. Take a high quality multi-vitamin/mineral |
| Excess additives/chemicals in diet especially aspartame and MSG (Avoid processed, packaged, fast foods) Pesticides and herbicides (in food/home use) Make home-made organic food | Eating damaged fats and oils (hydrogenated oils, partially-hydrogenated vegetable oils) Replace with extra virgin olive oil) | Eating conventional GMO non organic foods (sprayed with pesticides, and herbicides) Replace with organic foods | Unaddressed food sensitivities/allergies (especially wheat and dairy) Try food elimination diet for 1 to 3 months and then reintroduce with each meal for 3 days; observe symptoms |
| Poor digestion: Support digestion w/ digestive enzymes/HCL/zinc Pathogen waste products circulating in the body (candida, bacteria, parasites) Eliminate sugar/high starch foods/use antifungals, probiotics etc. | Medications: especially antibiotics-use only when necessary  Take NAC to combat effects of meds | Chemicals in personal care products (i.e. parabens-see Environmental Working Group's database: "Skin Deep" and replace with natural products) | Plastic container usage: Synthetic Bisphenol A (BPA) and pthalates, (replace with glass/stainless steel containers) |
| Indoor pollution from household cleaning agents, air fresheners, new carpets, and furniture, building materials, new cars. (Replace with organic or natural, or 2nd-hand products) Take chemicals/paints out of garage/open windows for fresh air | Excess stress (Try relaxation techniques-deep breathing etc.) Inadequate sleep: Try 1 hour quite time before bed | Lack of exercise (Walk at least ½ hour- 3-5 times a week, use a pedometer-goal 10,000 steps daily) | Lack of sunshine (Sun bathe for 20 min. midday from 10-2 pm from March to October without sunscreen in California time zone.) |
| Insufficient purified water intake (Drink 1/2 of your body weight daily) Use a water filter for faucet, bath and shower | Microwave, aluminum, and Teflon coated pan usage (Replace with stainless steel pots, minimize microwave use.) | Excessive negative thought patterns/chronic pessimism (Practice gratitude meditations, journal writing, yoga) | Eating large size fish which contain mercury (swordfish, shark etc.) Or farmed fish. (Replace with wild salmon, sardines, herring etc.) |

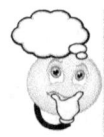

### Exercise 19a: Reducing Your Total Load

1. Make a list of your body's burdens and stressors, and determine which ones that you can eliminate or lessen in the next few months to bolster your energy and health.

2. Next, input health supportive diet and lifestyle substitutions (from the previous chart) in your plan to lighten your "total load." Be patient with this process, as it can take some time to fully incorporate all these changes.

---

### Liver Cleansing and Detoxification

The liver is our largest organ, and the primary organ of detoxification and elimination. Our liver's main role is to cleanse our blood and destroy toxic compounds. It acts like a large filter- sorting through, dismantling, and neutralizing everything that comes into our body. These toxins are then eliminated through the lungs, skin, intestines and urine. A very common issue as we age is that our liver can become overworked and overburdened by over-exposure to harmful compounds and destructive lifestyle habits. Especially burdensome are: environmental pollutants, heavy metals; chemicals in the household and personal care products; fried and processed foods; an excess of alcohol, stress and overeating. Once our liver is strained, it can't process toxins and fat proficiently. However, vibrant health and a long life rest on a well-functioning liver, and being able to eliminate toxins in an efficient and effective way.

Our liver is one of our most vital organs and has many other important functions besides detoxification. It activates our vitamins, antioxidants, fats, carbohydrates and proteins. It stores fat-soluble vitamins, iron, B12, blood and glycogen (glucose). In addition, it helps maintain healthy levels of blood sugar, synthesizes cholesterol, manufactures bile and 13,000 other chemicals, and maintains 2,000 enzyme systems.

Our liver is continuously working night and day; and is constantly removing drugs, heavy metals, air pollution, caffeine, alcohol, medications, chemicals, mucous, cholesterol, cellular debris, and hormones from our blood. For this reason it is important to incorporate daily detoxification measures to facilitate this process; as our liver can be overwhelmed when it is overloaded, and can become sluggish. A "sluggish liver" can't process toxins at a normal and required speed; which can cause a buildup of toxins in the blood, cells and organs. This build-up can lead to weight gain and ill health.

Having a sluggish weak liver in midlife will affect every other organ in our body; but by addressing the liver using detoxification measures that accelerate the elimination of toxins from the body, many conditions and health problems can be reversed. When our liver is working properly it is able to detoxify 99% of toxins from our blood before it is transported to other parts of the body.

*Signs of a sluggish/toxic liver include*

| Poor skin tone, and sallow coloring; liver spots on skin | Yellow coated tongue | Dark circles under eyes; yellow eyes | Reactions to food additives/chemicals and chemical induced smells |
|---|---|---|---|
| Acne, rosacea, rash on back | Itchy skin, itchy back, burning feet | Foggy thinking, headaches | Moodiness and irritability |
| Excessive sweating | Arthritis, flushed face or excessive facial blood vessels | Red palms and soles | Trouble digesting fats |
| Pain on right side of abdomen | Constipation or light tan stool | Pain under shoulder blades | Chronic Fatigue |
| Lack of appetite | Nausea | Feeling "sick" all the time | Edema and bloated belly |

*Liver Cleansing vs. Liver Detoxification*

It is important to gently detoxify the liver on an ongoing daily basis to reduce free radical damage. It is also very beneficial to do a more targeted, stronger cleanse a few times a year- ideally in warm weather (spring, summer, and early fall) to rest the digestive tract and aid in moving out additional toxins. The warmer months are the times when the body naturally wants to cleanse. A cleanse can also be performed after a period of poor eating; such as after the holidays or after a vacation.

Foods with bitter flavors are particularly important for detoxification, as the liver gets a positive jolt from them. Bitter tasting foods stimulate the liver to put out more fat emulsifying bile, which is needed to expel accumulated toxic waste. Traditional cultures regularly consumed bitters for this purpose. If we never eat anything bitter, our liver can become sluggish over time and retain the toxic buildup. Some bitter foods to try are: farm-grown dandelion leaf, arugula, parsley, escarole, mustard greens, endive, radicchio, rapini, bitter melon and bitter unsweetened chocolate. Artichoke also increases bile production.

Try to eat small amounts daily in salads, smoothies or as a cooked veggie. Larger amounts can be eaten while doing a seasonal cleanse.

Sour foods also have been shown to release excessive buildup of toxins in the liver. Additionally, they aid digestion, and stimulate normal bowel elimination. Sour foods include sour citrus, raw apple cider vinegar, real homemade fermented deli pickles and fermented veggies. Moreover, both sour and bitter flavors help to curb cravings for sweets. A morning ritual of drinking the juice of a half or a whole lemon can be a great liver supportive start to the day.

The following section provides general detoxification strategies that can be practiced daily. The second section provides a more intensive seasonal detoxification plan that ideally should be carried out in the spring, summer and/or early fall.

### *General Daily Liver Detoxification Support*

- Upon rising each morning: drink alkalinizing juice of ½ to 1 lemon in filtered water
- Eat adequate protein with specific amino acids for detoxification, growth and repair. (eggs, grass-fed undenatured whey protein, bone broth, organic free range foul, beef, lamb and fatty fish) Calculate your protein needs by multiplying your ideal weight by .36.
    - Example 130 lbs. x .36 = 46.8 grams of protein per day. Many people don't eat enough protein to efficiently detoxify their body
- Drink ½ of your body weight in ounces of filtered water.
- Eat at least 35 grams of fiber per day. Fiber pectin absorbs toxins in the intestines and aids in toxin elimination through the bowels: beans, whole grains, vegetables, fruit (apples), nuts, seeds, flax meal, ( 2-4 Tbsp. daily)
- Eat organic sulfur rich detoxifying cruciferous vegetables at least three times a week: arugula, bok choy, broccoli, Brussels sprouts, cabbage, cauliflower, collards, kale, kohlrabi, mustard greens, napa cabbage, radish, rutabaga, turnips
- Eat sulfur containing alliums-garlic, onions, shallots, scallions, and leeks
- Eat farm-grown dandelion greens
- Eat dark green leafy vegetables for chlorophyll
- Eat celery- For urine flow
- Eat beets-softens bile/ increases bile flow
- Eat organic detoxifying fruits: grapes, berries, citrus fruits (zest/pith and skin)
- Eat detoxifying herbs: cilantro-(heavy metal detox); parsley (blood cleanser),
- Eat detoxifying spices/herbs :cinnamon, rosemary, turmeric, dill, ginger

- Eat selenium rich foods: brazil nuts (no more than 2 a day), crimini mushrooms, seafood
- Drink liver supportive tonics: dandelion root, burdock root, ginger root, red clover
- Drink organic green tea: 2-4 cups daily. Use the tea bag several times; as the first steeping is the only one with caffeine.
- Eat gelatinous foods: (They bind to toxins) aloe vera/juice, flax, chia seed and sea weed
- Take heavy metal chelating agents: chlorella, cilantro, garlic, kelp, bladder wrack, sodium alginate, N-Acetyl-Cysteine (NAC), modified citrus pectin (Toxic metals most commonly associated with unfavorable health consequences include: aluminum, arsenic, cadmium, lead, mercury, and nickel.)
- Eat glutathione producing foods: asparagus, avocados, broccoli, cabbage, raw milk, undenatured whey protein powder, walnuts, and duck. (Avoid acetaminophen; it decreases glutathione)
- Eat cultured or fermented foods with "live and active cultures," or take probiotics to reduce waste products from bad gut bacteria.
- Lifestyle measures: exercise three times a week to sweat out toxins; practice yoga; dry brushing; sauna; lymph massage; rebounding; (activates lymph flow) stress reduction; thorough chewing; have one to two bowel movements daily. (Take magnesium citrate if constipated: 300-1,200 mg daily in divided doses)
- Use detoxification baths: Add 2 cups of unrefined sea salt and 2 cups of baking soda to the bath water. This also stimulates the lymph system. 1-2 cups of Epson salts can be added for magnesium and sulfur.
- To clear lymph: make a drink with one whole lemon, I Tbsp. lecithin, 1 Tbsp. olive oil, 4 oz. unsweetened cranberry juice diluted with 28 oz. filtered water (blend together) Drink 8 oz. of this once daily (note: lymph flow slows down as we age) Rebounding exercises are also excellent at moving lymph.
- Don't eat past 7 o'clock (It overworks the liver. The liver does much of its work while we sleep)
- Go to Sleep by 10 pm to facilitate liver detoxification processes.

See chart on next page.

## General Daily Detox Support

| Vitamin C- rich foods: citrus, berries, sprouts, peppers, salads<br><br>Ester- C supp. | Vitamin A/beta carotene: sea weed, dark leafy greens, orange veggies, eggs, liver | Folic acid (Folate): beets, dark leafy greens, nutritional yeast | N-acetyl cysteine (NAC) (600mg.) pharmaceutical detox support | Milk thistle |
|---|---|---|---|---|
| Sour foods lemon juice in water upon rising, apple cider vinegar, fermented veggies | Adequate protein to obtain amino acid antioxidants | Drink ½ your body weight in ounces of filtered water | 35 grams+ of fiber per day: flax meal etc. | Alliums: garlic (one raw clove daily) onions, scallions, leeks, shallots |
| Bitter foods: Dandelion greens, arugula, parsley, escarole | Eat well cooked cruciferous veggies (1 cup daily) | Dark leafy green veggies for chlorophyll | Celery | Beets |
| Detox fruits: grapes, berries, cranberries, pomegranate, citrus fruits (peel and pith) | Detox Herbs: cilantro, dill, arugula, dandelion leaf, rosemary and parsley | Detox Spices: cinnamon, turmeric, ginger | Selenium rich foods: Brazil nuts, crimini mushrooms, sea food | Liver Detox Teas or capsules:: dandelion root, burdock root, red clover, ginger Kidney support: parsley, uva ursi |
| Eat cultured or fermented foods: veggies, yogurt, kefir | Vigorous Exercise at least 3 x/wk. to sweat out toxins; also yoga, rebounding | Stress reduction<br><br>Don't eat past 7pm<br><br>Go to bed by 10pm | Glutathione producing foods: asparagus, walnuts, duck, undenatured whey protein, avocados, broccoli | Organic green tea: 1-4+ daily. It also supports kidney detox |
| Thorough chewing of food. 1-3 bowel movements daily (Take magnesium citrate if constipated (300-1,000 mg. daily) | Dry brushing, sauna, lymph massage <u>Herbs</u> to stimulate lymph flow: red clover, red root, stillingia, chaparral <u>Drink</u> lemon lymph beverage. | Detox baths with sea salt, baking soda, and Epson salts: 1-2 cups each | <u>Toxic metal chelating agents:</u> cilantro, spirulina, chlorella, garlic, kelp, bladderwrack, sodium alginate, modified citrus pectin, NAC | Gelatinous foods: flax meal, chia seeds, sea weed, aloe vera |

**Exercise 19b: Daily Detoxification support.** Input several foods and lifestyle routines that will offer daily detox boosting assistance.

**Detoxification in our body** is done through the activity of hundreds of detoxification enzymes in a two-step process called Phase I and Phase II Liver Detoxification. As we age, dysfunctions (either over-activity or under-activity) can occur in these systems.

In Phase I, through the cytochrome P450 enzymes, toxic elements (any substance that is foreign to the human body, and waste products that are produced inside our body) get biochemically transformed into secondary substances. Alcohol, medications, pesticides, sugar and refined carbohydrates are some of the substances that can interrupt or accelerate this process. If an individual has a dysfunction in Phase I processes, they may be intolerant to caffeine, perfumes, air fresheners, dyes, detergents and other environmental chemicals.

Conversely, when an individual has excessively over-active Phase I detoxification enzymes they are relatively unaffected by caffeine, and are able to sleep at night after drinking it. However, Individuals with an overactive Phase I detoxification system usually have had excessive exposure to a large amount of toxins or toxin exposure for a long period of time.

Phase I's detoxification process creates residual free-radicals that are even more noxious then the initial toxin. This is the reason that the compounds go through a second process (Phase II) in which the toxins are neutralized and eliminated. It is critical that the Phase II detoxification system works optimally in order to keep the process balanced. If Phase II isn't working properly or fast enough to keep up with Phase I, toxins will build up; resulting in oxidative damage. This can cause the whole system to shut down. (Termed pathological detoxifier) When Phase II, referred to as the conjugation pathway (meaning joining together in pairs) works properly, there is a more rigorous process of breaking down the toxic substances further; and then they can be excreted out through bile or urine.

**There are six Phase II pathways that need targeted nutrients to support their functioning.**

| Methylation | Sulfation | Glucuronidation | Glutathione | Acetylation | Glycine/amino acid pathway |
| --- | --- | --- | --- | --- | --- |

The glutathione pathway, as referred to earlier, is the key player in Phase II detoxification, as glutathione is the body's "master antioxidant." The liver is responsible for producing most of the glutathione needed by the body. It is pivotal in the breakdown of carcinogens and industrial waste. It also circulates in the bloodstream targeting cell destroying free radicals. Chronic illness, excessive exercise, high consumption of alcohol, and high toxin exposure can all deplete glutathione levels and cause a build-up of toxins in the body, resulting in a sluggish liver.

➡ Toxins accumulate in fatty tissues such as the brain, endocrine glands (adrenal glands etc.) and in fat layers causing:

| Brain dysfunction, brain fog | Hormonal imbalance | Exhausted adrenal glands |
| --- | --- | --- |
| Early menopause | Premature aging. | Obesity |

## Targeted Nutrients for Phase I and Phase II Detox

This next section is useful for people who may have compromised detoxification pathway concerns and want to carry out a more targeted "detoxification pathway" protocol: Note: cruciferous veggies, vitamin C rich foods, and limonene rich foods induce both Phase I and Phase II detox. * The top left square, on the following chart lists medications and other items that inhibit Phase I detoxification processes.

➡ Environmental chemical sensitivities (to caffeine, perfumes, dyes, detergents, air fresheners etc.) are all correlated with a dysfunctional Phase I detoxification system.

### Nutrients for Phase I Detox

| *Drugs that inhibit phases I: valium, Prozac, antihistamine, acid blockers<br><br>Alcohol, street drugs, charcoaled broiled meats and smoking etc.(induce excessive Phase I) | Cruciferous veggies (broccoli, cabbage, kale, cauliflower, mustard greens, collard greens, Brussel's sprouts, bok choy, radishes etc. | Vitamin C rich foods: tangerines, oranges, lemons, strawberries, peppers, sprouts, broccoli, kiwi, kale, leafy greens, tomatoes | Supplements/Herbs<br><br>Milk thistle herb:70-210 mg/day<br><br>CoQ10 (ubiquinone)<br><br>Vitamin C: 3,000+ mg. in divided doses |
|---|---|---|---|
| Limonene rich foods: citrus peel, caraway and dill seeds<br><br>(if sluggish phase I or 2) | *B-Vitamins: Dark leafy greens, yogurt, Brewer's yeast, nutritional yeast, organ meats, nori, tempeh, dried beans, eggs, sunflower seeds, avocado asparagus, mackerel, herring, shellfish, eel, dried beans, and peas | Vitamin E rich foods: spinach, nuts, seeds, olive oil, avocado | Flavonoid rich foods: buckwheat, green tea, berries, onions, apples, spirulina, chlorella |
| Glutathione rich foods: walnuts, asparagus, avocado, raw dairy, undenatured whey, garlic, onions, poultry<br><br>NAC, zinc, selenium supplements | Selenium rich foods: 2-3 brazil nuts, crimini mushrooms, shellfish | SOD rich foods: nuts, seeds, green beans, spirulina, oysters | Magnesium rich foods: greens, beans, nuts and seeds, sea weed. |

## Targeted Nutrients for Phase II Detox Systems/Phase II Pathway Dysfunctions

Spice extracts that stimulate Phase II: Curcumin extract, capsaicin extract, and cloves.

| Pathway/Inhibitors | Dysfunction | Supportive Nutrients |
|---|---|---|
| **Methylation**: inability to detox homocysteine effectively. Activators: B6, choline, betain, B12, and folic acid consumption | Depression, heart disease, estrogen dominance, allergies, dementia, cancer, toxic metal accumulation | Lecithin, tempeh, miso, egg yolks, dark leafy greens, garlic, onions, fish, organ meats, beets, meat, yogurt, beans, walnuts, nutritional or brewer's yeast, SAMe, lecithin supplements |
| **Sulphation**: NSAIDS and food dyes inhibit pathway. Activators: sulfur/cysteine foods | Medication and chemical toxicity | Egg yolks, cruciferous veggies (kale, broccoli, cauliflower, cabbage, collards) alliums (garlic, onions) dairy |
| **Glucuronidation**: Fluoride and aspirin inhibit pathway. Activators: fish oil, limonene | Medication and food additive toxicity; estrogen dominance | Fish, Fermented Cod liver oil, krill oil, citrus peels, dill, caraway seeds, Calcium D-glucarate and SAMe supplement |
| **Glutathione**: Deficiencies of zinc, selenium, B2 and B6 inhibit pathway. Avoid acetaminophen-decreases glutathione *If exposed to a high level of toxins or medications use vitamin C (3,000+ mg divided doses) and NAC (600 mg.) | Cancer and degenerative diseases | Proteins, eggs, beans, cruciferous veggies, citrus peel, undenatured whey, citrus, kiwi, peppers, strawberries, asparagus, avocado, walnuts, green tea Supplements: Vitamin C, NAC, milk thistle, zinc and selenium. Exercise is important! |
| **Glycine/Amino** Acid pathway: low-protein diet inhibits pathway, poor HCL levels inhibit pathway | Hypothyroid, arthritis, carcinomas, hepatitis, alcoholic liver issues, nausea during pregnancy | High protein, beets, home-made bone broths, HCL tablets with meals. |
| **Acetylation** Pathway: chronic stress inhibits pathway. Activators: Vit. C, B2, B6 | Migraine headaches from cheese and red wine, toxic reactions to sulfa drugs, caffeine intolerance | Sprouts, peppers, strawberries, broccoli, kiwis, organ meats, nutritional yeast, eggs, dried peas and beans, sunflower seeds, stress reduction |

Exercise 19c: Targeted Nutrients for Phase I and Phase II Detox Systems: Input any useful info or nutrients to boost these systems on your plan.

## Seasonal Cleansing Plans

Consider performing seasonal cleanses several times a year to accelerate toxin elimination, and to encourage optimal liver and elimination organ functioning. Cleansing also optimizes our defenses against diseases, and enhances whole body wellness and vitality. The best time for a cleanse is in the spring, summer or early fall when the body can get an extra boost from the sun and increased vitamin D synthesis. Resting is also important during a cleanse, and work should ideally be suspended at this time. Generally, most people who perform a cleanse experience temporary accelerated healing symptoms, such as headaches, fatigue, body odor, bad breath, diarrhea, or mouth sores.

Typically, after a few days of discomfort, most people will start to feel more energized, have clearer eyes, an upbeat attitude, and a sense of mental clarity; however, this is dependent on the level of toxin overload. It is important to use your own judgment when deciding to discontinue a cleanse. It is also important to do all cleanses under the care of a physician.

Caution: seasonal cleanses should not be carried out by individuals who are weak or fatigued; as they may not have sufficient energy to successfully neutralize and remove toxins, and may be subjected to serious side effects. Additionally, individuals who have been consuming the typical American SAD diet with overuse of sugar and refined products should not attempt a cleanse until they have successfully incorporated and maintained daily healthy eating routines for several months, as outlined in this book. Otherwise, the body may react too strongly to the abrupt transition.

### Levels One and Two:  1-14 day "Simplified Diet" Colon and Liver cleanse.

This is an excellent all around full body gentle detox. Try to rest during this cleanse to facilitate detoxification. **Designs for Health Paleo Cleanse kit** can also be used to support optimal detoxification while undergoing this cleanse.

### Foods to Remove from Diet

| Packaged/canned foods/processed foods/and oils. Extra virgin olive oil/coconut oil are permissible. Eat home-made meals and salads only | Non-organic foods | All sugars, sweeteners, artificial Sweeteners, and table salt. Organic green stevia, and unbleached sea salt or Himalyan salt are okay | Alcohol, coffee, tea, fruit juices, sugary drinks, un-filtered water. Organic green tea/herbal tea is fine | All meats, poultry, sea food, fish, eggs, dairy, and soy. (Soaked/ sprouted beans, nuts, and seeds, are okay) | Gluten containing foods, (wheat, rye barley, oatmeal) and all breads and pastas. (Soaked/sprouted quinoa, millet, amaranth, basmati brown rice and buckwheat are permissible) |
|---|---|---|---|---|---|

## Alkalinizing and Cleansing Foods to Include for a Level 1 and Level 2 Cleanse

| | | | |
|---|---|---|---|
| **Sour fruits**: berries, green apples, grapefruit, cranberries, Raw apple cider vinegar **Bitter veggies**: parsley, arugula, dandelion greens etc. | **Vegetables**: 80% raw, 20% cooked (cook the cruciferous veggies) You can puree your veggies into soups and smoothies to ease digestion. | **Ocean vegetables/ seaweed** (mineral rich): dulse, wakame, sea palm, hijiki, nori, arame, kombu, Irish moss etc | **Cultured vegetables and probiotics** (See recipe on page 275) or buy from health food stores |
| **Vegetable mineral broths**-drink as desired for strength and cleansing. (see recipe) | **Filtered water**: Drink a gallon per day to flush out toxins | **Fresh Lemon juice** in water-helps flush out toxins; drink upon rising and as desired | **Liver supportive herbs**- milk thistle, and *LivAmend*- helps increase flow of bile from the liver |
| **Colon Cleansers** Triphala: Ayurvedic herb: blood purifier, colon cleanser, liver cleanser. Dosage 1 or 2- 800 mg. caps 2 times a day with warm water at bedtime and upon rising. Or: *Sonne's #7 bentonite clay* or 3 charcoal capsules (once daily) | **Detox herbal teas**: dandelion root, milk thistle, burdock root, yellow dock, red clover, ginger, uva ursi (kidney, bladder support) Drink throughout the day **Detox spices/herbs**: cinnamon, ginger, turmeric, cilantro, parsley, rosemary, arugula, and dill | **Vegetable juices**- Juice celery, zucchini, parsley, carrot, beet, spinach and garlic or ginger together (rich in potassium) **For glycemic control**: no more than 2 carrots, and one beet. Drink several times a day. | **Eat soaked raw nuts, and seeds** for energy (soak 7-24 hours and then dry on lowest setting in oven or use dehydrator) **Eat sprouted seeds** and beans: alfalfa, clover, radish, sunflower, mung beans, lentils. Use sprouting jar, or buy from health store |

### Colon Detox

It is a good strategy to detoxify and unclog the colon before or during a liver cleanse; as the colon can have a large accumulation of hardened old fecal matter, chemical residues, E Coli bacteria, and parasite larvae. This can impede optimal detoxification. When we clean out the colon, we have an unobstructed course of elimination for all the stored toxins that we may have in our liver, blood and cells. The following compounds have been shown to absorb old fecal matter, chemical toxins, harmful viruses, parasite larvae, bacteria and aflatoxins (mold) which allows them to leave the body through the stool. It is suggested to take one bowel cleanser 1x each day of your cleanse.

**Bentonite Clay** (volcanic ash) *Sonne's #7* (wet form-directions on bottle) or dry clay: Put 1 tsp. in half cup warm water and let sit for 10 minutes; stir and drink. (Knoff, 2010)

**Activated Powdered Charcoal**: 1 tsp mixed in a cup of water or 2-3 capsules (Knoff, 2010)

The following chart is a **One Day Sample Meal Plan for Levels One and Two**. Olive oil and coconut oil should be the only oils ingested. Raw unpasteurized and unfiltered apple cider vinegar (with the mother) should be the only vinegar used on this plan; as it supports digestion, pH balance, and is high in enzymes and potassium. Drink one gallon of filtered water throughout the day, and drink detox teas as often as possible. Drink vegetable mineral broth as often as you like. (See recipe on pg. 217) Eat fermented veggies daily. If you have digestive discomfort with raw veggies or fruits; consider steaming them.

| On rising<br>16 oz. of filtered water with juice of 1-2 squeezed lemons | The Designs for Health <u>Paleo Cleanse kit</u> or Standard Process's <u>Purification Product kit</u> can also be utilized for detox. |
|---|---|
| Breakfast #1<br>1 cup mixed berry fruit salad with:<br><u>1/2-3/4 cup soaked and dried seeds and nuts:</u><br>Almonds, walnuts, flax, pumpkin, and/or sesame with a bowl of a soaked and cooked non-gluten grain. (You may add 100% stevia, coconut milk, cinnamon, ginger, or other spices to this)<br><br><u>Juice:</u> Juice celery, zucchini, parsley, carrot, beet, spinach and garlic or ginger together (rich in potassium)<br><u>For glycemic control</u>: no more than **2** carrots, and one beet. Drink several times a day<br><u>Liver support tea:</u> dandelion root etc. | Or Breakfast #2:<br>Fresh berry smoothie blended with 1 cup mixed berries, 2 celery stalks, 4 oz. green tea, ¼ banana, 2 Tbsp. flax meal, 1 Tbsp. nutritional yeast, cinnamon, ginger powder, and 1-2 tsp. chlorella or spirulina.<br><br>½ cup soaked seeds or nuts.<br><br>Dandelion root tea |

| Snack |
|---|
| **Raw** nori seaweed sheet topped with avocado slices, cucumber slices, grated fresh ginger and sesame seeds. Or choose avocado/tomato guacamole with celery sticks, and some sunflower seeds.<br><u>Drink</u>: 1-2 tsp. chlorella or spirulina in filtered water |
| Lunch<br><u>Salad</u> with ½ cup ea. cilantro and dandelion, and 1-2 cups spinach with 1/4 cup each: carrots, beets, celery, and alfalfa sprouts - top with fresh lemon juice, garlic and oil. Sprinkle with sea salt and fresh herbs.<br>**1-2** cups steamed broccoli with fresh herbs and olive oil drizzle.<br><u>Serve with ½ cup of seeds and nuts on a bed of:</u> quinoa, buckwheat or brown basmati rice. Add oil, garlic and spices/herbs for flavor.<br><u>Have a vegetable mineral broth with a sea vegetable</u> and ½ cup fermented veggies on the side |
| Snack<br>1 med. grapefruit, or med. green apple, or 1 cup berries, or pomegranate<br><u>¼ cup walnuts</u><br><u>Potassium–rich veggie juice</u> with: 2 carrots, 4 celery stalks, 2 zucchini, ½ beet, a bunch each: spinach, cilantro and dandelion; 1 raw garlic clove<br>Red clover tea |
| Dinner-Don't eat past 7pm<br><u>Salad</u>: 2 cup spinach/lettuce with 1/2 cup each: chopped beets, tomatoes, carrot, fennel, celery; a few sprigs of parsley/arugula, ½ cup lentil sprouts and 1/4 cup sunflower seeds. Top with fresh lemon juice and oil.<br><u>Spiced beans with quinoa or basmati brown rice</u><br><u>Steamed kale, broccoli, and red cabbage</u> w/ shredded ginger, garlic, sea salt, and drizzle of olive oil<br>Have 1-2 cups vegetable mineral broth with a sea vegetable, and ½ cup fermented veggies<br>Ginger root or dandelion root tea |
| Before Bed-Go to bed before 10pm<br>1-2 squeezed lemons in 8 oz. water. (Drink some vegetable broth if you are hungry.) |

### Level Three: 1-3+ Day Juice/Veggie Broth Fast:

This plan is for individuals who have stable blood sugar levels; are not weak; have performed cleanses before; and want to take their detoxification to the next level.

Juice/broth fasting is beneficial for optimizing liver and cellular detoxification as it gives the digestive system a respite; and as a result, the body's energy is diverted toward clearing toxins and waste at the cellular level. A moderate 1-3 day juice fast speeds up the release of excess mucous, old fecal matter, and debris from the body. Juice fasting essentially utilizes self-digestion to dismantle and burn-up compounds and tissues that are damaged and diseased.

Fasting hastens removal of toxins from the liver, kidneys, intestines, lungs, and skin; often causing remarkable changes as heaps of amassed waste products are driven-out of the body. There may be a short period of headaches, fatigue, body odor, bad breath, diarrhea, or mouth sores that accompany accelerated healing.

Juice fasting utilizes the benefit of a nutrient-dense food with a concentrated amount of phytonutrients. Fruits have a cleansing effect on the body, while vegetables have a cleansing and building effect on the body. (Rector-Page, 1990) Mineral rich broths are utilized to give warmth, energy and strength to the faster; and herbal teas support increased detoxification and elimination. Drinking a gallon of filtered water in addition to the juices and broths will hasten toxin removal.

Adding chlorella powder or spirulina to juices or filtered water is also recommended; as they contain added detox supportive nutrients such as: fiber, (binds to toxins) chlorophyll, (blood cleanser) and protein. (Eases hunger.) They also inhibit a blood sugar rise when using fruit.

A good detoxification plan should be done in three phases: cleansing, rebuilding and maintaining. After finishing the fasting detox plan, it is recommended to begin the "reentry week" by slowly re-introducing certain foods to give the body time to readjust. Begin with adding back fruits, vegetables, nuts, seeds and vegetarian meals the first few days. Then begin to build-up the body with high quality clean animal proteins and healthy fats. (If you are not a vegetarian) When adding back eggs, soy foods, dairy and grains; be mindful of any symptoms that may appear. Symptoms may indicate that you have a food sensitivity; and avoiding these foods for 3 months may be the best approach.

All recipes are on page 216 and 217. Bentonite clay or activated powdered charcoal can also be utilized for bowel cleansing prior to the juice fast. See page 212

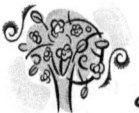

# Spring Juice Fasting Plan (Level 3)

| DAY ONE<br>Pre-Fast | DAY TWO<br>Bowel Cleansing | DAY THREE<br>Mucous Cleansing | DAY FOUR<br>Liver Cleansing | DAY FIVE<br>Post-Fast |
|---|---|---|---|---|
| **On rising**<br>16 oz. of filtered water with juice of 1-2 squeezed lemons | **On Rising**<br>16 oz. of filtered water with juice of 1-2 squeezed lemons<br>1 glass of water with Sonne # 7 Liquid Bentonite clay | **On rising**<br>16 oz. of filtered water with juice of 1-2 squeezed lemons | **On rising**<br>16 oz. of filtered water with juice of 1-2 squeezed lemons | **On Rising**<br>16 oz. of filtered water with juice of 1-2 squeezed lemons |
| **Breakfast**<br>2 cups green apple, strawberry, tangerine fruit salad<br><br>1/2-3/4 cup soaked and dried seeds and nuts: almonds, walnuts, flax, pumpkin, sesame<br>Fresh juice: 3 sour green apples, 1 lemon with rind, 2 cups celery, ½ in. piece ginger<br>Liver detox tea- (see next page) | **Breakfast**<br>8 oz. Fig, prune, raisin nectar (soak 1 cup each- dried figs, prunes and raisins in 8 oz. of water and cover overnight) Drink the strained liquid<br><br>Cup of veggie broth<br><br>Liver detox tea | **Breakfast**<br>8 oz. fresh grapefruit juice, blended with 2 cups spinach and dilute with water.<br><br>1 tsp. garlic/ onion/ honey syrup (mash 3 garlic cloves and slice lg. onion w/ 3 Tbsp. dark honey) cover for 24 hours. Take only honey infusion<br><br>Cup of veggie broth<br><br>Liver detox tea | **Breakfast**<br>12 oz. fresh juice: 4 tart green apples with skin, 4 oz. alfalfa sprouts, 4 sprigs mint-dilute with water<br><br>Cup of veggie broth<br><br>Liver detox tea | **Breakfast**<br>Fruit Smoothie: with 8 oz. almond milk<br>1 cup blueberries<br>1/4 ripe banana<br>2 Tbsp. flax seed meal, 1 Tbsp. nutritional yeast, and 1-2 tsp. chlorella powder<br><br>½ cups soaked seeds and nuts<br><br>Cup of veggie broth<br><br>Liver detox tea |
| **Snack**<br>Raw nori seaweed sheets topped with avocado and cucumber slices- sprinkled w/ sesame seed and sea salt<br>Water with 1-2 tsps. chlorella | **Snack**<br>8 oz. organic aloe vera juice<br><br>8 oz. potassium juice | **Snack**<br>12 oz. fresh juice: apple/carrot/alfalfa sprout juice w/ ¼ tsp. fresh ginger, and 1 tsp. spirulina | **Snack**<br>12 oz. Potassium Juice | **Snack**<br>12 oz. Potassium Juice<br><br>½ cup fermented veggies<br><br>Handful of nuts/seeds |
| **Lunch**<br>Salad:1/2 cup each Cilantro/ dandelion and 1 cup spinach with 1/4 cup each: Carrots, beets, celery, sunflower sprouts topped with 1 Tbs. olive oil and lemon juice<br>1-2 cup steamed broccoli with ½ cup steamed mung bean sprouts, ¼ cup seeds<br>Liver detox tea | **Lunch**<br>12 oz. Potassium juice<br><br>8 oz. water w/ 1 tsp chlorella granules<br><br>ginger tea | **Lunch**<br>12 oz. Potassium juice<br><br>1 tsp. garlic/onion honey infusion<br><br>Liver detox tea | **Lunch**<br>12 oz. Potassium juice<br><br>Cup of veggie broth<br><br>Liver detox tea | **Lunch**<br>Salad with ½ bunch each: dandelion greens, cilantro and spinach and ¼ cup each carrots, celery, beets, alfalfa sprouts and sunflower seeds with lemon/ oil dressing.<br><br>1-2 cups steamed broccoli, dulse seaweed and onions<br><br>Liver detox tea |

| DAY ONE | DAY TWO | DAY THREE | DAY FOUR | DAY FIVE |
|---|---|---|---|---|
| **Snack**<br>1 med. Tangerine w/ skin or 1 cup berries<br><br>½-¾ cup soaked walnuts<br><br>12 oz. fresh juice: Carrot/green apple/spinach diluted with water<br><br>Red clover tea | **Snack**<br>8 oz. fresh juice: 3 cucumbers, 2 Tbsp. apple cider vinegar and 1 in. piece of fresh ginger<br><br>Cup of veggie broth<br><br>Red clover tea | **Snack**<br>12 oz. fresh juice: 3-green apples, ½ cored small pineapple, 4 oz. alfalfa sprouts, 1 tsp. chlorella, 4 sprigs mint. Dilute with water<br><br>Cup of veggie broth<br><br>Red clover tea | **Snack**<br>8 oz. fresh juice: 1 beet, 2 carrots, 4 celery stalks; one bunch each: kale and parsley w/1 in. piece of ginger<br><br>Cup of veggie broth<br><br>Red clover tea | **Snack**<br>Medium green apple<br><br>2 tbsp. almonds with nori seaweed sheets<br><br>Cup of veggie broth<br><br>Red clover tea |
| **Dinner**<br>Salad: 2 cups spinach with 1/4 cup each: beet, carrot, fennel, celery and clover sprouts-topped with one Tbsp. each: olive oil, lemon juice and sunflower seeds.<br><br>Cooked veggies: 2-3 cups steamed bok choy, cauliflower, and red cabbage w/ minced ginger (salt to taste)<br><br>½-cup brown rice or quinoa | **Dinner**<br>16 oz. veggie broth<br><br>8 oz. potassium juice<br><br>8 oz. aloe vera juice<br><br>Ginger tea | **Dinner**<br>16 oz. veggie broth<br><br>12 oz. glass green apple/pineapple/ alfalfa sprout juice (see above)<br><br>1 tsp. garlic/onion/honey infusion<br><br>Ginger tea | **Dinner**<br>16 oz. warm veggie mineral broth<br><br>8 oz. of potassium Juice<br><br>Ginger tea | **Dinner**<br>2-3 cups steamed mixed veggies: broccoli, cauliflower, collard greens, kale, and carrots etc.<br><br>1/2-3/4 cup quinoa, with sesame seeds and dulse seaweed flakes.(sea salt to taste)<br><br>Cup veggie broth<br><br>Ginger tea |
| **Before Bed**<br>2 squeezed lemons in 8 oz. water<br><br>Liver detox tea | **Before Bed**<br>8 oz. Sonne' Liquid bentonite<br><br>Liver detox tea | **Before Bed**<br>2 squeezed lemons in 8 oz. water<br><br>Liver detox tea | **Before Bed**<br>2 squeezed lemons in 8 oz. water<br><br>Liver detox tea | **Before Bed**<br>2 squeezed lemons in 8 oz. water<br><br>Liver detox tea |

\*This plan can be modified to focus on liver cleansing, and omit the bowel/mucous cleanse.

\***Liver detox teas**: You can choose a liver detox blend tea with the following herbs, or use these herbs singly in teas: dandelion root, burdock root, milk thistle, and yellow dock.

\***Organic Potassium Juice Recipe** (Juice in a juicer) 2 carrots, 5 stalks celery, 1 beet, 2 zucchini, ½ bunch each: dandelion and spinach; a handful of cilantro, parsley or arugula, and one garlic clove.

\***Drink Plenty of Filtered Water** to dilute toxins: consume 7 cups before noon; 7 cups before dinner; 1-2 cups in the evening.

\***Vegetable Broth recipe on next page.** Drink more broth if you feel hungry.

\*Add more chlorella or spirulina powder to water or juice if you become fatigued.

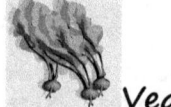 ## Vegetable Mineral Broth

This mineral broth is excellent for cleansing, neutralizing acids, and strengthening and rebuilding the body. It is an excellent source of energy, electrolytes, and minerals. Drink it often and as an afternoon pick-me-up; and to optimize your mineral status.

Fill a large stainless steel pot with purified water. Add (chopped up) any selection of seasonal organic vegetables, such as:

Vegetables: celery*, carrots*, nettles, beet root,* spinach, kale, swiss chard, daikon radish, burdock root, cauliflower, broccoli, turnip*, dandelion (leaf and root), sweet potato, onions, garlic, leeks etc.

Add some spices or herbs such as: rosemary, thyme, parsley, oregano, sage, cilantro, bay leaves, peppercorns, ginger, arugula, and cilantro.

1 tsp. sea salt and a few pieces of kombu seaweed.

Simmer with lid on for 1-3 hours or longer, strain out the veggies, and drink the warm liquid throughout the entire fast.

(*include leafy tops)

---

**Exercise 19d: Plan and Schedule a Seasonal Cleanse:** Print out Seasonal cleanse information, and vegetable mineral broth recipe. Attempt a liver and colon cleanse one to three times a year. Some enthusiastic individuals fast once a week.

Chapter 20

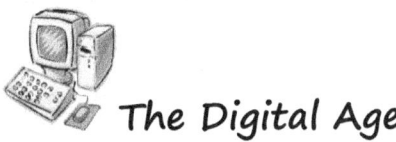 The Digital Age:

EMF's, Electro Pollution and Electro Sensitivity

Within a little over 15 years our 21st century society has moved from a media intake of merely cable television, stereos and radios to an inundation of digital media, and a rapidly expanding telecommunications network. Over-exposure to all of these new gadgets and technologies however has contributed to increasingly more free-radical forming electromagnetic frequencies (EMF's) and electromagnetic radiation (EMR's) in our daily lives. Both produce an unnatural form of radiation, termed electro pollution.

Electro pollution is attributed to the electric and/or magnetic fields generated from wireless or radio frequency fields; cell phones; high tension power lines; wiring in the walls of our homes; common household appliances, and other communications technology. Unfortunately, electro pollution has been linked in many studies to childhood leukemia, brain tumors, sleep problems, depression, allergies and many other conditions.

EMF's, the most widely known form of electro pollution, are derived from power lines and electric appliances. EMF's are generated when an electric current flows through a conductor or wire. This subsequently creates a magnetic field. (All electricity produces a magnetic field) When we are exposed to EMF's, an electrical charge essentially passes through our body. EMR's are created by mobile cell phones, Wi-Fi, microwave ovens and other technology.

Many experts believe that the sudden increase of technology and EMF's/EMR's in the world has produced an inordinately high and unmanageable toxic load for our bodies. A number of individuals are highly affected by EMF's/EMR's (electro sensitivity) and may experience a collection of bewildering symptoms; while others may be less sensitive.

Ann Louise Gittleman, author of *Zapped*, a book on the subject of electro pollution, writes that our society is potentially experiencing 100 million times more electromagnetic radiation than our grandparents experienced. She also asserts that exposure to this massive amount of electro pollution is a subliminal stressor on our body that agitates our nervous system and raises our stress hormone-cortisol. She makes the case that this chronic stress on our body can accelerate our aging and weaken our immunity.

Biophysicist and electro-medicine expert, Dr. James Oschman Ph.D., contends that we are energetic beings; and as a result our physiology and our body's own bioelectric fields are extremely sensitive. This receptiveness, he claims, is why we are easily affected by the cycles of the moon and the ubiquitous EMF's in our modern digital world.

Dr. Ross Adey, past chairman of the *National Council on Radiation Protection and Measurement,* evaluated the potential health risks of EMF's. He found that EMF's, and higher radio frequencies used by cell phone and broadcast towers exert harmful biological effects; and can adversely affect human health. He also made the case that EMF's damage our cell membranes and may interrupt the electrical impulse that carries messages across our cell membranes. EMF's, according to experts also change the shape and growth of our cells- leading to cell death and alteration of our genes. Due to these findings, the late Dr. Adey called for strong action to curtail the excessive EMF exposure that the U.S. population was experiencing. However, his warning has since gone unheeded.

Electromagnetic radiation has also been shown to alter the behavior of calcium ions which affect our brain function. These changes are associated with cancer and melatonin depletion. Melatonin is an essential hormone and a powerful antioxidant, and also regulates our sleep cycle. A deficiency in melatonin will create sleep difficulties.

Other studies have shown that EMF exposure interrupts the functioning of our endocrine system and hormone production; most notably our thyroid, pineal, pancreas, and adrenal glands; also our insulin and sex hormones.

Countless other studies over the past decade have additionally concluded that EMF's and other frequencies pose a threat to our health. Although there is sizable evidence, the U.S. safety organizations such as the F.C.C. and the F.D.A. don't find the evidence convincing enough; therefore they aren't altering U. S. safety standards.

However, in 2012, an international group of concerned experts (scientists, researchers, and public health policy professionals) published a report known as the *Bioinnitiative Report,* concluding that the existing standards for public safety are completely inadequate to guard our health. They have called for a large scale safety standard implementation. You can read this report at bioinnitiative.org.

## Sources of EMF's/EMR's

| Wireless technology, WiFi | Cell phones/cordless home phones | Cell and broadcast towers | Power lines/transformers | Nuclear power plants |
|---|---|---|---|---|
| Fluorescent lights | Electrical appliances/devices: T.V's, computers, ipads, ipods, digital alarm clocks, refrigerators etc. | Dimmer switches | Microwave ovens | Electric blankets |
| Electric razors, Hair dryers, electric toothbrushes etc. | X-rays/ EKG's/ CT scans | Dirty electricity: spikes in a building's electric currents from old electrical infrastructure | Device chargers | Jobs: electrical line workers, electrician, welder, T.V repairers, cashiers, radiology lab workers |

Another concerned expert, Dr. Ollie Johnson has studied for numerous years the effects of radiation on people who suffer from electromagnetic hypersensitivity. He has found that the effects of EMF's are cumulative and can get worse over time. Many individuals who are unable to handle environmental chemicals also have an increased sensitivity to EMF's. Hundreds of other studies have found that chronic electric and magnetic field exposure may cause a myriad of adverse effects on the body.

Due to this abundant evidence, a number of organizations have officially recognized the condition of "electro sensitivity," and the impact it has on its sufferers. They have also recommended precautions to reduce EMF exposure. Among the organizations are the *World Health Organization* and the *European Parliament,* along with the Canadian and Swedish governments. Several states in the U.S. also have recognized the month of May as *Electromagnetic Sensitivity Awareness Month*. However, many medical authorities still do not believe that the condition exists.

## Conditions Associated with Electrical Technology & Symptoms of Electro sensitivity

| Brain tumors, salivary gland tumors (cell phone use) | Insomnia (suppresses melatonin production) | Chronic fatigue, CFS | Mood disturbances (depression/anxiety/irritability) suppresses serotonin production ADD/Poor concentration | Ringing in the ears, ear pain, dizziness |
|---|---|---|---|---|
| Decreases antioxidant production (SOD) | Decreases production of thyroid hormones: (EMF's and radiation target the thyroid gland) | Creates DNA damaging free radicals | Free-radical eye damage from UV blue light emitted from computer, T.V., tablet, and smart phone screens. | Headaches, Eye problems, vision difficulties, light sensitivity, |
| ALS, Type -3 diabetes | Heart arrhythmia's/ Heart disease | Allergies | Infertility | Digestive disorders |
| Skin redness, tingling, burning, itching | Parkinson's | Breathing problems, worsening asthma | Poor memory/Alzheimer's | Leukemia in children |

Fortunately there are helpful dietary and lifestyle measures that we can take to reduce the harmful effects of EMF's and radiation, and protect our sensitive bodies.

## Phone Protection Measures

- Keep cell phones out of bedroom (don't use as alarm clocks they emit radiation.)
- Keep cell phones as far away from head as possible, (4") or use speaker phone, or hands free kit w/ a wireless air tube near the ear piece, or buy a cell phone wire guard; as the microwaves penetrates 2" into your brain and other organs.
- Don't text in your lap,
- Don't keep cell phones in your pocket. (Radiates reproductive organs-danger to testicles) Put in purse or holster case.
- Turn cell phone off when not in use/turn Wi-Fi off of cell phone when not in use
- Switch cell phone to both sides of head often.
- Don't use cell phone in car. (Power levels increase when in metal)

- Don't use phone when signal is weak. (Power levels increase)
- Keep phone conversation short.
- Spend less time on PDA's (blackberry, iPhones etc.; they have a higher ELF)
- Replace wireless or cordless phone with corded landline phone.
- Install an RF filter on your phone line (around $20 at electronic stores) or an anti-EMF phone shield
- Reduce exposure by avoiding overuse

### *Other EMF and Radiation Protection Measures*

- *Keep electrical equipment out of the <u>bedroom</u> to protect melatonin levels/keep alarm clocks or sound machines at least 3 feet away from bed. Take out DVR's laptops, iPads and Bluetooth. Unplug the T.V.
- Book an EMR home assessment appointment from a specialist
- Install KVAR power units on electrical panels (refrigerator, washers, fans, motors)
- Install power strips on computers
- Get rid of wireless connection or turn off wireless router at night and when not in use. Go back to DSL and Ethernet connection.
- Unplug electrical appliances when not in use
- Assess whether there are cell, antenna or broadcast towers near you at antennasearch.com. Studies have found that antennas closer than ¼ mile from your home or work can impair your health. Use EMF shielding paint on the exterior and interior of home if close to cell towers.
- Check for leaks in microwave oven (if older unit) or eliminate microwave.
- Don't use laptop on lap; buy a laptop EMF shielding pad and screen.
- Only have medical radiation when necessary-avoid full body scans/EKG's/CT scans in routine checkups (ionizing radiation is cumulative and weakens immune system) Mammography and mouth X-rays are not as potent.
- Install a Qu Wave USB harmonizer to neutralize EMF's from any device that uses a USB port. (Computer, T.V. etc.)
- Test and Install micro surge filters in your home to neutralize dirty electricity from power surges (Stetzerizers) stetzerelectric.com
- Reposition beds and desks away from meter boxes as they are the highest source of house emitting EMF's, and can travel through walls. (Or buy meter box shields.)
- Don't locate bed on the other side of wall from refrigerator or hot water heater.
- Keep bed away from dimmer switches and ceiling fan control boxes.
- Select a low emissions computer.

Studies have established that antioxidants are helpful in reducing the damaging effects of EMF's and EMR's:

### Antioxidant Rich Foods that Combat EMF/Radiation/Blue light Damage

| Artichokes | Asparagus | Blueberries | Cinnamon | Cranberries/or diluted 100% juice |
|---|---|---|---|---|
| Cruciferous veggies | Cumin | Sulfur-rich foods: Garlic, onions, eggs | CoQ10 foods: organ meats, grass-fed beef, bison | Asian mushrooms (shiitake, reishi) |
| Pomegranate juice diluted | Prunes | Red beans | Rosemary | Seaweeds: iodine reduces EMF/radiation absorption in gut |
| Tart cherries: contains melatonin | Turmeric | Astaxanthin-rich foods: wild Alaskan Salmon, (sockeye) red colored seafood | Walnuts | Yogurt /kefir |

(Sourced from Dr. Gittleman, 2010; L. McLean, 2011; and Dr. Al Sears, 2014)

### Supplements/Herbs to combat EMF's/EMR's/Blue Light

| Sea Buckthorn tea | Honeybee propolis | Superoxide dismutase (SOD) *Designs for Health Brain Vitale* powder | Alpha Lipoic Acid | Milk thistle |
|---|---|---|---|---|
| Ultra-H-3 | Undenatured whey protein powder | Vitamin D3 | N-acetyl-L-cysteine (NAC) | Melatonin (Radio protective) |
| Zinc | MSM | Calcium | Magnesium | Iodine |
| Selenium | Vitamin E | Chaparral herb | Vitamin C | Eye protection: Astaxanthin, CoQ10 |

(Sourced from Dr. Gittleman, 2010, L. McLean, 2011; and Dr. Al Sears, 2014)

*Take an EMF/Radiation Neutralizing Bath*

Add one pound of unbleached sea salt and one pound of aluminum-free baking soda to very hot bath water and soak for at least 20 minutes. (Gittleman, 2010)

Other EMF technology products can be found at:

- Less EMF Inc.
- LowBlueLights.com
- emfsafetystore.com

**Exercise 20: Input any useful electro pollution information** or EMF combating foods, herbs/supplements/activities/devices to your plan.

Chapter 21

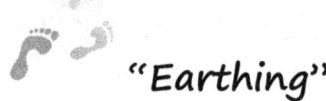

# "Earthing"

## The Ultimate Anti-Aging Agent

Throughout millennia traditional cultures have recognized that the earth held sacred healing energy. These cultures honored their connection to the earth and rested on its surface or walked barefoot in order to absorb its restorative powers. Unfortunately, our current society lives a mostly earth-evading life-style and as a consequence, we have lost our stabilizing connection to the earth and our innate natural grounded state.

According to integrative cardiologist Dr. Steven Sinatra, author of the book, *Earthing,* our planet is one giant electric battery that is constantly being replenished by heat from its molten core via solar radiation and from lightening. He theorizes that since we humans inhabit a bioelectrical body that is constantly transmitting and receiving energy from biochemical reactions; the electric energy abundant on the earth's surface, (specifically negative charged free electrons) is transmitted throughout our bodies by direct skin contact with the ground. He claims that when we wear synthetic soled shoes and sleep in elevated beds with insulated energy blocking materials, we cut off this life-giving earth energy.

It appears that our ancestors' intuition about the curative energies of the earth is now backed by solid scientific evidence. Over the last fourteen years scientific experts from an array of disciplines have been gathering significant scientific proof about the "Earthing" theory. Proponents of this theory believe that the earth's free electrons stabilize and restore our natural rhythms and electrical state when we make skin contact with the ground. They assert that this aids us in being better able to self-regulate and self-heal; and thus benefits every aspect of our physiology.

Two renowned scientists, biophysicist James Oschman, and electrophysiologist-biophysicist Gaetan Chevalier have studied and written extensively about earthing. These scientists believe that earthing produces an anti-aging effect in our body. They have observed that the earth's free electrons effectively neutralize our free-radicals, and strengthen our immunity. These discoveries encourage authorities to see great promise and far reaching benefits to our health and quality of life.

As a result of these inspiring findings, the "Earthing" or "Grounding" movement is in full swing. Thousands of people have applied the concept of earthing in their daily lives, and thousands of studies have documented the wealth of health benefits that it confers. Earthing entails sitting, or laying on the ground with direct skin contact or walking barefoot on the soil or grass for a recommended 20 minutes to a half hour or more to absorb or "conduct" the earth's negatively charged free electrons; whereby the body immediately equalizes to the same electrical level as the earth.

Walking on wet grass or soil supplies further conductivity; and bathing in the ocean, lakes or rivers is also highly conductive. Interestingly, the salt and minerals in the ocean increase the conductivity one hundred times further than freshwater sources. Unpainted concrete (even in the basement or garage) can also conduct the earth's free electrons; as well as rocks and stones. Slightly wetting the concrete can enhance the effect. Wearing thin leather shoes moistened by sweat or dew (similar to moccasins) can also conduct free electrons when walking on concrete, grass or soil. Asphalt, wood, glass, plastic, rubber and vinyl are non-conductive insulating surfaces however, and won't transfer free electron currents.

There are also conductive devices (sheets, foot pads, auto seat pads, computer desk pads, electrode patches, mats, knee bands, and shoes etc.) that one can connect to while in bed, sitting, walking or working. These devices can transmit the same natural healing energy of the earth into our bodies. They are becoming increasingly popular as they can expand the amount of time that individuals receive grounding health benefits; especially when a busy life or inclement weather limits its feasibility. When most people earth or ground, they report almost instant feelings of calm, revitalization and wellbeing. They also report better sleep, less pain and a more youthful appearance.

According to the authors, "Earthing remedies an electron deficiency and an electric imbalance; and replenishes and recharges our body." Numerous scientific studies have established that earthing diffuses chronic inflammation; which as mentioned earlier, is the causative factor in more than 80 chronic diseases. Interestingly, recent research has demonstrated that inflammation is actually an electron deficiency in the body. Investigations have also found that when we are chronically ungrounded and disconnected from the earth, our body is vulnerable and prone to inflammation related diseases and accelerated aging.

Numerous health experts are excited about the many health applications that earthing can provide; especially for the cardiovascular, immune, respiratory and digestive systems. Another important finding is that earthing increases our powerful antioxidant, and sleep regulator known as melatonin. Melatonin is cancer-protective as well. In addition, earthing normalizes our stress hormone cortisol, and cools down our nervous system; which is a great resource for our stressed-filled society.

A landmark earthing study published in the journal *European Biology and Bioelectromagnetics,* (known as the *Applewhite Study)* demonstrated that when the human body is grounded to the earth, it is flooded with health enhancing electrons; and simultaneously is shielded from damaging electro pollution. Yes, you heard that right- earthing trumps EMF's. (Ober, Sinatra, Zucker, 2010)

Many top athletes also regularly earth themselves, including NFL football players, swimmers, and triathletes. Even the American cycling teams were grounded after daily competitions at a past *Tour de France*; and reported impressive recovery from the day's races.

Grounding has been shown to slow down the aging process as evidenced by ninety year old Arnold Beldon Ph. D., featured in the book *Earthing*. Dr. Beldon claimed that he had been sleeping grounded for over eight years, and maintained that he was in excellent health. His doctor also reported that his exceptional health is remarkable given his advanced age.

*Research also indicates the following health benefits of Earthing:*

| Premature aging prevention | Indigestion, GERD prevention | Anxiety relief | Reduces exhaustion, increases energy | Thins the blood and improves blood pressure, arrhythmias, reduces risk of metabolic syndrome |
|---|---|---|---|---|
| Relieves muscle tension and headaches | Reduces jet lag | Protects the body against EMF's | Lessens PMS and other hormonal menopausal symptoms | Chronic pain reduction: backache, arthritis, tendonitis, etc. |
| Accelerates recovery from athletic activity and injuries | Improves circulation, reduces varicose veins | Dramatically improves healing and helps prevent bedsores | Normalizes the body's biological rhythms | Improves respiratory illnesses and breathing improvement |
| Detoxification effects/immune system enhancement | Food/environmental allergy improvement | Skin improvement: eczema, psoriasis | Eye health for Itchy, smarting eyes | Improved male performance |

(Ober, Sinatra, Zucker, 2010)

According to Dr. Sinatra, earthing confers "dose-related effects." He believes that the more earthing that we do, the better our health and body functions will be. He recommends connecting to the earth two to three times a day for fifteen to thirty minutes, (with devices also) and if feasible- sleeping grounded. He also suggests that the more compromised a person's health is, the more earthing should be done. Given all the health advantages of earthing, it would behoove us to make it part of our daily healthy-aging arsenal.

*Exercise 21: Consider performing "earthing" or grounding daily, or as often as possible and/or purchasing grounding devices (for sleeping and everyday use.) This may mitigate inflammation, EMF exposure, and insomnia; and promote high level health. Input any pertinent information into your plan.*

Chapter 22

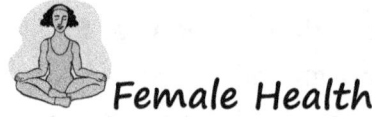

# Female Health

## Perimenopause/Menopause & Hormonal Health

As women reach middle-age they enter the stage known as perimenopause, which initiates a transition between a woman's fertile years and the end of her menses at *menopause*. This is a period in which women's hormone levels naturally begin to shift; and many women at this time begin to dread the changes that they may go through. However, menopause is a natural rite of passage for women, not a dysfunctional condition, and can be an enriching time.

Many women's-wisdom teachers believe that menopause is meant to be a significant, sacred and transformative life-passage that heralds the beginning of a woman coming into her true power; a time to speak her truth, and a time to release whatever is not serving her anymore. Dr. Christiane Northrup, author of several books on menopause, claims that the menopausal transition actually changes a woman's brain chemistry; resulting in amplified creative energy and intuition. Due to the fact that menopause is so life-altering, it is beneficial during this period for women to take some private time for self-reflection and nurturance. With proper self-care, menopause doesn't have to be a difficult or uncomfortable transition, but a time of liberation, expansion and wisdom.

Menopause occurs in a two-stage process. Perimenopause, the first stage, begins with dropping progesterone hormone levels and ends with fluctuating and decreasing estrogen levels. A woman's period becomes irregular at the end of perimenopause; and menopause itself is identified as the cessation of a woman's period for a one year period. The average age for menopause onset is age 51; however, the age of an individual's menopause is correlated with her mother's age at menopause. The accurate scientific term after this period is called postmenopause, and I will be referring to this period by using the popular term of "menopause" to describe all the phases of this transition.

Throughout the stages of menopause the ovaries go through a shift in which there is a reduction in active egg follicles. This egg follicle decline results in a diminishment of the production of the female hormones estrogen (estradiol) and progesterone; however our ovaries and body fat will still make another form of estrogen called estrone. Additionally, the adrenal glands become responsible for taking over the dwindling production of estrogen. Estrogen production will be far below normal reproductive levels however- postmenopause; and progesterone levels will as well be lower than previously. Testosterone hormone levels may decline or increase, depending on the woman. This life-changing time can be a rocky period for many women due to sudden and erratic shifts in their hormones, and from emotional upheavals.

Many menopausal women experience various physical symptoms of low or imbalanced hormones including: irregular bleeding, hot flashes, night sweats, palpitations, insomnia, mood swings, and mild cognitive changes. Other symptoms include headache, vaginal dryness, hair thinning, facial hair, low libido, weight gain, dry skin, and urinary incontinence. With proper self-care however, common menopausal disturbances can be minimized.

Hormone health and balance is the foundation of a woman's lifelong wellness; and therefore it is important during menopause to keep the body's hormones at their best possible levels. According to Dr. Sarah Gottfried, author of *The Hormone Cure*, hormone imbalances can be one of the top reasons for accelerated aging.

The key to a smooth menopausal transition and optimal hormone levels is to optimize or restore the health of three critical organ functions: the adrenals, the liver, and the thyroid. Poor functioning in these areas is typically the underlying cause of hormone imbalances, and distressful menopausal symptoms. One of the first areas of decline common to many menopausal women is with the thyroid and adrenal glands. If the liver is overwhelmed it too will cause problems during menopause. Additionally, if a woman has experienced prior PMS issues, she is more prone to an increase in menopausal symptoms.

Chronic stress of any kind, as mentioned previously, impairs the adrenal, liver and thyroid glands. It is important to note that the more emotional stress a woman experiences, the more PMS and menopausal symptoms she will experience; as stress decreases estrogen and progesterone production.

Normally at menopause the adrenal glands are designed to compensate for the declining ovarian hormone production; but a poor reaction from weakened adrenal and thyroid glands will not produce adequate estrogen and progesterone. This hormone depletion will trigger hot flashes, night sweats, heart palpitations and other related symptoms. Studies have shown that simply incorporating stress-reduction techniques reduced hot flashes in women by 41-92%.

Poor nutrition also plays a role. Sugar, gluten, excess caffeine, alcohol, refined carbs, rancid and trans-fats and overeating can trigger hot flashes and other menopausal symptoms. Mineral deficiencies also create problems for menopausal women. Zinc, magnesium, vitamin C, and B complex are common nutrient deficiencies at menopause. Toxins (also known as endocrine disrupters) and poor liver detoxification also have a detrimental effect on our hormone levels. Additionally, poor digestion and probiotic status are involved in menopausal difficulties. Lastly, a lack of exercise can trigger imbalances and symptoms.

Dr. Louise Gittleman, author of *Super Nutrition for Menopause, also* asserts that a copper/zinc imbalance is the most prevalent mineral imbalance that she finds in women of menopausal age, and with patients who have low thyroid conditions. (A low thyroid status is very common during menopause). She claims that the adrenal glands take over the estrogen production from the ovaries, and when under stress, zinc levels drop. When this happens, copper tends to accumulate (since zinc and copper compete for absorption.) The result is a copper excess and a zinc insufficiency. In addition, she explains that in perimenopause a progesterone deficiency or an estrogen-dominance can also encourage copper to accumulate.

Copper overload is frequently accompanied by an underactive thyroid and a sluggish liver which makes it difficult to metabolize hormones or toxins; and as a result can worsen menopausal symptoms. Copper overload also can trigger mood problems such as anxiety, and a racing mind. Supplementing with zinc, vitamin C, and NAC can often reverse copper overload. (See dietary supplement section.)

Mary Shoman also asserts in her book, "The Menopause Thyroid Solution," that a thyroid condition can worsen any menopausal problems, and can deplete the body's ability to cope with stress so much so that a woman can feel extremely tired, but wired. She claims that many conditions associated with menopause can be thyroid related, such as: brain fog, a racing brain, a slow metabolism, hot flashes and anxiety.

Fortunately, there are many strategies we can utilize during perimenopause/menopause to support our body through this momentous life transition.

*Lifestyle, Foods, Botanicals and Nutrients to Ease the Menopause Passage*

Stress Reduction: The more stress that a woman experiences, the more hormone imbalances she will have. Stress is often the causative factor in menopausal symptoms such as hot flashes, anxiety and insomnia because stress decreases levels of the calming and sleep-promoting hormone, progesterone. Reducing stress will additionally help to support increased estrogen production. (The adrenal glands are the source of postmenopausal estrogen production.) Learning how to center, relax and calm ourselves is very important during the menopausal years. Learn relaxation and stress reduction techniques; reduce work load; go to bed earlier (by 9 pm); rest more; reduce excessive exercise; take deep breaths; and get massages etc. See "Stress" chapter.

Exercise 3-5 x a Week: But do not exercise excessively as it weakens the adrenal glands and promotes oxidative stress.

Eating and Hydrating well are vitally important during menopause: Eat 5-10+ servings of fruit and veggies. (no more than 3 fruits daily) Eat adequate protein at every meal. Cruciferous and leafy green veggies are important for magnesium and liver detox. Eat high fiber and fermented and cultured foods. Have omega-3s in fish and fermented cod liver oil. Drink green tea. Eat hormone-free and organic meats and produce. Limit high fat consumption, sugar, coffee, gluten and alcohol. Support digestion with HCL/digestive enzymes.

- Sea weed: Nutritionist Dr. Annemarie Colbin believes that it is the seaweed and fish that contribute to lower rates of menopausal problems in Japanese women. She suggests eating a Japanese meal: fish, miso soup and seaweed salad, at least several times a week. Sea weed will also benefit thyroid function for those with low thyroid conditions due to its high iodine content. Good sources include bladder wrack, wakame, nori, sea palm and dulse.
- Selenium-rich brazil nuts for thyroid support (2 daily)
- Phytoestrogen-rich foods: Work in a similar way to our estrogenic hormone, and can act as a substitute for decreased estrogen production. (estrogen mimics) They also stimulate sex hormone binding globulin in the liver. (Weed, 2002) Eat on a regular basis: *fennel, *fermented soy, *freshly ground flax seed, sunflower and sesame seed, yellow split peas, baby lima beans, red lentils, parsley, dandelion greens, *seaweeds, alliums, olives, pomegranate seeds, citrus-peel, red kidney beans, black turtle beans, sun chokes, and burdock root. (Phytoestrogenic plants in whole form are thought to be safe, but not those in isolated and concentrated forms as in soy supplements. Cancer risk)
- Menopause symptom relief can be a bit of a moving target for some women due to biochemical individuality. Susan Weed has observed that some women respond favorably by increasing phytoestrogenic foods/herbs; while others need to utilize "liver helpers," such as milk thistle and dandelion root. Others may need to decrease their stress hormone levels; whereas others need to increase cooling foods and herbs, (chickweed, elder) and cooling activities.

Additional Menopausal Support Botanicals:

- For low estrogen causing hot flashes and night sweats (in peri/menopause) use mineral-rich Isoflavone estrogen mimics in combination: black cohosh, red clover, and kudzu.
- For low progesterone particularly in perimenopause (causing PMS, anxiety, bone loss and insomnia) use progesterone mimics in combination: Passion flower, chaste berry and wild yam. These stimulate the synthesis of progesterone receptors. Use passion flower alone during postmenopause. (Boosts the calming brain chemical GABA- depleted due to low estrogen/progesterone levels.)
- Organic Maca is a very effective remedy for menopausal patients, especially with low thyroid. It is a highly nutritious food that has been used by the native Peruvians

for menopausal symptoms. It is rich in minerals, especially selenium, calcium and magnesium, and also fatty acids. Maca is an adaptogen. It supports the hormone system to adapt and balance itself, and is known to reduce or eliminate menopausal symptoms such as hot flashes, vaginal dryness, and depression. It also provides nutritional support for the endocrine system, including the adrenals, the thyroid, and the ovaries. Maca stimulates the body to produce its own hormones, and as a bonus supports a healthy libido. Dosage: Take 2 Maca capsules daily with breakfast. After a week gauge your symptoms. If not feeling substantially better, add a capsule. When the symptoms are 80% improved, remain at that dose. Maca has an accumulative effect over time. Contraindications: prescription estrogen treatments, estrogenic herbs like black cohosh and red clover, soy isoflavone supplements, or ginseng. (Shoman, 2009)

- Phytoestrogen Food-like Herbal Infusions: nettles, hops, chamomile, licorice root, (adrenal support) dandelion root, (liver detox) red raspberry leaf, oat straw, (calming) sage, (foggy brain), alfalfa (mineral rich) *red clover; (blood cleanser with 10x more phytoestrogens than soy) seeds of fennel, coriander, cumin, celery, caraway, poppy, anise and fenugreek. Drink freely. (Weed, 2002) (See herbal chapter and below for dosage)

- Other Menopause Support Botanicals: Motherwort, burdock root, ashwagandha, holy basil, ginger, dong quai, hawthorne, sarsaparilla, saw palmetto, and peppermint. Use in combinations or alone. Dosage: 2 to 3 cups a day; effects after 3 months. All above herbs are known to reduce hot flashes, mood changes and insomnia. Dong quai also stimulates the proliferation of bone cells. Ashwagandha is an adaptogenic herb that stimulates thyroid activity and may help fight fatigue. It also supports the adrenal gland. Holy basil is also an adaptogenic herb that supports the adrenals, and is very calming. Oat straw (nervine) and nettle tea help restore minerals in the body due to stress. Nettles also supports healthy liver functioning. Sage tea diminishes brain fog, hot flashes, and night sweats. Take in tea/infusion, tincture, standardized extracts or freeze dried capsules.

- To Prevent Bone Loss Due to Low Estrogen Levels: nettles, oat straw, horsetail, red clover and comfrey infusion. (Drink freely)

Menopausal Support Supplements

- Take high quality multivitamin/mineral supplements/trace mineral supplements. *Innate Response's Women+40 Greens* also aids in balancing hormone levels.
- Increase Zinc levels: Zinc functions in the body to manufacture thyroid hormones. A deficiency of zinc reduces the amount of thyroid hormone produced. Zinc supplementation restores normal thyroid function in zinc deficient hypothyroid menopause women. In addition zinc is needed for proper hypothalamic function.

Increasing zinc levels can repair the HPA (Hypothalamus, Pituitary, Adrenal) axis and support healthy adrenal function. Improving these gland functions will in turn improve menopausal symptoms. (Zinc also promotes mental alertness, and improves sleep. In addition, zinc decreases lead levels, owing to the fact that lead replaces zinc in the body if zinc levels are low. Dosage: 15 mg/daily.

- Increase Vitamin C and Bioflavonoids: Vitamin C is a water soluble vitamin that acts as a powerful antioxidant to help reduce inflammation and hot flashes. Vitamin C has been shown to reduce the elevation of cortisol, a stress hormone. Vitamin C is essential for optimal functioning of the adrenal glands due to the fact that it is stored in these glands. The adrenals are an important source of post-menopausal estrogen hormone synthesis. Balancing the hormone production helps regulate hot flashes. Hot flashes also deplete our stores of vitamin C, therefore it is important to increase our vitamin C consumption. Vitamin C also supports bladder problems and vaginal dryness common in menopause. Bioflavonoids (often paired with vitamin c) also have a slight estrogenic effect on the body. The Dose of vitamin C for adrenal fatigue is 3,000mg/day (divided doses). The preferred form of supplementation for vitamin C is Buffered C or Ester C with bioflavonoids or Acerola cherry.

- Increase Vitamin B5 and B-complex vitamins: Vitamin B5, also called pantothenic acid, is known as the "anti-stress vitamin." Vitamin B5 plays an important role in healthy adrenal gland functioning as It supports the adrenals by acting as a precursor for cortisol and adrenal hormones. While stress can weaken adrenal functioning and deplete B vitamins, supplementing with extra B5, along with B-complex (to maintain balance) can aid the adrenal gland to regulate and synthesize hormones throughout menopause. Regulating the hormones- estrogen and progesterone can reduce the likelihood of hot flashes. Hot flashes also deplete the body of B vitamins; therefore one needs to ensure there is a good supply of vitamin B-rich foods in the diet, especially with the onset of hot flashes. Vitamin B5 can also support hippocampus brain repair; thus improving brain fog and poor short term memory- common in menopause. In addition, it is also helpful for reducing fatigue. B5 supplement: 500 mg daily (divided doses) with whole food vitamin B-complex or nutritional yeast.

- Gamma-oryzanol (ferulic acid) Enhances pituitary function and supports the hypothalamus in releasing and raising endorphins which plummet with hot flashes. It is also known to lower cholesterol and triglyceride levels. Dosage: 300 mg daily. Effects after 2-3 months

- Vitamin E has been shown to relieve hot flashes. It also improves blood supply to the vaginal wall, thus improving menopausal vaginal dryness. Dosage: 400-800 IU daily. Effects after 2 months.

- Natural Desiccated Thyroid contains a full spectrum of thyroid hormones as well as nutritional co-factors that naturally mimic the action of human thyroid function. Desiccated Thyroid raises thyroid hormones to normal levels. Healthy thyroid function supports menopausal symptoms and helps one deal with stress more efficiently. Many classic menopause symptoms are often actually low thyroid symptoms. Determine need through thyroid testing. Best forms are: prescription Nature-Throid, and Westhroid.
- Iodine Supplementation for thyroid hormone production: Iodine deficiency is widespread in our society. 3-6 Kelp capsules (600 mg.) daily or Iodoral Iodine tablets. (Take iodine loading test to determine need/dosage)
- Melatonin is known as the "queen of all hormones" because it monitors and directs the whole hormonal system. Melatonin acts like a hormonal adaptogen; helping to moderate-adrenal, thyroid and reproductive hormones. It also aids in thyroid T4 to T3 conversion. Dr. Pierpaoli, M.D. of the book "The Melatonin Miracle," believes that melatonin is an important supplement to utilize during menopause because of its hormone balancing effect. He also states that it increases the density of estrogen receptors in the uterus, breast and ovaries and improves their sensitivity. It also prevents atrophy of the ovaries, vagina, and uterus. Melatonin also has an adaptogenic effect on cortisol levels. In addition, melatonin supports sleep by resetting the body's sleep clock; which is often disturbed during menopause. Dosage is 1- 3mg daily.
- Phosphatidyl Serine lowers excessively high cortisol levels, especially at night when trying to sleep. It induces calm, and quiets an over active mind. 100 mg 2x a day. Increase to 200 mg if no effect.
- Desiccated Adrenals to support adrenal fatigue. (Enzymatic Therapy's Adrenal Stress End.)
- Vitamin D functions as a hormone, and it is essential for the pituitary gland to produce thyroid hormone. It may also play a role in T 3 binding to its receptor. In addition, it enables conversion of T4 to T3. It is also vital for healthy immune function. Vitamin D (with calcium, magnesium, and vitamin K2) also decreases hot flashes and depression at menopause. Best form: cholecalciferol (D3) Take a Vitamin D lab test to check on vitamin D status.
- 5-HTP supports insomnia. Night sweats and hot flashes cause frequent waking and many women find it difficult to fall back to sleep after waking. Women may suffer from exhaustion, memory problems, and depression as a result. Decreasing estradiol levels are associated with trouble falling asleep and frequent waking. Elevated FSH is also linked to frequent waking. 100-300 mg 45 min. before bed.
- Liver Detoxification: N acetyl-cysteine, milk thistle, and dandelion root.

- Pregnenolone: sex hormone precursor by **Apex Energetics**/ or Bio-identical hormones if necessary.
- **Metagenics Estrovera** has been clinically found to relieve hot flashes and insomnia.

*Menopause Supportive Nutrients, Supplements and lifestyle Measures*

| *Stress reduction: yoga, baths, soft music, deep breathing, massage, meditation etc. Homeopathic remedies: Lachesis, Pulsatilla, Belladonna, Amyl Nitricum | High quality multi vitamin/mineral Women's +40 Greens Oat straw/red clover Infusion for mineral depletion Vitamin E: nuts, seeds, vitamin E supplement 400-800 mg daily Gamma oryzanol: 300 mg daily | *5-9 servings of fruit/veggies; cruciferous/green leafy veggies/ high fiber/ fermented foods/ Omega-3's in fish/ fermented cod liver oil/ green tea/ organic meats and produce. Support digestion with: HCL/ dietary enzymes | *Zinc rich foods: oysters, liver, eggs, crimini mushrooms, red meat. Zinc aspartate- 25 mg daily Magnesium rich foods: leafy greens- 1,000 mg. magnesium citrate | *Vitamin C rich foods: bell peppers, nori sea weed, strawberries, kiwi, bok choy, kale, tangerine, parsley. Ester-C 3,000 mg. daily in divided doses |
|---|---|---|---|---|
| *Vitamin B-5 rich foods: nutritional yeast, sunflower seeds, chicken liver, egg, Vitamin B5 supplement for adrenal fatigue: 500 mg. w/b-complex. | Additional support herbs: *motherwort, *sage, licorice, alfalfa,*ashwagandha, holy basil, nettles,*oat straw, ginger, dong quai Use tea, infusion, or capsules | Phytoestrogenic-infusions:*Red clover, hops, chamomile, red raspberry leaf, seeds of fennel, fenugreek, coriander, poppy, celery, cumin, anise, caraway | Progesterone promoters: *chaste berry- 225 mg/day, passion flower, wild yam (infusion also) L-theanine for anxiety | To Boost Libido: Maca: 2 capsules daily with breakfast, and Support NO levels For insomnia and anxiety: passionflower |
| For hot flashes: Black Cohosh 40 mg; kudzu: 100 mg; Red Clover: 80 mg a day (or infusions) | Thyroid Support: *Sea Weed: bladder wrack, dulse, nori, wakame, sea palm etc. | Natural desiccated thyroid: If lab test reveals hypothyroid: Nature-throid | Thyroid support *Iodine Supplementation with kelp or Iodoral | Thyroid Support: *Brazil nuts: 2 daily for selenium; Eggs for vit. A. |
| Sleep aid: *Melatonin: 1.5 to 3 mg 5HTP: 100-300 mg | Cortisol reduction: *Phosphatidyl Serine: 100 mg. 2 x daily (sleep/stress) | Adrenal support: dessicated adrenals | *Vitamin D3: 4,000-10,000 IU with vitamin K2 (under Dr.'s care) | Pregnenolone or or Estrovera, or Bio-identical natural hormones |
| Phytoestrogen rich foods: (estrogen mimics) fermented soy, fennel, flax meal, dandelion, parsley, beans | *Liver detox: N acetyl cysteine, vitamin C, milk thistle, dandelion root, oat straw, yellow dock, burdock root | Limit coffee, sugar, alcohol, overeating, gluten and very high fat diets; but avoid a low fat diet | *Exercise at least 3 times weekly *Drink half your weight in oz. of water | Bone support: nettles, comfrey, oat straw, and red clover infusions |

➡ **Lab tests:** home zinc tally test, thyroid testing, Iodine loading test, hormone panel

See exercise 22 on next page.

**Exer. 22: Female Health.** Input/print out any gender specific information and supportive nutrients, supplements and lifestyle measures to enhance your hormonal and general health.

Chapter 23

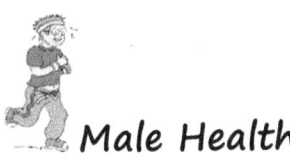

# Male Health

## Andropause, Hormone Balance, & Prostate Health

Although it is not widely recognized, research since the 1940's has shown that men between the ages of 40-65 undergo a gradual decline in hormones somewhat similar to what women experience in menopause. Andropause, the term used for this male hormone shift, involves the lessening of testosterone and cortisol hormone levels. Men also experience ongoing increases in estradiol, sex hormone binding globulin (SHBG) and dihydrotestosterone. (DHT) These hormone shifts can for some men cause a few undesirable symptoms. The following chart shows some common symptoms of andropause.

### Common Symptoms of Andropause

| Abdominal weight gain | Memory loss | Diminished sex drive | Hair Loss | Night sweats |
|---|---|---|---|---|
| Muscle Loss | Fatigue | Male breasts | Sleep Apnea | Depression/irritable male syndrome |

As men age, they may additionally experience problems involving the prostate gland including: benign prostatic hyperplasia, (BPH-an enlargement of the prostate gland); frequent urination; chronic pelvic pain, and prostate cancer. Studies confirm that 30%-50% of U.S. men ages 50-59 develop an enlarged prostate, and 50% of men over age 70 develop BPH. Erectile dysfunction is another frequent condition that can manifest in midlife.

However, in many instances research has revealed that diminishing testosterone levels, prostate issues, and erectile dysfunction can be linked to poor nutrition and unwise lifestyle choices. Some habits that particularly impact male health at midlife are chronic unmanaged stress; excess calorie intake; obesity; overindulgence in alcohol; and a sedentary lifestyle.

Fortunately, it may be possible to prevent the decline in male health that can occur with aging. It may also be possible to achieve male hormonal balance by adopting healthy lifestyle choices. There are many strategies that can be employed for this purpose. See the chart on the following page.

## Strategies to Support Male Hormonal Health

| Eating a whole foods diet containing cold-water fish, healthy fats, whole grains, squashes and tubers, and plenty of veggies. | Reducing caloric intake: Drink a glass of water ½ hour before eating and then eat until 80-90% full. | Balancing blood sugar with adequate protein at every meal. Eating low glycemic foods, and avoiding sugar |
|---|---|---|
| Limiting alcohol to only one glass of red/white wine daily (if desired): Alcohol is a diuretic that creates free-radical formation and inflammation | *Getting regular physical activity: the highest erectile dysfunction rates were associated with a sedentary lifestyle. | Avoiding toxins/ xenoestrogens (plastics, pesticides, food additives, chemicals in personal care products etc.) |
| *Decreasing body fat | Stress reduction and management | Increase antioxidant-rich plant foods (colorful foods) |

Recent studies completed on male health have revealed that erectile dysfunction, a common issue for men in middle-age, may be the first visible indication of underlying health problems; and is very often a sign of cardiovascular disease developing within a man. In a study published in *The Journal of the American Medical Association,* men who had developed erectile dysfunction over 5 years had a 45% greater risk of a heart attack or stroke then those who did not have erection problems.

Dr. Ballentine Carter, director of adult urology at *John Hopkins University,* makes the case that high blood pressure, obesity, inactivity and metabolic syndrome are all associated with male sexual performance problems. He also states that drug treatments for cardiovascular disease can additionally trigger erectile dysfunction. Dr. Ballentine believes that men who suffer from erectile issues can improve their performance into their later years if they implement a regular exercise program; particularly a daily half hour brisk walking program.

Engaging in regular vigorous physical activity will also protect men from heart disease; the number one killer of men. Studies find that exercise also has a profound influence on maintaining optimal prostate health and in reducing a man's risk for prostate cancer. Dr. Carter believes that both working-out and weight-loss combined improve blood flow to the pelvic region and diminish inflammation in the prostate gland. As a bonus a regular fitness program can decrease body fat, reduce stress, and revitalize the body.

Dr. Carter suggests purchasing a pedometer to fulfill daily walking goals. Studies suggest that walking 10,000 steps per day will reduce the risk of prostate issues and prostate cancer, and also the risk of all chronic diseases. (See exercise section for more details)

Our Western diet is additionally often to blame for erectile dysfunction and prostate impairments. The chemical-laden Western (SAD) diet, coupled with male obesity is responsible for up-regulating inappropriate estrogen production in middle-aged men. (also known as aromatase.) Due to this nutrient-poor diet, the death rate from prostate cancer is 4-5 times higher than in Asian countries.

Western men often tend to eat some of the worst western dietary offenders including:

| Fried Foods: French fries, fried fish, fried chicken, and onion rings | Salty Snack Foods: chips, pretzels, peanuts | Sugar/fat or flour desserts: cake, candy, ice cream, pies | Fast Food Burgers | Meat-topped Pizzas |
|---|---|---|---|---|
| Beverages: regular/diet sodas, tap water, energy drinks, coffee drinks, alcohol | Fat-free/sugar-free desserts: frozen yogurt, breakfast bars, cookies | Excess commercial/cured meat consumption | Eating large meals at night | Overeating anytime |

Fortunately many men experience improvements in their sexual and prostate health and quality of life when they improve their eating and lifestyle habits. The following table offers nutritional and lifestyle information to support male hormone and prostate health.

(See next page)

| Male Hormone/ Erectile Dysfunction Support | Enlarged Prostate Gland Support |
|---|---|
| **Avoid or limit** alcohol, caffeine, sugar and smoking<br>**Avoid toxins** (xenobiotics) in plastics; personal care and household products; packaged and non-organic foods<br>**Reduce carbs (breads and pasta) and excess fat** (fried foods/dairy etc.)<br>*Eat Lycopene containing foods daily: esp. tomatoes/tomato sauces (cooked and raw) spinach, kale<br>*Zinc rich foods: (vital for testosterone/male health) oysters, pumpkin seeds, herring, ginger root, egg yolk, liver, brazil nuts, chili powder | **High vegetable intake:** 5+ daily<br>**Concentrated tomato products** (lycopene) daily<br>Tomato-sauce based dishes eaten for 3 weeks- PSA concentration decreased by 17.5%<br>**Green tea** inhibits PSA (instead of coffee)<br>2 Tbsp. Flax meal daily (inhibits aromatase)<br>**Tempeh/miso (in moderation)** lowers PSA<br>**Pomegranate fruit extract:** lowers PSA<br>**Onions/garlic:** lowers BPH<br>**Decrease Carbs:** lowers BPH (50% of calories)<br>Cold-water fish/ O-3's<br>Avoid commercial red meat consumption<br>Use *Innate Response's Men+40 Greens* |
| Eat beets for Nitric Oxide support<br>Eat Miso and tempeh in moderation<br>Flax seed meal: 2 Tbsp. daily<br>Eat cold water fish 3x/wk or take fermented cod liver/krill oil<br>Liver Detox: citrus, onion, garlic, cooked broccoli, kale, cabbage, cauliflower, greens<br>Medicinal mushrooms (boosts testosterone) | **Supplements that reduce aromatase:** (Down regulates male estrogen production)<br>Resveratrol/ red wine<br>Grape seed extract<br>Mangosteen<br>Chrysin |
| **Sexual Function Enhancers:**<br>Catuaba and yohimbe bark (some side-effects)<br>Fo-ti<br>Tribulus :increases testosterone and male performance- 1,000 mg. twice a day<br>Red Ginseng<br>Maca | **Supplements to support the prostate gland/ BPH:**<br>Zinc: 15-50 mg daily<br>Saw palmetto: 320 mg daily<br>Pygeum: 75-200 mg. day<br><br>Or use *Designs for Health Prostate Supreme* |
| **Hormone Supportive Supplements/Herbs:**<br>High quality multi vitamin/mineral<br>*Saw palmetto: 300 mg. 1-2x daily<br>Pygeum bark extract<br>Zinc: 25 mg<br>Vitamin E: 400 IU<br>Pumpkin seed oil<br>Vitex (supports progesterone metabolism)<br>DIM (supports xeno-estrogens metabolism)<br>Ashwagandha, astragulus (boosts testosterone) | **Lifestyle Changes that lower proliferation of prostate cells**<br>Adequate protein (see protein section)<br>Lose weight (obesity-high risk for BPH)<br>Keep blood sugar stable (avoid sugar/starchy carbs, protein at every meal)<br>Exercise daily<br>Manage stress |

➡ The Prostate Specific Antigen (PSA) is the main prostate cancer biomarker and can be assessed through lab testing.

## Male Pattern Baldness

Many men as they reach middle-age may start to see signs of hair loss. This can be very disconcerting for a lot of men. However, there may be help in sight. New research links an abnormal amount of a protein called prostaglandin D2 (PGD2) to be the main stimulus for male pattern baldness; as PGD2 has been shown in clinical studies to block hair-growth on the scalp. As luck would have it- cutting-edge research performed in Italy points to the use of two anti-inflammatory compounds used jointly to halt the production of PGD2; and thus arrest hair loss. They are resveratrol and curcumin. It appears that taking the two together, according to the research, is more effective, owing to their synergistic effects. It might be worth a try if you would like to keep your youthful head of hair.

Additionally, the traditional Chinese "longevity tonic" known as fo-ti has been highly regarded for thousands of years to restore hair growth and color. Use fo-ti under a Chinese medicine practitioner's supervision, as high doses can cause side-effects.

**Exer. 23: Male Health**. Input/print out any gender specific information, supportive nutrients, supplements and lifestyle measures to enhance your hormonal and general health into your wellness plan.

*Chapter 24*

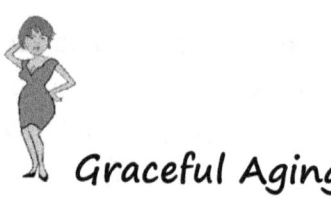

*Graceful Aging*

*Delaying the Visible Signs of Advancing years*

Middle age is the stage of life when we typically start bemoaning that we are losing our youthful looks. Our skin may start to show wrinkles or lose its tone; or we may see the first signs of sun damage. This can be a discouraging time for us and we can start to develop a defeatist attitude that: "it's all downhill from here."

But we don't have to lose heart. According to dermatologists, our skin renews itself every two weeks; and therefore they claim it is possible to reverse and repair some of our skin damage if we improve our lifestyle habits. Additionally, it is feasible to control the rate at which our physical appearance ages. Just as it is with all areas of our health, we can gain an understanding of how our diet and lifestyle can support or spoil our youthful looks, and modify our habits if need be.

An important point to be aware of is that our body directs its limited nutritional resources first and foremost in making sure that our vital organs are functioning properly. It doesn't waste precious stores on parts of the body that are not necessary for our survival. After fortifying our vital organs, if there are any nutrient reserves left, the body will then direct the surplus to non-vital areas of the body, such as our skin, hair and nails. Declining youthfulness in midlife therefore may be the result, in part, due to inadequate nutrient stores. Fortunately, it is possible to delay this degeneration by simply boosting nutrient levels.

*There are other factors that can play a role in premature skin aging. They are:*

| Glycation | Toxins/free radicals | UVA damage | Shortened telomeres | Poor hydration, poor digestion, low protein consumption |
|---|---|---|---|---|
| Poor blood circulation | Poor sleep | Chronic stress and poor thyroid function | Hyaluronic acid and HGH depletion (see HGH section) | Waning estrogen hormone levels |

## Living a Skin-Healthy Lifestyle

Our skin also reflects our internal health. When our bodies are healthy, we have a vibrant glowing radiance about us. However our skin can start to age and lose this radiance when we receive too few nutrients and experience too much damage. This can ruin our once youthful skin. A study carried out by British researchers that was published in 2007 in *the Journal of Clinical Nutrition* sought to determine whether the quality of our food effects how our skin looks. They discovered that subjects who ate a higher intake of trans fats, (hydrogenated oils) and processed carbohydrates had more pronounced wrinkles; while those participants who had a high intake of vitamin C had fewer wrinkles as they aged.

Another study titled: *Food Habits in Later Life*, spanning from 1989-1996, inspected the diets of 2,000 people to see whether their diet influenced the youthfulness of their skin. It was determined that those with the least wrinkling had a diet higher in vegetables, olive oil, fish, and legumes; with lower intakes of sugar, margarine (trans fat), and processed foods.

These studies confirm another large body of research that affirms that glycation, (mentioned earlier) a process where renegade sugars bind with proteins, is a key player in premature skin aging. Glycation causes protein fibers to become deformed, hard and inflexible. (Cross-linking) This process causes wrinkles, sagging skin, discoloration and dullness. If you recall from the earlier chapter- a high carb and high sugar diet, especially high fructose corn syrup speeds up glycation. An excess of carbs from grains, pasta and bread (even whole grain) can also accelerate the process. Thus, if you long to keep your youthful looks, it's best to limit all forms of sugar, and to cut down on flours, and an excess of fruit.

Additionally, foods cooked over 250 degrees (stated previously) have also been implicated in generating glycation reactions. Barbequing, frying, grilling, or broiling foods should be minimized. As an alternative, it would be advantageous to eat more raw foods, or use slow cooking, steaming, simmering, poaching or stewing.

The supplement carnosine, and the spices- cinnamon, ginger and cumin have also been demonstrated to inhibit glycation reactions. These might be of help to you and your skin if you have been habitually indulging in carbs, and want to remedy its harmful effects.

As the above studies confirm, optimal nutrition, especially a high intake of vitamin C is essential to keep skin youthful. Collagen is the most important component of the skin; as it maintains the skin's structure, and gives skin a plump, smooth, young looking appearance. Vitamin C is the key nutrient for synthesizing collagen and is therefore vital to maintain the skin's collagen levels. Without sufficient vitamin C, the skin loses its tight structure and begins to loosen, sag and wrinkle. Vitamin C also protects our skin from free-radicals. Vitamin C is not stored in the body, (accept in adrenals) so it is important to keep a steady supply in our blood; and to try to consume vitamin C rich foods at every meal. Cooking however depletes vitamin C levels in foods; so eating vitamin C rich foods in their raw state will supply greater quantities. (Citrus, strawberries, peppers, kiwi, spinach, sprouts, rose hips, camu camu, acerola cherry, salad greens, tomatoes, berries and steamed broccoli) Supplemental vitamin C (Ester C) is also recommended (3,000 mg. daily in divided doses.)

Gelatin, a compound formed when slow cooking the bones and skins of meats, poultry or fish is another excellent source of collagen. Cooking chicken bones or any other bone stock for 12-36 hours will break down gelatin into the broth; which then can be synthesized into skin-strengthening collagen. Gristle is another gelatin source which is formed from the breakdown of connective tissue of slow cooked roast beef. A gelatin mold termed aspic additionally contains quite a bit of skin-nourishing collagen.

Hyaluronic Acid, a natural moisturizer synthesized in our body, is also important for keeping our tissues and skin moist; and for maintaining skin elasticity and speeding up the healing process of wounds and scars. Unfortunately our hyaluronic acid levels decrease as we age; thus maintaining optimal levels in our body could decrease skin aging. As luck would have it, hyaluronic acid also can be derived from connective tissue of animals, and can additionally be obtained from boiling the bones and skin of chickens or other animals into a broth. It seems that bone broth is a "twofer"! (two-for-one) when it comes to preventing wrinkles! Bone broths are easy to make. See the recipe section in the back for details.

Another key component of skin health is keratin. Keratin gives skin (also hair and nails) its strength. Keratin also helps prevent sagging and wrinkles. Sources best for keratin production are foods high in iron-rich proteins such as: beef, liver, lamb, clams, oysters and egg yolks. Keratin can also build up and produce dull skin as we age. A dry brush or a papaya enzyme facial mask can remove this excess keratin.

Elastin is another key element of healthy skin. Elastin promotes skin firmness. As elastin production decreases in middle age, areas of decreased firmness develop, especially along the jaw line, neck and around the eyes. Eating vitamin A-rich foods has been shown to increase elastin production by 300%. (Leafy greens and yellow/orange colored foods) Copper-rich foods have also been found to slow elastin breakdown. (Calves liver, spirulina, shiitake mushroom, sesame seed, soy, chocolate, crab, and sunflower seeds.) Grape seed extract is another nutrient shown to protect and promotes elastin production.

Free-radicals, our ever-present nemesis, according to research, jeopardize and damage our skin health as well. In fact, the average woman applies about 515 free-radical generating chemicals to her skin every day from personal care products (make-up, creams, perfumes, deodorants, sun screens etc.). If we wish to forestall the signs of aging on our skin, it is important to endeavor to abstain from free-radical forming activities and substances whenever possible.

There are many organic and natural skin care lines that are free of harmful chemicals on the market now. In order to decrease the damaging impacts to our body and skin, it is best to avoid chemical laden skin-care products. The most harmful chemicals are: parabens, isopropyl alcohol, propylene, sodium benzoate, mineral oil, alcohol, and fragrances etc. (For more info. see the *Environmental Working Group's "Skin Deep"* web site, and the "total load chapter" in this book)

## Premature Skin Aging Sources and Support

| | | |
|---|---|---|
| Inadequate nutrition (see above) Food allergies also are the cause of dark circles under eyes | Glycation Avoid sugar and refined grains Eat cinnamon, ginger and cumin Take carnosine supplements | UVA sun damage: Use zinc oxide SPF 30 for prolonged exposure-reapply every 2 hours. Wear a hat when in the sun |
| Toxins/Free radicals: Chemicals in household products (cleaning products etc.) cause lipofuscin-age spots, under eye bags and accelerated aging. Use chemical-free products. | Poor hydration: Causes deep wrinkling, gauntness and under eye hollows Drink half of your body weight in oz. of filtered water | Poor blood circulation: Exercise; eating spicy foods and taking the herb- hawthorne can improve poor circulation |
| Sleep deprivation: Produces free radicals; sleep restores and repairs your skin. Go to bed before 9 or 10pm | Psychological stress: Produces free radicals; depletes nutrients; causes glycation. Use stress reduction strategies. | Estrogen depletion Causes collagen reduction and dry skin (see menopause section) |
| Excess Caffeinated drinks: Reduces minerals, dehydrating; limit to one small coffee daily or drink decaf green or herbal tea instead | Excess alcohol: reduces minerals; free radical overload; overwhelms liver Drink only one glass of red wine daily or less | Poor thyroid function: Creates bags under eyes.(see thyroid section) |

*Our skin needs additional vitamins, minerals and phytonutrients to build up its support structure; help repair damage; slow its aging; and keep it radiant. Other components of an anti-aging skin-healthy diet and lifestyle include:*

| | | | |
|---|---|---|---|
| Adequate protein (cysteine and methionine): egg yolks, yogurt, poultry | Selenium: nutritional yeast, brazil nuts, liver, sea food, mushrooms | Silicon (hair/ nails also): horsetail herb, alfalfa, cucumbers, asparagus, avocado, rice bran, oat bran, drink diluted watermelon juice | Zinc: oysters, herring, beef, lamb, egg yolks pumpkin seeds, ,ginger root, peas |
| Sulfur: the "beauty mineral:" egg yolks, meat, fish, poultry, legumes, onions, garlic, kale, cabbage, cruciferous<br><br>MSM supplement | Lycopene: In studies women with higher concentrations of lycopene had smoother skin: Tomatoes and sauce, watermelon, pink grapefruit | Gamma linoleic acid (GLA) moisture retention, fluidity and flexibility to skin cells: evening primrose oil, borage oil, red current, hemp seed oil, organ meats, spirulina, chlorella | B-Complex vitamins: nutritional yeast, organ meats, beef, eggs, fish, sweet potato, avocado. Vitamin B5 can be taken to decrease skin aging |
| Preventing/reducing age spots from sun damage (photo-aging): aloe vera- (topically) Boswellia cream, Selenium, vitamins A, C and B | Hyaluronic acid: a natural internal moisturizer: homemade chicken bone broth simmered for 24+ hours | Mineral-rich foods/teas: sea vegetables, leafy greens, soaked sunflower seeds, horsetail, alfalfa and nettle teas | Telomere lengthening: People who look younger have longer telomeres (See telomere section) |
| Moisturizing Foods: eat avocado, olive oil, olives, coconut oil, borage oil, grape seed oil, omega-3s, and vitamin A rich foods: eggs, butter, liver, cod liver oil | Hydrating Foods: filtered water, green tea, mineral waters<br><br>herbal teas: calendula, chamomile, witch hazel, rose hips, peppermint | Skin Tighteners: asparagus, black eyed peas, celery, rhubarb, peanuts.<br>Facial exercises have also been found to aid in maintaining skin tightness (See Facial Magic program) | Foods to prevent skin sagging: chickpeas, clams, rosemary, dates, eggs, brazil nuts, green peas, spirulina, shiitake mushrooms, crab, chocolate, sesame, sunflower seeds, leafy greens, yellow/orange foods |

## Topical Everyday Natural Moisturizers for Mature Skin

| Raw Extra Virgin Coconut Oil or Red Palm oil: Moisturizing cooking oils found in natural food stores. Dab on your skin. | Vitamin E: Prick open a vitamin E capsule and apply to skin at night.<br><br>Rosehip seed oil has been shown to regenerate skin and reduce wrinkles. | Aloe Vera Gel: The famed youthful beauty of Cleopatra came from aloe vera usage. (obtain from whole plant)<br><br>Also known to reduce photo-aging dark spots. | Green tea: As a skin toner. Many youthful looking Japanese women apply it to their face. Anti-inflammatory, antioxidant protection, tightens pores. Dab on with cotton ball or put in spray bottle. |
|---|---|---|---|

## Hydrating/Toning Herbs to Steam Face With

(Put in a bowl with steaming water, cover head with a towel and lean over bowl)

| Chamomile flowers | Eucalyptus leaves | Rosemary leaves |
|---|---|---|

## Mature Skin Facial Mask

Use 1-2 tsp. dark *Manuka* honey from New Zealand. Apply to your face for 10 minutes or more, then rinse. The honey encourages skin to make hyaluronic acid; a compound that plumps up skin owing to its ability to absorb 3,000 times its weight in water. The honey then forms a delicate mesh like collagen structure on the skin.

See chart on next page for other youth enhancing ideas.

## Delaying Other Visible Signs of Aging

| Varicose Vein Prevention/Support | Hair Loss/Graying Hair/Dry Hair | Nail Splitting, Soft Nails | Menopausal facial Hair |
|---|---|---|---|
| Causes: Decreased ability to breakdown fibrin; poor diet; low fiber; long periods of standing; straining on the toilet; Vitamins E, C and A deficiency; essential fatty acid deficiency; poor circulation; liver malfunction, and constipation (see digestion and liver section) | Hair Loss: usually indicates a sluggish thyroid or liver. Unhealthy dry hair: Can be due to low thyroid/poor liver function/or nutrient depletion. (see sections) Hair growth aids: B vitamins, alfalfa | A zinc deficiency often causes weak nails Low thyroid and digestive functioning also can trigger weak and splitting nails Take silica tablets or alfalfa, horsetail, cucumbers, asparagus, avocado Biotin-rich foods: Nutritional yeast, eggs, legumes, mushrooms, salmons, sardines Biotin suplm't: 2.5 mg | Hormonal Estrogen/Testosterone Imbalances often are the cause of facial hair in mature women. (see hormone section) High levels of DHT (testosterone conversion) promotes facial hair. Take saw palmetto: 160 mg twice daily. Also useful for hair loss on head during menopause. |
| Supportive activities: Walk, bike ride, jog or swim to push pooled blood back into circulation. Increase fiber and berry consumption; elevate legs when possible; go barefoot on wet grass; walk in ocean; take Epson salt baths; Increase fibrinolytic activity of the blood: cayenne, garlic, onions, ginger, bromelain (on empty stomach) Herbs: hawthorne, horse chestnut, butcher's broom Supplements; Pycnogenol/grape seed extract (protects capillaries) vitamin C-3,000mg. in divided doses | Graying hair has been found to be triggered by diminishing catalaze enzyme activity, stress, and mineral and vitamin B depletion, (eat beef liver, organ meats, avocado, nutritional yeast, leafy greens, alliums) and/or take Pantothenic Acid 500 mg Paba: 1,000 mg Folic acid 800 mcg For high minerals: Molasses, (1 Tbsp.) Seaweed, horsetail, nettle root, oat straw. Cured fo-ti herb capsules or tea to maintain/restore hair color (use under professional supervision) | A poor digestive system is also linked to weak nails, as necessary minerals for the nails may not be properly absorbed (See digestive section) | |

## Graceful Aging and the Mind-Body-Spirit Connection

It appears that negative emotions can also accelerate the visible signs of aging. According to Dr. Hema Sundaram, dermatologist, and author of *Face Value, the Truth about Beauty-and a Guilt Free Guide to Finding It*, there are seven emotions that age us. They are:

| Envy | Guilt | Fear | Anger | Self-Criticism | Pessimism | Perfectionism |
|------|-------|------|-------|----------------|-----------|---------------|

Dr. Sundaram asserts that these seven emotions are hurtful to our inner spirit; and as a result can age us prematurely. She speaks to the fact that letting these negative emotions have power over our lives can destroy our beauty by dwarfing our inner spirit. However, as mentioned earlier, if we can redirect the energy that we are expending on these negative emotions, and reframe our thoughts into positive perspectives, we can then express the loftiest aspects of our soul; which inherently radiates beauty.

Practicing positive affirmations daily and having a gratitude practice often can change our unbecoming attitudes; and help our inner beauty to shine through. These activities also have been found to slow down the aging process. Additionally, Dr. Sundaram emphasizes that feeling happy and having a positive opinion about ourselves really can make us look good.

In fact, there is an old saying that wisely states: "There is no cosmetic for beauty like happiness." It is a wonder how a warm self-assured smile or a contented feeling from within can truly light up a person's eyes and face. This is what makes us truly beautiful. If truth be told, some women feel that they become more beautiful as they age; as their face reflects the growth of their soul. It is time for us in middle age to embrace our inner and outer beauty. We can look and feel beautiful (or attractive) at any age! A helpful approach to use when we find ourselves criticizing our looks as we age is to immediately find one aspect of ourselves that we like; and dwell on this aspect instead.

- ♥ Affirmation: I can feel and look vibrant and beautiful (or attractive) at any age. My inner beauty shines through!

**Exercise 24: Graceful Aging:** *Input/print-out any useful charts or information to help delay the visible signs of aging. If I criticize my looks, I will immediately find one aspect of myself that I like.*

# Chapter 25

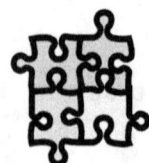 ## Putting it All Together: Key Vibrant Aging Takeaways

I have taken you through a tremendous amount of health information in the course of this book, and it may be daunting to try to adhere to all the recommendations. However, the material put forth in this book is just a framework to work with. It is not designed to be a hard and fast rulebook to be followed rigidly or compulsively. You will have much more success if you notice what suggestions call to you; and then follow them in a balanced and relaxed manner.

Similarly, what you will want to do is to cultivate an intention to eat well, and to stay in balance by keeping physically active; managing stress well; and ensuring adequate relaxation and sleep. You will also want to strive to eat as close to nature as possible by choosing foods that are whole, unprocessed, or minimally processed, and locally grown. These clean foods are higher in nutritional value, and are foods that our genes and biochemistry are adapted to; and which our ancestors ate for millennia. If you follow your ancestors lead and eat in a similar manner, you will be able to sustain good health as you age. By eating this way your body will allow you to live up to your full potential as a vibrant, creative human being. You will also be pleasantly surprised at the powerful changes that you will witness in your life when you decide to take control of your health.

I wish you all the best on your path to long-lasting health. Remember, our best years are not behind us, but in front of us!

*Die young at a very old age!* Vikram Khanna

---

### Tips to Cultivate a Health-Enhancing Lifestyle

- Wake up in the morning with grateful thoughts. Cultivate optimism.
- Develop a sense of meaning and purpose to animate your inner life.
- When you notice yourself having unproductive or stressful thoughts: practice a few rounds of deep breathing and some positive affirmations. Reframe the thoughts.
- Nurture a sense of humor. Don't take yourself too seriously!
- Walk barefoot on grass whenever possible for 20-30 minutes or more when the weather is warm- to absorb inflammation-fighting free-electrons.

- Sun bathe for 20-30 minutes between 10 and 2 pm. from spring through fall to obtain about 10,000 IUs of vitamin D. The sun is the best source of vitamin D.
- Keep active. Try to do some form of exercise in the morning. Yoga, stretching, strength training, or walking. Stand up every 20 minutes if seated for a long period of time. Exercise maintains balance and mental and psychological health; and reduces risk of chronic health challenges and degenerative diseases.
- Try to address addictive coping behaviors.
- Develop an inner life. Take a few minutes several times a day to regain mindfulness. Repeat affirmations or perform some deep breathing.
- Take time out for yourself every day.
- Keep your mind active and involved. Our brain has regenerative capacity and can make new neurons if we use it.
- Take therapeutic baths with Epson salt, sea salt and baking soda.
- Stress management. Find out what calms and centers you. Most of us have stressful lives; we just have to find positive ways to cope with it.
- Maintain a strong social network and rely realistically on the support of family and friends. Enhance social connections by being involved in group activities or doing service work. Spend time with positive supportive people. It can reduce your risk for heart disease and other degenerative diseases.

---

## Get Organized

Many of us make poor food choices due to a lack of high quality food on-hand; or because there is nothing already prepared in the refrigerator. That is why it is important to take the time one day each week to spend a few hours writing up a weekly meal plan; shopping for food; and cooking some meals beforehand. The meal plan does not have to be rigid. The idea here is to have prepared food on hand whenever you get hungry.

- Write up a shopping list that you determine from your meal plan for a week's worth of food. Write this up before you head to the store.
- Have on hand (in car/office etc.) an emergency food bag that you can eat if you get hungry when you're-on-the go. This will keep you from eating poor quality food. Examples: a small bag of nuts; a can of sardines or salmon; a bag of nori sea weed; veggie sticks etc.
- Chopping up vegetables for your meals and salads will be a major part of your food preparation. Ideally you should chop up your veggies right before your meal- as chopped vegetables loose nutrients if not eaten right away. However, many people

find chopping very time consuming. In this case, when there are time constraints, cutting up veggies ahead of time will provide you with prepared salads and snacks to have on hand to grab and go. It's suggested to prepare one big covered container of crunchy salad, and another container of veggie sticks such as celery, carrots, jicama, red peppers, or cucumbers. You can add the leafy veggies to the salad (lettuce and spinach) when you are ready to leave; as they wilt easily when mixed into salads. You may also want to cut up some vegetables for your meals so they are ready to go when you make dinner after work. Having organic frozen veggies on-hand is another time-saving meal prep option.

- Cook-up a big pot of soup, grains or beans at the beginning of the work week to have for lunches, snacks and meals for that week.
- Another recommended time saver is to double or triple recipes and freeze some for later use.
- Use a crock pot: prepare recipe in the morning. It will be done when you come home from work.
- Make up a quick salad dressing to have on hand. This will stand-in for most commercial salad dressings on the market that use bad oils and high fructose corn syrup. Blend 2 parts olive oil with 1 part raw apple cider vinegar; add 1-2 tsp. of Dijon mustard (optional) and 1-2 chopped cloves of garlic. Season to taste with sea salt and pepper. Add some of your favorite herbs: oregano, basil, and thyme are good. You can even add a couple anchovy fillets. Substituting lemon juice for the vinegar is also a tasty option.
- Multi-task in the kitchen: soak or sprout beans, grains, and nuts and seeds while you are unpacking your groceries. Cook soups and grains, or bake some meat or winter squash for the future while you are making dinner.
- Once a month plan to prepare a big pot of bone broth that can be stored for later use by pouring in ice cube trays. Use as a base in soups and other dishes. You can also purchase bone broths in the refrigerated section of health food stores.
- Once a month plan to prepare a 2 quart glass jar of fermented vegetables. (or buy from health food store in refrigerated section)
- Make a pot of marinara sauce once a month (lycopene rich) to top veggies, grains and meats. Freeze in ice cube trays and use when needed.
- Once or twice a month plan to prepare some probiotic dairy, almond or coconut yogurt or kefir. *Cultures for Health* or *Body Ecology* sell many starter cultures. You can also buy an inexpensive yogurt maker at Cultures for Health. Alternatively, you can purchase unsweetened "Live and Active" yogurt and kefir at health food stores.

- Soak grains, nuts, beans and seeds in filtered water to release mineral binding phytates. You can also sprout these for additional enzymes and nutrients. Many health food stores are also starting to sell sprouted grains.

---

### *Nurture Healthy Eating Routines: Eat as Close to Nature as Possible.*

- Drink the juice of ½-1 fresh lemon with water upon rising, for alkalinity after sleeping and for liver cleansing.
- Periodically check your digestion and stomach acid status upon rising with the baking soda home assessment. If HCL levels seem to be low: eat bitter foods or apple cider vinegar and water before meals to stimulate production and aid absorption of protein and minerals. Additionally, it may be advantageous to use stress reduction strategies. Supplements may also be needed. (See protein digestion section.) Check you digestive enzyme status periodically by taking the digestion self-assessment quiz. Digestive enzymes may be called for if symptoms exist.
- Increase intake of fresh organic foods. They are higher in antioxidants, vitamins and minerals and free of toxic chemicals. Shop at farmers' markets or join a CSA.
- Eat a varied and diverse diet to provide a large selection of different nutrients in different ratios.
- Eat a protein-rich breakfast within an hour of rising for blood sugar control. The old adage "Eat breakfast like a king; lunch like a prince; and supper like a pauper" recently has gotten scientific backing.
- Drink half your weight in ounces of filtered water daily to support detoxification and circulation. Bring a glass or stainless steel water bottle with you to work etc.
- Make small changes to your diet. Reduce one type of vitamin robber that you consume on a regular basis such as white flour products, sugar, coffee, alcohol etc. Example: eliminate one can of soda or one cup of coffee or one drink a week. Be an informed consumer; read labels to minimize consumption of artificial and draining ingredients. A healthy product should contain 5 ingredients or less on the label. (Unless there are some natural herbs)
- Practice portion control and calorie restriction. Slowly readjust your portion sizes. Starchy carb servings should be about the size of your fist or less (or ½ cup); meats should be about the size of your palm. Practicing calorie restriction (by 10-30%) without malnutrition has been shown to consistently extend lifespan and improve health. It has also been revealed in research studies to improve a number of biomarkers of aging by as much as 70%, including reversal of glycation; reduction in inflammation; reduction in oxidative stress; improved brain function; and a

beneficial effect on DHEA and Human Growth Hormone. Practicing portion control can take some time if you suffer from leptin resistance or blood sugar imbalances. (See weight management section) It becomes easier, however when you eliminate all grains; high glycemic fruits; and cashews- as these trigger overeating.

- Eat clean protein at every meal for immunity, growth, repair and maintenance of skin, blood, organs, neurotransmitters, and hormones etc. Eat protein to curb sugar cravings. (See protein formula)
- Eat healthy fats at every meal for heart and brain health, immunity, inflammation control, energy production, fat soluble vitamins and satiety. Fat doesn't make you fat, sugar does! (Avocados, olive oil, olives, nuts, seeds, butter, coconut oil, omega-3 sources etc.)
- Eliminate all trans fats and partially hydrogenated oils.
- Decrease or eliminate consumption of polyunsaturated oils such as soy, corn, sunflower, safflower, peanut, and canola. Inflammation promoting
- Eat non-starchy carbohydrates at every meal; such as leafy and crunchy veggies and low-glycemic fruits for detoxification, minerals, vitamins and antioxidant protection. Try to eat 5-10+ veggies daily and 1-3 low-glycemic fruits daily. (unlimited lemons and limes) Have a leafy and crunchy salad with olive oil dressing and raw apple cider vinegar daily. Cover half of your plate or more with veggies.
- Eat three portions of veggies in a meal for every serving of protein for alkalinity; and one serving of a healthy fat per meal.
- Eat several small snacks daily to stabilize blood sugar and to prevent fatigue, especially if you suffer from blood-sugar imbalances.
- Decrease consumption of gluten-containing grains (wheat, rye, barley, and commercial oatmeal) to decrease digestive issues and inflammation. Increase consumption of easily digested, mineral-rich gluten-free grains. (Basmati rice, millet, quinoa, buckwheat, amaranth, organic corn etc.) Don't eat the same grains at every meal. Mix them up to avoid immune reactivity. Levels 2 and 3: Decrease grains and substitute with winter squashes, cooked root veggies, sweet potatoes, and yams etc.
- Increase fiber consumption to 35+ grams daily. Have 2 Tbsp. flax meal daily. Add fiber-rich beans, avocado, nuts, seeds, berries, coconut flakes and kale to your daily routine.
- Decrease consumption of grain flour products (breads, pasta, baked goods, chips, crackers etc.) and substitute with nut or bean flour products or eat starchy carbs in their whole form; such as whole grains, winter squash, and sweet potatoes.
- Invest in a sprouting jar: sprouted food contains more nutrients- especially enzymes and vitamin C. Sprout beans, seeds and grains. Sprouted grains are now sold in bulk bins in health food stores. Add bean and seed sprouts to salads and in smoothies.

- Plan to add at least one liver-boosting <u>bitter food</u> such as: arugula, dandelion greens, or parsley daily to your meal plan.
- Add booster foods (aka superfoods) to your daily routine to increase antioxidant protection, detoxification, energy and cancer prevention such as: seaweed, green powder algae, nutritional yeast, cultured and fermented foods, fermented cod liver oil, flax meal etc.
- Add spices and herbs to all of your meals and snacks: anti-inflammatory, antioxidant, anti-viral, antibacterial, cancer and cardio protective.
- Drink health and longevity-enhancing teas regularly: green tea, rooibus, nettles, horsetail, oat straw, comfrey, dandelion root and tulsi. (hot or cold) Liver, bone, stress and cancer protective.
- Carry out a simplified diet cleanse or fasting program seasonally (in hot weather) to support digestion and liver function.
- Aim to get in at least one source of the antioxidants vitamin A, C, E, selenium and zinc at each meal. Strive to eat at least one blue/purple colored fruit daily and several servings of carotenoids at each meal. Consume carotenoids with some form of fat to facilitate absorption. Eat B-vitamin sources at each meal. Try to get in a vitamin K2 source daily.
- Eat slowly and peacefully. Take at least a half hour to eat your lunch and dinner and take 15 minutes to eat your snacks. Savor your food, and be grateful.

## Daily Food Servings

| Proteins: 3-4 servings<br>3 oz. animal<br>6 oz. vegetable | Nuts and seeds:<br>2 -6 Tbs. | Booster foods: 2-4+ servings daily.<br>(n. yeast, seaweed, algae, spices/herbs) | Fruits: 1-3 servings<br>½ cup or 1 medium<br>(unlimited lemon and lime) |
|---|---|---|---|
| Crunchy/leafy veggies:<br>5-10+ servings daily<br>1 cup raw leafy, ½ cup cooked leafy, ½ cup crunchy | Starchy vegetables: 1-3 servings daily-<br>½ cup | Whole grains: 1-3 servings daily (or none)<br>½ cup | Fluids: ½ your body weight in oz. of water, tea, broth, or veggie juice |

## Tips to Increase Veggies and Fruits in Your Daily Diet:

For all-day antioxidant protection and cancer and disease prevention, plan to eat 5-10+ servings of organic veggies a day. (3-6 plus cups) Vegetables are nutritional powerhouses, and shouldn't be short-changed. Purchasing organic vegetables will provide you with tons more vitamins, minerals and antioxidants than conventionally grown produce. Arrange to have veggies at breakfast, lunch, snacks and dinner to neutralize free-radicals throughout the day.

High chlorophyll leafy greens are especially powerful as they help cleanse the blood, and provide significant amounts of magnesium, calcium, vitamins A, C and E, plus vitamin B6. Cooked cruciferous veggies such as broccoli, kale, collards, cabbage, turnip greens and bok choy etc. help neutralize toxins and defend the body against hormone related cancers such as breast, ovarian, and prostate. Adding sprouts to meals also increases our nutrient status.

Don't forget to eat from the rainbow: orange, yellow, red, purple and green fruits and veggies. Strive to get in 5 different colors a day and try to eat a vegetable and a fruit for breakfast. Additionally, aim to eat three different colored fruits/vegetables at lunch and at dinner or more! Have veggies raw, steamed, sautéed, baked and fermented. In the summer or in hot climates attempt to have about 80% raw veggies and 20% cooked veggies. In the winter or in cold climates it is advised to eat more cooked veggies and less raw. According to food scientist Shirley Corriher, mineral loss from cooking is minimal, but vitamin loss from cooking varies. Many vegetables only lose 20% or less vitamins from cooking; however if vegetables are cooked above 105 degrees- vitamin C and vitamin B2 will be lost. Conversely, cooking increases nutrient and antioxidant availability of carrots, tomatoes, spinach and mushrooms.

* <u>Level one</u>: Eat 5 veggie servings daily. Levels 2 and 3: eat 7+ veggie servings daily.

*<u>All levels</u>: Eat 1-3 fruit servings daily. (Emphasize low glycemic) High glycemic fruit is okay in small amounts. (Mango, pineapple, papaya etc.) Limit dry fruit to a small quantity. You can have an unlimited amount of lemon or lime juice.

- Vegetable serving size is ½ cup crunchy or ½ cup <u>cooked</u> leafy or 1 cup <u>raw</u> leafy
- Fruit serving size: ½ cup or one medium piece of fruit
- Have a breakfast salad with ½ cup cucumbers, ½ cup tomatoes, a sliced fig, and red onion to taste. Top with lemon and olive oil. Shredded jicama, raisins, and carrots with lemon/oil dressing is also a tasty breakfast salad.
- Keep a covered bowl of cut-up veggies in the fridge to grab easily; also to bring to work to use with dips. This will help you avoid office snacks.
- Have a big antioxidant-boosting tossed salad daily. Besides the usual mixed leafy salad greens and spinach; add crunchy veggies: grated beets, grated fennel bulb, celery, carrots, shredded jicama, raw green beans, raw zucchini, red peppers, tomatoes, radishes, chopped raw garlic clove, dulse sea weed, chopped red onions, scallions, or shallots. Consider adding herbs such as: grated ginger, dandelion, fresh basil, fresh rosemary leaves, fennel leaf, dill leaf, arugula, parsley, and cilantro. Some

other nice additions are: sunflower seeds, nuts, olives, fresh figs, artichoke hearts, avocado slices, sprouts, (sunflower, mung, pumpkin seed, alfalfa, lentil etc.) snow peas and garbanzo beans. Keep salad in a large covered glass container to grab and go for lunch. It will keep for several days. Leafy greens wilt-put them into your salad before you leave the house.

- Add mushrooms to your dishes. Asian mushrooms such as shiitake, maitake, reishi, cordyceps and lion's mane are considered both a food and a medicine, as they are packed with protein, B-vitamins, minerals and immune boosting compounds. Regular consumption is known to reduce cancer risk. However it is recommended to not eat mushrooms raw, as they are poorly digested and contain small amounts of toxins. The toxins are destroyed by cooking or drying however. Cooking also boosts their nutrients.
- Increase veggie consumption by adding leafy greens to soups, stir fries, casseroles, beans and stews. They shrivel up and are barely noticeable after cooking.
- Grate carrots, zucchini, beets and summer squash into sauces, stews or in casseroles.
- Make a pot of marinara tomato sauce and pour over cooked veggies.
- Stock up on organic frozen veggies for easy meal prep when you are strapped for time. They don't need to be chopped up. You can add them to beans and meat dishes.
- Substitute mashed avocado for mayonnaise (rancid oils) on breads and in tuna salads, or make your own.
- Make vegetable based guacamoles, pesto's, pates and salsas as a dip for veggies or crackers; or to put into romaine lettuce wraps or nori seaweed wraps.
- Buy or make crispy kale chips with coconut or olive oil, instead of potato or corn chips.
- Go to restaurants with salad bars when going out for lunch or dinner.
- Steam veggies, then top with melted butter, garlic powder, sea salt, lemon and dill. (Dried or fresh.)
- Make quick creamy vegetable soups by sautéing in oil for five to ten minutes: onions, garlic, dark leafy greens, broccoli and carrots etc. Add herbs such as parsley, thyme, rosemary etc. Include broth, cream, yogurt or water and blend in a blender. The choices are endless. Have fun experimenting!
- Add veggies, such as onions, tomatoes, spinach and mushrooms to egg dishes (scrambled, poached, omelet etc.)
- Add sea veggies (sea weeds) to soups, salads, casseroles, grains or eat plain. Top nori seaweed- sushi style with avocado, sliced carrot, cucumber and tamari sauce.
- Have a bowl of fruit on the counter or desk for easy access at home or work.

- Buy frozen berries to add to smoothies. They are also a good ice cream replacement alone or blended with coconut milk, or yogurt and stevia. Use instead of sugary deserts.
- Cut up raw fruits such as apples for easy access. Squirt with lemon or lime juice to keep from browning. Dip apple slices in almond butter and sprinkle with cinnamon.
- Squeeze lemon and lime juice onto steamed or sautéed veggies; squeeze juice into filtered or sparkling water or green tea. Squeeze lemon or lime juice onto salads.
- Grate the peel or pith from lemons, tangerines, or oranges and add the zest to smoothies, salads and cereals etc. (Antioxidant rich)
- To easily boost your veggie intake; make fresh veggie juices using carrots, celery, spinach, parsley, garlic and beets etc. (daily or weekly) Dilute with water.
- Sauté kale and tomatoes in coconut oil with a clove of garlic and red pepper flakes
- Steam broccoli with 1 T. fresh ginger; add 1 T. tamari. Top with red pepper flakes; 1 tsp. of toasted sesame oil and 1 tsp. toasted sesame seeds. (toast raw seeds on a dry hot pan for a minute)
- Slow roast root veggies such as beets, carrots, daikon radish, and turnips; toss with coconut oil, sea salt and ½ tsp. rosemary, or 1 tsp. thyme or oregano. Bake for about 1 hr. or until soft at 250 degrees.
- Make a quick whole grain salad using left over quinoa or brown rice. Add diced veggies and onion or garlic with the herbs- parsley, basil or cilantro. Dress with olive oil and vinegar or lemon juice.
- Sauté dark leafy greens in oil with garlic or onion, and add a splash of apple cider vinegar (very tasty with Swiss chard)
- Cut in half any winter squash, and sprinkle pumpkin pie spice, or sage on top. Bake.
- Make a shredded beet and carrot salad: add chopped cilantro or parsley and top with some sunflower seeds. Cover with a lemon/olive oil dressing and garlic.
- To ensure the removal of thyroid suppressing goitrogens from selected vegetables thoroughly steam, bake or sauté the following goitrogen containing veggies: bok choy, broccoli, broccolini, Brussels sprouts, cabbage, cauliflower, Chinese cabbage, choy sum, collard greens, kai lan, kale, kohlrabi, mizuna, mustard greens, radishes, rapini, rutabaga, tatsoi, turnips. Note: a small amount eaten raw occasionally will not hamper thyroid function.

## Breakfast Ideas

- Try to include vegetables in your breakfast: celery stalks and carrot sticks; breakfast salads; cooked greens with eggs; pumpkin and celery in smoothies etc.
- Organic butter (raw and pastured-best) is a high quality fat and can be used in small quantities in your breakfast dishes.
- Green smoothies are one of the most nourishing breakfasts and a wonderful start to the day. They are high in protein, phytonutrients, minerals and fiber. See smoothie recipe on the healthy aging meal plan in the next section. If you are still hungry after drinking the smoothie- have a breakfast salad; nut butter on a celery stick, oatmeal, steel cut oats or buckwheat hot cereal on the side.
- "Live and Active" yogurt or kefir- Add cinnamon and nutmeg; a handful of fresh raspberries; nuts and seeds; and a Tbsp. of flax meal.
- Buckwheat cereal (Pocono brand) with berries, nuts, whey protein powder and almond milk
- *Food for life Ezekiel* sprouted grain granolas with ½ c. kefir or yogurt and berries
- Quinoa flakes from *Ancient Harvest* or in bulk section of health food store. Add nuts, flax meal; and kefir, yogurt or raw milk.
- Oat meal or steel cut oats with 1 T. flax meal; 1 T. unsweetened coconut flakes, a handful of raw nuts; and ½ cup berries, with stevia (levels 1 and 2) Soak cereal and nuts overnight.
- 2-3 Poached eggs with garlic and steamed greens or pesto sauce on top. You can also put the eggs over oatmeal. (Savory style) with salt and pepper.
- 3 oz. salmon, halibut or sardines with 1 cup sautéed veggies and ½ cup quinoa
- Sprouted buckwheat cereal with almond milk, 1/4 tsp. nutmeg and 1/2 tsp. cinnamon; add ½ cup berries, ¼ c. nuts, 1 T. flax meal and stevia.
- Chai spiced grain cereal (½- ¾ c. buckwheat, amaranth, quinoa, or millet soaked overnight/then cooked) with 1 cup coconut milk. Add spices: ½ tsp. cinnamon; 1/8 tsp. ginger; 1/8 tsp. each: nutmeg, cloves, and cardamom. Add ¼ c. nuts and 1 T. flax meal. Stevia to taste.
- Cold cereal: Lydia's Sprouted Cinnamon Cereal with raw milk, berries and flax meal or *Go Raw* Simple granola with almond milk, cinnamon and stevia
- Turkey bacon or chicken or turkey sausage (without sugars, preservatives, or hormones) with sautéed veggies.
- Homemade chicken bone broth soup with chicken bits and greens (common breakfast in Asian cultures.)

- Red bean and egg bowl or burrito. Sauté in oil: onion, garlic, cumin and oregano with previously cooked red beans. (small red, kidney or aduki) Pile bean mixture on top of eggs; add salsa or hot sauce.
- Quick scrambled eggs with spinach, tomato, dill, onion. Sprinkle with cheese or nutritional yeast.
- Whisk the French herb combo: fresh chervil, chives, parsley and tarragon into an omelet or scrambled eggs
- Add rosemary to ½ c. cooked sweet potatoes, or small red potatoes. Top with poached eggs and shredded beets or carrots.
- Whisk sage into a veggie frittata
- Egg omelet or scramble- topped with onion, cilantro, ½ sliced avocado and 1/2 cup pico del gallo sauce
- Note: to increase your vegetable consumption, consider adding a raw veggie (carrot, celery etc., at the end of your breakfast.

---

## Lunch and Dinner Ideas

- Remember: A serving of grains is only ½ cup or one slice of bread.
- A daily raw veggie salad is recommended for superior antioxidant protection and vitamin C.
- Have dinner leftovers for lunch.
- You don't always need a recipe to make delicious food. Just sprinkle organic garlic powder, sea salt, and fresh or dried oregano, rosemary, sage, or basil on meats or poultry for a quick and delicious meal. Lemon juice also works well with this. Dill, basil, parsley, chives, or tarragon taste great with garlic powder, lemon juice and sea salt on fish and seafood.
- Level one: Have sprouted grain bread or millet and flax bread (*Sam's Deli*) sandwich with avocado, sprouts, and organic turkey or chicken breast, (from Applegate farms or sliced from whole turkey or chicken) with a leafy and crunchy salad and olive oil vinegar dressing. Level 2; use 1 piece of bread; level 3: wrap this in a large seaweed sheet or romaine lettuce leaves.
- Basmati brown rice or quinoa and bean bowl cooked with onion, veggies, and tomatoes; seasoned with sage, sea salt, cumin, oregano or cilantro. Have it with a small salad.
- Substitute salmon for tuna in salmon salad sandwiches. Mix in mashed avocado, sea salt, and cut-up onions and celery into the salmon. Just as good as tuna salad!

- Homemade bean or meat vegetable soup with mixed green salad and a lemon, olive oil, garlic, cilantro or basil dressing.
- Poached, or baked fish (wild salmon, halibut, cod etc.) and a yam with veggies and a small salad.
- Top a large leafy and crunchy salad with a lump of chicken salad; or hummus, sardines, or salmon. Add *Annie's Natural's* salad dressings, or better yet make your own.
- Chicken or turkey chili with kidney beans, and a salad.
- Chicken, ground beef, fish or turkey taco seasoned with garlic, cumin and red pepper; placed in brown rice or teff tortillas, topped with lettuce, guacamole, and cilantro. Add a side-salad or steamed greens.
- Hearty meat or bean veggie stews with a salad.
- Chicken salad made with chopped chicken, mashed avocado, parsley, chopped celery and onions- on a bed of greens.
- Baked chicken leg with sautéed veggies and two small baked sweet potatoes. (Small potatoes eaten together contain more fiber than one large potato.)
- Turkey, chicken or ground beef bunless burgers served with oven baked sweet potato fries (tossed in coconut oil, garlic and rosemary) served with steamed greens, tomato and broccoli.
- Stir- fried veggies made with tamari, garlic, ginger, and sesame oil- combined with chopped tempeh or meat; with ½ c. quinoa or basmati brown rice.
- Poached salmon topped with a spinach-dill puree: 1 T. olive oil; 1 T. lemon juice; 1 clove garlic; a cup of cooked spinach, fresh dill, salt and pepper. Puree in blender.
- Slow roasted chicken sprinkled with fresh/dried sage and sea salt. (220 degrees for at least 2 hours) Done when bones lift out.
- Thai inspired sautéed ground turkey (1 lb.) made with 1 medium onion; 1 can of coconut milk; 2 tsp. (or more) green curry paste; 2 tsp. fish sauce; a bunch of basil or cilantro; and juice from 1 lime added at the end.
- Seafood Tacos: fish, shrimp, or scallops sautéed in butter with onions, garlic, oregano, cumin and salt. Add cilantro and squeeze of fresh lime at the end. Serve with organic stone ground corn or brown rice tortillas.
- Lentil or other previously cooked bean made into a salad with chopped onion, garlic, oregano, celery and parsley. Mix with ¼ cup olive oil and 2 T. lemon juice.
- Make a nut butter sauce to top fish, tempeh, veggies or grains: Blend ¼ c. nut butter with 1- 2 tsp. tamari; ¼ tsp. cayenne; clove garlic; a tsp. fresh ginger; and Tbsp. water. Pour over fish.

- Make a Moroccan inspired poultry or meat dish: Mix about a pound of meat with ½ tsp. each ground cumin, coriander, cinnamon, garlic powder, and ½ tsp salt. Add chopped leeks and carrots to pan. Bake as usual.
- Make a macadamia cream sauce to top veggies, seafood and grains: blend until creamy in blender: about 1/3 cup macadamia nuts with 1 garlic clove; the juice of ½ lemon; ¼ cup basil; and ½ tsp. sea salt. Add more lemon juice to thin.
- Make a curry poultry or vegetable dish with coconut milk, turmeric, cumin, ginger and garlic
- Make sage, oregano, basil or tarragon butter to pour on veggies, grains or meats. Simmer 1 stick of butter with ¼ cup chopped herbs until slightly browned. Pour over meal.
- Pesto is very versatile and quick to make, and can top meats, grains, eggs, fish, and veggies. Pesto also can be wrapped in romaine lettuce leaves or tortillas for lunch. Consider making pesto with basil, cilantro, spinach or sorrel.
  **Basil pesto**: Blend together in food processor: 3 cups fresh basil with ½-¾ cup olive oil; 4 garlic cloves; ½ cup walnuts; ½ cup parmesan cheese or nutritional yeast; and salt to taste. **Cilantro pesto** can be made with 3 cups cilantro; ½ cup olive oil; 4 cloves garlic; ½ cup sunflower or pumpkin seeds; 1 T. lemon juice; ½ cup parmesan or nutritional yeast; and salt to taste. **Spinach or sorrel pesto** can be made with 3 cups of the greens; ½ cup olive oil; 4 cloves garlic; 1/2 cup almonds or cashews; ½ cup parmesan cheese or nutritional yeast, and salt to taste.
- One easy and delicious way to get seaweed in your diet is to make a nori seaweed and grain salad with 8 cups cooked brown basmati rice, millet or quinoa; 2-4 cups nori seaweed; 1 tsp. grated ginger; scallions or onions; 1-2 tsp. brown rice vinegar, minced garlic cloves; and a large handful of cilantro or parsley.
  Dulse is also a versatile sea vegetable when added raw to dishes. It can add a unique flavor accent to potatoes, eggs, veggies, rice, quinoa, soups and salads. Or just eat it plain.

---

## Soup Ideas

Soups are a nice accompaniment to lunch or dinner, eaten with a large salad. **Bone stock** can be a very nutrition-packed base for any soup. Bone broths are easy to make. Simply put bones and skin from any animal in a large pot of filtered water with 2 Tbsp. of apple cider vinegar to draw out the minerals. You can add onions, garlic, carrots, celery and herbs such as parsley, thyme, rosemary, and bay leaf. Bring to boil; then skim off the scum on the top layer. Simmer it from 1-3 days. After cooking, strain out the liquid and freeze the broth in ice cube trays to add to other dishes to increase their nutrient levels. (Instead of water) It is invaluable as a base for soups. Don't forget the traditional immune-boosting chicken soup made with bone broth.

- o  Miso soup can be very quickly made. Just boil 1-1/2 cups water or bone broth with scallions, garlic wakame seaweed, carrots and tempeh or fish. Add 2-3 tsp. miso paste at the end and mix in.
- o  Bean soups are also easy. Just put soaked and drained dry beans (lentil, pea, black, pinto, aduki or cannellini) in a pot of water or bone broth. Add garlic, onions, carrots, celery and herbs such as oregano, bay leaf, parsley and thyme. Cook until beans and veggies are tender.
- o  Tomato soup is packed with heart-healthy lycopene. Cook one sliced onion; 3-4 garlic cloves; 2 large carrots; and 2 stalks celery in 4 Tbsp. butter until tender. Then stir in 2 (28 oz.) cans of tomato sauce or crushed tomatoes; 4 cups bone or vegetable broth; 2 Tbsp. chopped fresh basil; (1 Tbsp. dried) 1 Tbsp. chopped oregano; (1/2 Tbsp. dried) and 1 tsp. sea salt. Cook for 20 minutes. Pour soup into blender and puree until smooth.

---

## Snack Ideas

Snacks are important to help maintain blood sugar and energy levels throughout the day. They also give you an opportunity to add some extra antioxidant-rich veggies and fruits to your day.

- o  Celery sticks with almond butter or macadamia nut butter
- o  Baked apples with cinnamon and walnuts
- o  A mineral packed hummus dip made with garbanzo beans is an easy and great tasting snack to help you get over the afternoon slump. Just use 1- 15 oz. can of garbanzo beans or 2 cups cooked chickpeas; ½ cup sesame tahini; 5 Tbs. olive oil; ¼ cup fresh lemon juice; 4 medium cloves garlic; ½ tsp salt and a bunch of cilantro or artichoke hearts. Blend in a food processor. Eat ¼-½ cup hummus dip with 1 cup steamed or raw cut veggies. (carrots, celery, fennel, jicama, or red pepper sticks)
- o  Sardines have a strong fishy flavor, but can be made more palatable and tasty in a pate. Blend one 3.75 ounce can of sardines (in spring water) with 3/4 avocado; 2 cloves garlic; the juice of 1 lime and a bunch of cilantro or parsley. Blend in food processor. You can use it as a dip for celery sticks or wrap it in romaine lettuce leaves. It is also tasty on *Mary's Gone Crackers* crackers.
- o  Artichokes are also tasty as a pate. Blend a 14 oz. can of artichokes (rinse to remove citric acid) with ¼ cup broth; ¼ cup olive oil; 1/4 cup lemon juice; 1 cup walnuts; 1/4

cup red onion; 2 cloves of garlic; ½ tsp salt and 1 Tbsp. fresh basil or oregano. Puree until creamy. Use with veggie sticks.
- Kale chips are a great alternative to high carb grain chips. You can buy them in a package or make your own. Simply tear one bunch of thoroughly dried lacinato kale into small pieces and massage 1 Tbsp. of coconut oil or olive oil into the kale. Add sea salt to taste. You can add spice combinations to it, such as cumin, chili pepper and garlic powder; or dill, lemon and garlic powder. Mix everything together in a bowl. Spread the kale mixture flat on a baking sheet and bake for about 35 minutes (until crisp) at 300 degrees. Turn the leaves over half-way through baking.
- Make a guacamole paste: Mash one medium avocado; a chopped onion; 4 tsp. lemon or lime juice; one chopped medium tomato; fresh cilantro and sea salt to taste. Eat with a few baked blue corn chips (level one) or with whole grain crackers or with veggie sticks.
- Make homemade salsa with 2 cups tomatoes; a Tbsp. each of olive oil and lemon or lime juice; 1 medium onion; and chopped hot pepper or hot sauce to taste; add a handful of cilantro and sea salt. Eat with a few baked blue corn chips (level one) or on top of *Mary's Gone Crackers* crackers, or top beans with it.
- Make a bean and nut pate using cannellini beans. Blend a 15 oz. can or 1-1/2 cups cannellini beans with 2 Tbsp. lemon juice; 2 cloves garlic; 2 tsp. olive oil; 1 cup nuts; (almond or walnut) 1 bunch parsley; and sea salt to taste. Blend in a food processor. Put on whole grain crackers, nori sea weed wraps, lettuce wraps or use as a dip with veggie sticks
- Liver pate is also a great nutrient powerhouse to support flagging energy levels. Simply cook in a pan one large red onion (about ¾ cup chopped) with 2 cloves of garlic in 3 Tbsp. butter until tender. Add 1 lb. of organic chicken livers and cook for about 10 minutes. And ½ tsp. of salt and 1/8 tsp each ground cloves, nutmeg, ginger and black pepper. You can change up the spices and use 2 tsp. each thyme and sage instead of the clove/nutmeg combo. Cook for 5 minutes, and then blend in food processor. Great on whole grain crackers or wrapped in nori sea weed or lettuce wraps.
- Have ½ cup of berries with a small handful of almonds, walnuts, or pumpkin seeds.
- Have one cup of homemade buttered popcorn with 1 Tbsp. nutritional yeast and sea salt or tamari sauce to taste.
- Have a medium green apple sliced and topped with one Tbsp. almond butter and cinnamon.
- Have a small fruit with 3 dice-sized cubes of raw cheese. (if no sensitivity to cheese)
- Have a cup of veggie or bone broth.
- Have a small unsweetened fruit yogurt or kefir drink.

- Have a freshly juiced veggie juice.
- Have a glass of water with ¼ to 1 tsp. spirulina or chlorella blended in. (a great energy boost)
- Make a sea weed and nut snack mix. Mix ½ cup sunflower seeds; 1/2 cup almonds and ¼ cup walnuts with tamari sauce to taste. Tear 5 large sheets of raw nori seaweed into small pieces; add ½ tsp. sea salt and mix with the nut mixture. Spread mixture on a tray and put in oven on its lowest setting until the mixture is dry.
- Note: also refer to carb substitute chart for more snack examples.

## Dessert Ideas

A great deal of recent scientific research has proven that our physiology is not intended to tolerate an abundance of concentrated sugars and sweet tasting food. Our early hunter gatherer ancestors rarely consumed sweets or even fruits, as they had very little access to them. Occasionally, they might come upon raw honey, but their access to sweets; mostly berries, was seasonal and not steady or usual. However, our modern Western culture makes sweets too readily available; and for many of us this temptation is too hard to resist. Nevertheless, as I have pointed out many times in this book, the key to quality aging is to keep blood sugar levels stable, as sugar (any kind) raises triglyceride levels; increases belly fat; and drives multiple disease processes.

Strive to gradually cut-down on your consumption of sweets. The healthiest option to satisfy a sweet-tooth is to emphasize consumption of organic fruit. Fruit comes already packaged with health enhancing substances such as fiber, vitamins and antioxidants. Additionally fruit doesn't spike blood sugar levels at the level that concentrated sugars do. However, it is advised to make the majority of your fruit choices low-glycemic. Low-glycemic fruits, such as berries, cranberries, acai, sour green apples, kiwis, feijoas, and grapefruit should be the mainstay of your daily diet. Eating this way will retune your taste buds to enjoy the natural sweetness of lower sugar foods. You will even find that foods you never thought were sweet actually have a slight sweetness.

When you do desire a sweeter dessert, stevia is a healthy non-caloric natural sweetener option. It is extracted from the stevia rebaudiana plant and has been the subject of hundreds of studies over several decades. These studies have attested to stevia's health benefits such as regulating blood sugar; therefore it is a very beneficial sweetener to use when endeavoring to keep blood sugar levels stable and when attempting to avoid age-accelerating glycation. It has an outstanding safety profile and can be purchased as whole leaves, a green powder, a liquid extract, or a white powder. Ensure that the stevia is alcohol and additive free. (Level 3 can use the less processed stevia green powder or whole leaf stevia to naturally sweeten foods) Additionally, it has been found in studies to even lower blood pressure.

Individuals at Levels 2 and 3 can rely more on stevia when desiring to sweeten their foods. Individuals at level 1 may not be able to tolerate the taste of stevia, and can add a small amount (I Tbsp. or less) of buckwheat, manuka or tupelo honey; black strap molasses or Grade B or C maple syrup to their foods; as these sweeteners contain minerals and dietary antioxidants that help support their metabolism. (Sugar and high fructose corn sweeteners do not.) However, they do raise blood sugar if in high doses. Additionally, the darker the honey is, the higher the ORAC value. Other more healthful sweet alternatives for level one that provide some nourishment are: sorghum, amazake, barley malt, brown rice syrup, organic cane sugar, rapadura, date sugar, fruit juice concentrate, or palm sugar. (Eat infrequently, however,)

---

The following desserts can help you to satisfy your sweet tooth and assist you in steering clear of other more unhealthful temptations. Other options are in the high-glycemic swap-out chart.

- Frozen blueberries: A handful is very satisfying.
- Frozen blueberries w/ plain yogurt or coconut milk blended together w/stevia (to taste) in a food processor or blender. Similar to ice cream.
- Berry ice: blend until smooth- 2 cups frozen berries with 1-1/2 cups water and 2 Tbsp. lemon or lime juice in a food processor or high speed blender.
- Small frozen banana with cinnamon and crushed walnut pieces
- Chilled can of full fat coconut milk blended with 2 tbsp. cocoa powder and stevia. Blend in a blender.
- Fruit and plain yogurt smoothie with stevia
- Instant frozen yogurt: Blend 1 pound bag of frozen fruit with about ¾ cup Greek yogurt, and a dash of stevia in a food processor or high powered blender. Blend until smooth. No need to freeze, it is ready to eat.
- Cranberry, blueberry, raspberry or strawberry sorbet w/ stevia: Put berries, stevia and a cup or two of ice in a high speed blender or food processor. Blend until thickened.
- Avocado chocolate mousse: blend one avocado with ½ tsp. vanilla extract; 3 Tbsp. cocoa powder; and ½ cup of raw milk, or almond milk; plus stevia (to taste) in a food processor.
- Baked apple with cinnamon and chopped nuts.
- Drizzle a little raw honey on chopped nuts and toss. Roast on low temperature.

- o Baked figs with a sprinkle of cinnamon and nutmeg.
- o Organic antioxidant-rich dark chocolate with 70%+ cocoa content sweetened with stevia. (one square)
- o Pumpkin pie pudding: Blend together 1 cup chilled canned pumpkin w/ ½ cup chilled coconut milk; ½ tsp. of pumpkin pie spice, vanilla extract and stevia.

---

## Top Anti-Aging Foods

Making smarter food choices in midlife can regenerate our health, and add years to our life. That is why it is important to include food in our daily meal plan that offers the highest concentrations of easily digestible nutrients, vitamins, minerals and antioxidants. Adding foods recognized for their exceptionally high nutritional value beneficially affects one or more target functions in our body, and will support a healthy internal environment. This will make a big difference in our health; resulting in a reduction in disease risk factors and a slowing of the aging process.

I have provided a chart, and an explanation of some of my top picks for vibrant aging and longevity. Of course the book addresses many others. Consider emphasizing these foods in your daily or weekly health-promotion plan.

Note: some foods are very strong detoxifiers, and should be eaten in small amounts initially if you have not eaten them before; as they can result in uncomfortable detoxification symptoms. You can work up to higher quantities as your body stabilizes.

### Top Anti-Aging Nutrient Dense Foods

| Spirulina and chlorella powder or tablets | Seaweed | Fermented foods: veggies, kefir, yogurt etc. | Nutritional yeast | Fresh veggie juices<br><br>Sprouts | Green tea | Bone stock |
|---|---|---|---|---|---|---|
| Spices: Cinnamon Ginger | Undenatured, grass-fed Whey protein powder | Egg yolk and white (with DHA) | Parsley | Organ meats/ Liver | Cold water fish/ cod liver oil | Flax seed meal |
| Raw garlic | Turmeric | Fresh lemon juice | Beets | Cooked cruciferous veggies | Dark leafy greens | Carrots |
| Avocado | Tomato | Asian Mushroom | Cultivated Dandelion | Cranberry | Blueberry | Celery |

1. Algae Green Powders: (spirulina or chlorella) blood builders, detoxifiers, heavy metal removal, energy enhancing. Have ¼ tsp. - 1 Tbsp. daily. Start out slowly.
2. Cultured and fermented foods: (fermented veggies, cultured "live and Active" dairy or coconut/almond yogurts and kefirs) probiotics, immune boosting, aid digestion, antibiotic, anti-carcinogenic. Have 1 tbsp.-1/2 cup or more of fermented veggies at each meal. (Sauerkraut should be eaten in smaller amounts due to its anti-thyroid activity.) Start out slowly.
3. Sea vegetables (arame, kombu, dulse, wakame, nori, hijiki, sea palm etc.) youth enhancing, detoxification boosting, anti-carcinogenic, anti-biotic, anti-viral; thyroid health supportive; radioactive element detoxifier; degenerative disease prevention. Eat daily. Begin with nori sheets, as they are universally liked.
4. Nutritional Yeast: youth enhancing; stress supportive; energy, heart health and immune system boosting. Eat ¼ tsp.-2 Tbsp. daily. Start out slowly.
5. Green Tea: immune system booster; powerful anti-carcinogenic compounds; glycation preventative; anti-inflammatory; and anti-viral. 1-4 cups daily. Start out with one. Make sure to decaffeinate it later in the day by steeping the tea bag for 10 seconds in hot water; then pour out the water and refilling hot water into the cup with the leached tea bag.
6. Freshly juiced Vegetable juices: energy boosting; alkalinizing; liver cleansing; anti-carcinogenic. Daily or weekly. Start out with a glass one time a week.
7. Homemade bone stocks: youth enhancing, immune boosting; bone and joint supportive; calming; improves stomach HCL levels; repairs inflamed intestinal lining caused by leaky gut. Make a pot monthly and store in ice cube trays to add to your dishes. Eat bone broth soups for lunch and dinners on a regular basis.
8. Cinnamon: detoxification support; bone building; and blood sugar regulation support; prevents damaging protein glycation. 1 tsp. daily. Start out slowly.
9. Turmeric: anti-inflammatory; anti-carcinogenic; protects liver from toxins; lowers blood sugar; rheumatoid arthritis support. 1 tsp. daily. Start out slowly.
10. Organ meats/liver: The most nutrient-dense food! Anti-fatigue factor; bone, brain, nerve, heart, and eye health protection; slows aging process; ATP and cell mitochondria enhancer; anti-cancer agent; hormone production supporter; mood health and blood sugar balancer. Eat several times a week or more.
11. Wild cold water fish (canned or fresh): salmon, herring, cod, sardines, anchovy etc. or fermented cod liver oil: heart health supportive; anti-inflammatory. Take fermented cod liver oil daily in the winter for added vitamin D. Eat 3-4 times a week.
12. Flax seed: (ground into a meal at home with coffee grinder/freeze) richest source of fiber lignans: anti-carcinogenic; (especially breast and colon) digestive tract anti-

inflammatory; heart attack and stroke preventative; constipation supportive. 2 Tbsp. daily.

13. Raw garlic: Broad spectrum anti-biotic; anti-viral (combats viruses, parasites, bad bacteria) cardiovascular health supportive; anti-carcinogenic; immune booster; a good cold remedy. 1-3 cloves daily. Start out slowly. Eat more when coming down with a cold. You can also take aged garlic extract (supplement) for better breath.

14. Raw ginger: digestive tract tonic; anti-inflammatory; liver detoxifier; cardiovascular and arthritis supportive; glycation preventative. 1-4 ginger teas daily if have joint pain. (Boil a 1-2 inch fresh ginger piece for 20 minutes in several cups of water) Grate fresh ginger in foods.

15. Parsley: anti-carcinogenic; blood purifier; blood building; brain boosting; and eye health aid. A few leaves daily.

16. Fresh lemon/and juice: high medicinal value; high vitamin C levels; blood, lymph and liver purifier; aids in removal of residual toxins from medications. ½ to 1 freshly squeezed lemon with filtered water in the morning daily. Add lemon or peel to water throughout the day. Eat pith, and grate zest into foods.

17. Avocado: High fiber; cardiovascular health aid; balances blood sugar; blood and tissue renewal support; glutathione production support. ¼- 1 whole avocado throughout the day.

18. Tomatoes/tomato sauces and salsas: anti-cancer agent; (especially prostate, cervical, and pancreatic) detoxifier; male health aid; digestive disorder support; neutralizes animal based uric acid. (Avoid if have nightshade-sensitive arthritis.) 4 times a week or more.

19. Cooked cruciferous vegetables (glucosinolates): (broccoli, kale, Brussels sprouts cabbage etc.) Numerous anti-cancer compounds: exceptionally high in cancer combating activity; accelerates removal of toxic estrogen; suppresses colon polyp growth; immune system booster; and eye health support. Cook thoroughly to remove anti-thyroid goitrogens. Have three times a week or more.

20. Blueberries (especially wild) fresh or frozen: anti-carcinogenic; brain, memory and nervous system supportive; cardiovascular health aid; blood sugar regulation; degenerative eye health support. Stimulates genes that promote our longevity. (sirtuin genes) ½-1 cup daily.

21. Cranberries: anti-inflammatory; anti-carcinogenic; liver detox and bacterial infection support. Lung and breathing support. Eat fresh during the winter season. Eat frozen or juiced weekly in summer.

22. Dandelions (and other bitters-arugula, citrus peel etc.): liver cleanser; bile flow aid which supports detoxification; gall bladder support. Eat several times a week or daily. Start out slowly.

23. Asian mushrooms: (Shiitake, maitaki, lion's mane, reishi, cordyceps) fresh, (cooked) or sun dried; immune booster, anti-carcinogenic, CVD preventative, longevity tonic. Sun dried shiitake contain vitamin D. Eat several times a week or daily.
24. Red beets: aid lymphatic, gall bladder and liver function; circulation support; CVD prevention; male performance aid; brain health support. Eat several times a week or daily.
25. Leafy greens: (Kale, collard greens, spinach etc.) mineral, antioxidant and vitamin rich; packed with anti-cancer compounds; liver, nervous system and eye health support. Eat three servings daily. <u>Sprouts</u> are also a nutrient packed superfood, as the quality of the protein, fiber, vitamins and essential fatty acids is boosted after sprouting seeds and legumes.
26. Carrots: anti-carcinogenic; immune-boosting; infection fighting; stroke and heart disease preventative; eyesight supportive; (cataract and macular degeneration support) healthy skin booster. Eat 1-2 daily
27. Celery: high blood pressure prevention; (2-4 stalks a day) anti-cancer agent; aids kidney, liver and digestive functions; blood sugar regulator; eases water retention. Eat 1-4 daily.
28. Undenatured grass-fed whey protein powder: powerful immune booster; detoxifier; and muscle builder/repairer. 1 scoop- a couple of times a week or daily.
29. Eggs (with yolk) are considered the perfect food due to their exceptional protein profile and amazing storehouse of nutrients. They are mineral and B vitamin rich and contain the richest source of eye protective lutein and zeaxanthin. Eggs have a number of other health applications including: boosting memory; decreasing blood vessel damaging homocysteine; and enhancing thyroid and hormone balance.

See meal plan on next page. Meal plan recipes are all in <u>meal ideas</u> section on pages 260-266, or on pages 273-275.

# Vibrant Aging Meal Plan

**(Levels 2 and 3: Try to add a veggie to breakfasts/snacks. Add fermented veggies and sea weed.)**

|  | Day One | Day Two | Day Three | Day Four | Day five |
|---|---|---|---|---|---|
| Breakfast | Undenatured whey fruit smoothie w/ booster foods & hot buckwheat | 2-3 poached eggs topped with pesto sauce or steamed greens<br><br>Green apple | "Live and active" yogurt or kefir w/ raspberries, nuts, seeds, flax meal, shredded coconut, and cinnamon | Sprouted grain granola w/raw goat, or nut milk; whey protein, strawberries, flax meal, and seeds | 2-3 lightly scrambled eggs w/onion, spinach tomato and dill<br><br>3/4 cup of berries |
| Snack | Nori seaweed and nut snack mix | ½ cup berries and a handful of almonds, sunflower, or pumpkin seeds | Medium green apple (sliced) w/cinnamon, and spread w/ 1 Tbsp. almond butter. | Drink a cup of vegetable juice or mineral or bone broth.<br><br>½ c. cranberries | Small "live and active" kefir or beet kvaas drink.<br><br>Medium kiwi |
| Lunch | Baked chicken on a bed of mixed raw, leafy and crunchy veggies w/arugula & raw garlic clove. Dress with oil, basil and vinegar | Bone broth lentil and veggie soup<br><br>Serve with whole grain and nori seaweed salad<br><br>Fermented beets, carrots and ginger (pg. 275) | Ground turkey and kidney bean chili<br><br>Serve with a large leafy and crunchy green salad w/ cilantro, sprouts and oil and vinegar dressing | Tomato veggie soup<br><br>Serve with Mock tuna salad (canned salmon) on a bed of leafy and crunchy veggies with parsley and lemon oil dressing. | Stir-fried tempeh and bok choy dish seasoned w/tamari, garlic, sesame oil and ginger<br><br>Serve with miso and wakame seaweed soup<br><br>Carrot/beet salad |
| Snack | Humus dip w/ carrot, fennel and red pepper sticks | Sardine pate w/ veggie sticks, or romaine wrap, or *Mary's Gone Crackers* crackers | Tomato salsa w/ kale chips, *Mary's Gone Crackers* crackers, or carrot sticks | Nori seaweed sheets topped w/ avocado, carrot and cucumber slices; topped with tamari and ginger | Liver pate on a romaine lettuce wrap or on *Mary's Gone Crackers* crackers w/ carrot stick |
| Dinner | Wild poached salmon w/ spinach- dill puree, served w/ ¼ avocado and quinoa or 2 small sweet potatoes<br><br>Steamed mixed veggies with lemon/oil/dill<br><br>Small salad w/ parsley, sprouts and dressing | Grass-fed beef with sage-butter sauce and sautéed shiitake or other mushrooms w/ Br. basmati rice Served w/ steamed kale, carrots, swiss chard, and zucchini (dress with sage butter)<br><br>Small salad w/dandelion, shredded beets, sprouts and dressing | Black or red beans sautéed with onions, garlic, oregano, cumin, tomatoes and mixed veggies. <u>Serve on top of</u> basmati brown rice or quinoa w/ guacamole.<br><br>Baked butternut squash w/oregano<br><br>Small leafy and crunchy salad w/ rosemary, and lemon/oil dressing | Baked Chicken with marinara sauce<br><br>Sautéed broccoli raab with garlic and basil<br><br>Spaghetti squash - top with marinara<br><br>Small leafy and crunchy salad w/ arugula, sprouts and dressing | Steamed oysters or halibut served w/ macadamia cream sauce<br><br>Quinoa or baked kabocha squash sprinkled w/sage<br><br>Sautéed garlicky broccoli, carrots, and spinach<br><br>Small dandelion tossed salad w/dressing |

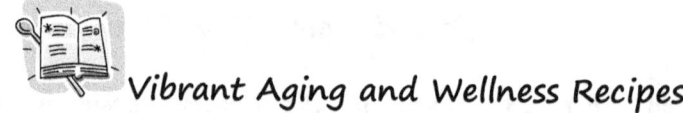 **Vibrant Aging and Wellness Recipes**

### Whey Protein Powder Smoothie

Undenatured whey protein smoothies are a superior breakfast alternative to acid-forming breakfast cereals, toast, pancakes or muffins. When we get up in the morning we are often dehydrated and have low blood sugar. Our body is also often overly acidic. Whey smoothies are particularly beneficial because the high protein liquids, and alkalinizing constituents alleviate all these issues. Whey also boosts our glutathione levels, immunity, and muscle development and repair: very important for healthy aging.

<u>Directions</u>: Blend together in a blender: 8-12 oz. almond milk, raw milk, kefir, coconut milk or green tea; ½ tsp.-3 tsp. spirulina or chlorella powder; ½ c. to ¾ c. blueberries; 1 tsp.-2 Tbsp. nutritional yeast; 1 tsp. cinnamon; and 2 Tbsp. flax meal. (To avoid rancidity ground the seeds in a coffee grinder and freeze in small batches). Add one scoop of non-denatured grass-fed whey just before you stop blending to preserve its immunoglobulins and lactoferrin. If you like it sweetened, you can add 1/3 banana, a few dates, or green stevia powder or liquid concentrate.

Additional nutrients can be added such as: 1-2 Tbsp. antioxidant-rich sour cherry, pomegranate, acai or cranberry concentrate; probiotic powder or liquid; chia seeds or raw nuts; 1 tsp. cod liver oil or coconut oil, or shredded coconut; 1/2 avocado; or some spinach, sprouts, canned pumpkin, or a couple of celery sticks. Some anti-inflammatory herbs can also be added such as ½ tsp. turmeric or ginger.

A number of individuals also like to add super-foods to provide powerful antioxidant protection such as: wheat grass juice, mangosteen, moringa, noni powder, aloe vera, rose hip powder, camu camu, bee pollen, royal jelly, propolis, maca, alfalfa, nettles, oat straw, citrus peel zest, cocoa powder, or nopal cactus etc. Have fun and experiment with it! Smaller quantities (¼ tsp) will not alter the flavor of the smoothie.

---

### Home-Made Almond Milk

Forgo the packaged and processed almond and nut milks and make your own! Commercial nut milks (even organic) contain youth-depleting rancid oils, sugars and additives. You can quickly and effortlessly whip-up your own.

Just place one cup of any nut or seed into a high speed blender or food processor with 3-4 cups of filtered water. You can add cinnamon, vanilla extract, a few dates or stevia, and blend on high until nuts are liquefied. Strain through a cheese cloth or strainer, and store in a glass bottle in the refrigerator. Enjoy!

---

### Vegetable Mineral Broth

This mineral broth is excellent for cleansing, alkalinizing, and building up and rejuvenating the body. It is an excellent source of electrolytes, and minerals. Drink it for breakfast or as an afternoon pick-me-up; and to optimize your mineral status.

Fill a large stainless steel pot with purified water. Add (chopped up) any selection of seasonal organic vegetables, such as:

Vegetables: celery*, carrots*, nettles, beet root,* spinach, kale, swiss chard, daikon radish, burdock root, cauliflower, broccoli, turnip*, dandelion (leaf and root), sweet potato, onions, garlic, leeks etc.     (*include leafy tops)

Add some spices or herbs such as: rosemary, thyme, parsley, oregano, sage, cilantro, bay leaves, and peppercorns. Add one tsp. sea salt and a few pieces of kombu seaweed. Simmer with lid on for 1-3 hours or longer; strain out the veggies, and drink the broth.

---

### Anti-Aging Homemade Bone Stock

Bone stock is a nutrient packed super-food! Bone stock is easy to make. Simply put bones, and skin (necks/backs/feet etc.) from any animal in a large pot of filtered water with 2 Tbsp. of apple cider vinegar to draw out the minerals. You can add onions, garlic, carrots and celery; and herbs such as parsley, thyme, rosemary, and bay leaf. Bring it to a boil then skim off the layer of scum that forms on top. You can simmer it from 1-3 days. Refrigerate the broth or freeze the broth in ice cube trays to add to other dishes and sauces later. And of course it is invaluable in soups.    Note: Chicken feet are especially collagen-rich.

---

### Fermented Vegetables

One of the most important things we can do to boost our chances of enjoying vibrant health in midlife, and in our senior years is to maintain a healthy balance of friendly bacteria in our gut. Unfortunately most people by the time they reach middle age have an elevated quantity of disease causing bacteria due to a high sugar acid-producing diet, chronic stress, and anti-biotic usage. Additionally, researchers at Rice University estimate that 70% of Americans may suffer from an overgrowth of candida fungus.

Many people are now relying on probiotic supplements to enhance their bacterial profile and to ameliorate candida and bad bacteria overgrowth. However, many probiotics can't survive harsh stomach acids, and many vary in quality and potency. Additionally, researchers at Bastyr University found that four out of twenty probiotic products tested had no sign of living beneficial bacteria present at all.

Fermented foods are far superior to lab-made probiotic supplements as they are guaranteed to contain "live and active" bacteria, and to contain a much higher and diverse profile of beneficial bacteria. In fact, merely adding ¼ tsp. of a culture starter to a 1 gallon container of shredded vegetables can supply a whopping 100 billion colony forming units (CFU) of probiotic bacteria. (Mercola, 2014) A really great component of fermented veggies is that they contain the much need vitamin K2 that our bones and blood vessels so greatly need.

### Fermented Beets, Carrots and Ginger

<u>Makes about 2 Quarts</u>:

4 large beets

3-4 pounds carrots

1 large red onion

3 inch piece of raw ginger

2-3 cloves garlic

2 Tbsp. sea salt (prevents growth of bad bacteria)

(Optional): 2 cups soaked wakame seaweed, chopped

Directions: Thoroughly wash and dry veggies. In a food processor, shred beets, carrots, onion, garlic and ginger. Place shredded veggies in a large bowl and thoroughly mix with 2 Tbsp. sea salt. Pound the mixture with a wooden pounder or meat hammer until juices come to the top of the mix. Pack mixture into a wide mouth 2 qt. mason jar. Tamp mixture down to press out the air and to further force the brine out. Leave 1 inch space below the top of the jar. Cover tightly and keep at room temperature for 3-7 days depending on the temperature. Hotter conditions will speed up the culturing process. The ferment is ready when it bubbles. Place a towel under the jar to absorb brine if it overflows. The tissue of vegetables naturally contains lactic acid bacteria, and when allowed to ferment with salt they will reproduce and proliferate. Many people like to add a starter culture to their veggies to ensure certain strains of bacteria (add an additional 1/2 tsp. of the culture blended with some brine in a 2 qt. jar) Body Ecology and Kinetic Culture are two highly regarded cultures. Have ¼ - ½ cup of the fermented veggies 1-3 times a day with meals. Start out very slowly however, with 1 tsp. of the juice and slowly work up to give bacteria time to adjust; otherwise you may have uncomfortable digestive and detox symptoms.

# Vibrant Aging Supplements and Nutraceuticals

Regenerative medicine now knows that certain supplements and botanicals can slow or reverse the progression of aging and chronic diseases. Taking a <u>few</u> select nutraceuticals under a medical professional's guidance; along with following an antioxidant-rich whole foods diet is one way to fast track your wellness and vitality, and to support quality aging. The following are my top picks:

Take a high quality food-based multi vitamin-mineral along with a <u>few</u> of these:

| | | |
|---|---|---|
| Curcumin: anti-aging, anti-cancer, anti-inflammatory, and anti-oxidant properties. | Acetyl-L-Carnitine: boosts brain, memory and heart health. Telomere lengthener. | Vitamin C (liposomal or buffered Ester C) antioxidant, detoxifier; skin and cancer protective |
| B-complex vitamins or 2 Tbsp. nutritional yeast: reduces high homocysteine levels; boosts brain and heart health. | Vitamin E (mixed tocopherols) prevents fat oxidation; heart/vascular system protective. Telomere lengthener. | Omega-3 Essential Fatty acids: Fermented cod liver oil or krill oil- essential for overall good health. |
| Magnesium/Calcium Citrate combined: stress, bone, muscle, nervous system, and mood protective. | Astaxanthin: powerful anti-inflammatory, antioxidant for brain, eye, and joint health. Aids stamina. | Vitamin D3: vital for immune, mood, cognitive, and bone support etc. Take in winter. |
| N-Acetyl-Cysteine: boosts glutathione levels, liver detoxifier. Telomere booster. | Probiotics: supports gut and immune health. | Melatonin: antioxidant; supports sleep, telomere protection, and general well-being. |
| Vitamin K2: eliminates excess damaging calcium in arteries and joints. Bone protective. | EGCG (green tea extract) Immune booster, cancer protective. Telomere lengthener. | Betaine HCl/pancreatic enzymes with meals: supports digestion and absorption of nutrients. |
| Carnosine: reduces damage from glycation. Eye protective. Telomere lengthener. | Resveratrol: anti-aging antioxidant; heart and cancer protective. 200-300 mg. Take w/ <u>Pterostilbene</u>: activates longevity genes, boosts SOD, and mitochondrial function. | Co Q10: (ubiquinone) increases cellular energy; heart protective. |

**Anti-aging/Brain-boosting supplements** from <u>Designs for Health</u>: Brain Vitale, Kre Alkalyn Pro, Resveratrol, Acetyle-L Carnitine, XanthOmega krill oil and Metabolic Synergy.

**Anti-Aging/Brain boosting supplements** from <u>Metagenics</u>: COQ10ST-200, Celapro, MitoVive, Women's Wellness Essentials Prime, and Men's Wellness Essentials Vitality.

**Anti-Aging/Brain-boosting supplements** from <u>Apex Energetics</u>: Glutathione Recycler, Super Oxicell, NeuroFlam, Neuro-PTX, NeuroO2, Acetyl-CH Active, DHEA

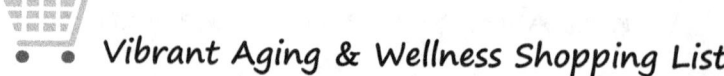

# Vibrant Aging & Wellness Shopping List

This shopping list can be printed and taken with you food shopping. I have supplied a general list of foods that benefit overall aging, and on the back you can write specific foods for your particular health needs.

### Healthful Fats:

___ Extra virgin coconut oil

___ Extra virgin olive oil

___ Organic butter/ghee

___ Red palm oil

___ Olives

___ Avocado

### Proteins: Meat/Fish/Soy:

___ 100% grass-fed beef

___ Grass-fed buffalo meat

___ Organic liver/organ meat

___ Wild fish (canned okay)

___ Organic poultry/lamb

___ Organic Tempeh/miso

### Dairy: (if no sensitivities)

___ Organic DHA eggs

___ Organic raw cheese (cow/goat)

___ Organic unsweetened yogurt/kefir

### Legumes/Beans: (canned okay)

___ Lentils

___ Red beans (all)

___ Black/pinto beans

### Condiments: Spices/herbs also

___ Apple cider vinegar/Stevia

### Starches-Grains & Veggies:

___ Quinoa

___ Basmati brown rice/wild rice

___ Millet

___ *Mary's Gone Crackers* crackers

___ Amaranth

___ Gluten-free oats

___ Whole grain sprouted bread

___ Gluten-free whole grain bread

___ Paleo bread

___ Winter squash

___ Sweet potato/yam

___ Pumpkin (canned also)

___ Red/purple potatoes (small)

___ Peas/corn (frozen okay)

### Fruits (fresh/frozen):

___ Blueberries (wild is best)

___ Purple/red berries (all)

___ Green sour apples

___ Lemons/limes

___ Kiwi

___ Grapefruit

___ Tangerine

___ Cherries

### Vegetables:

___ Dark leafy greens

___ Broccoli & all crucifers

___ *Beets*

___ Carrots

___ Celery

___ Salad greens

___ Mushrooms

___ Red peppers

___ Sprouts

___ Tomatoes-canned ok

___ Artichoke -canned ok

### Booster Foods:

___ Sea weed/nori sheets

___ Spirulina/chlorella

___ Nutritional yeast

___ Flax seed

___ Nuts/seeds

### Beverages

___ Sparkling water

___ Green tea

___ Grass-Fed Whey

___ Rooibos or herb tea

___ Coconut water/milk

**My Personalized Food, Supplement, Herb, and Health Supply Shopping List**

*(Print-out on the back of the shopping list)*

| FOODS | SUPPLEMENTS | BOTANICALS | OTHER |
|---|---|---|---|
| | | | |

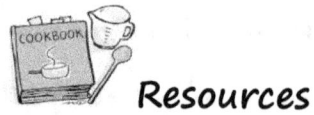

# Resources

## Cookbooks

**Mediterranean Diet:**

Against the Grain: 100 Low Carb Mediterranean Recipes; Diane Kochilas

Mediterranean Paleo Cooking: Over 125 Fresh Coastal Recipes for a Relaxed, Gluten-Free Lifestyle; Nabil Boumrar, Caitlin Weeks

The New Mediterranean Cookbook: A Delicious Alternative for Lifelong Health; Nancy Harmon Jenkins

The GI Mediterranean Diet: The Glycemic Index Life-Saving Diet of the Greeks; Fedon Alexander Lindberg

Conquer Diabetes and Pre-Diabetes: The Low-Carb Mediterranean Diet; Steve Parker M.D.

My New Mediterranean Cookbook: Eat Better, Live Longer by Following the Mediterranean Diet; Jeanette Seaver

**Okinawa Diet:**

The Okinawa Program: How the World's Longest-Lived People Achieve Everlasting Health; Bradley Wilcox

The Okinawa Diet Plan: Get Leaner, Live Longer, and Never Feel Hungry; Bradley Wilcox, and M. Suzuki

**Paleo:**

Make It Paleo: Over 200 Grain-Free recipes for any occasion; Bill Staley

Practical Paleo: A Customized Approach to Health and a Whole Foods Lifestyle; Dianne San Filippo

Paleo Slow Cooking: Gluten-Free Recipes Made Simple; Chrissy Gower

The Everything Paleolithic Diet Slow Cooker Cookbook; Emily Dionne

The Primal Blueprint Cookbook: Quick and Easy Meals You Can Make in Under 30 Minutes; Jennifer Meier, Mark Sisson

The Paleo Kitchen: Finding Primal Joy in Modern Cooking; Julie Bauer; George Bryant

Against All Grains: Delectable Paleo Recipes to Eat Well and Feel Great; Danielle Walker

**Traditional Cultures:**

Nourishing Traditions: The Cookbook That Challenges Politically Correct Nutrition and the Diet Dictocrats; Mary Enig, Sally Fallon

Odd Bits: How to Cook the Rest of the Animal; Jennifer McLagan (organ meat recipe book)

The Complete Nose to Tail; Fergus Henderson

**Gluten-Free/Dairy-Free**

Cooking with Coconut Four: A Delicious Low Carb, Gluten-Free Alternative to Wheat; Bruce Fife

The Dairy-Free and Gluten-Free Kitchen; Denise Jardine

The Gluten-Free Bible; Jox Peters Lowell

**General Health Cookbooks**

The Great Cholesterol Myth Cookbook; Dr. Steve Sinatra (Cardiovascular Health)

The Glycemic Load Diet Cookbook: 150 Recipes to Help You Lose Weight and Reverse Insulin Resistance; D. Carpenter, and R. Thompson

The Stevia Cookbook; Donna Gates, and Ray Sahelian, M.D.

Flavors of Health; Ed Bauman, and Lizette Marx

Clean Eats: Over 200 Delicious Recipes to Reset Your Body's Natural Balance and Discover what it Means to be Truly Healthy; Alejandro Junger

The Blood Sugar Solution Cookbook: More Than 175 Ultra-Tasty Recipes for Total Health and Weight Loss; Mark Hyman

The Ultra-Wellness Cookbook: 200 Delicious Recipes that Will Turn on Your Fat Burning DNA; Mark Hyman

The Good Herb: Recipes and Remedies from Nature; Judith Benn Hurley

The Summer Garden Cookbook; M. Kaplan

The Grass-fed Gourmet Cookbook; Shannon Hayes

Pasture Perfect; Joe Robinson

Tender Grass-fed Meat; Traditional Ways to Cook Healthy Meat; Stanley Fishman

Long Way on a Little; Shannon Hayes (Budget cooking)

Healthy Gourmet for Everyday Cookbook: Eat Drink Be Glad; Rebekah Fedrowitz

**Fermented Foods:**

Real Food Fermentation: Preserving Whole Fresh Food with Live Cultures in Your Home Kitchen; Alex Lewin

Fermented Food for Health: Use the Power of Probiotic Foods to Improve Your Digestion, Strengthen your Immunity and Prevent Illness; Deidre Rawlings PhD.

---

## Lab Tests for Optimal Aging

Lab testing is useful to help accurately measure our present state of health and/or to find the underlying root cause of complex health issues. Testing would then help us determine what modality would effectively remedy the problem. Retesting, after a period of time, would allow us to monitor how well the targeted foods, supplements, botanicals and lifestyle changes are improving the condition.

*Physician Referrals:* The following lab tests can be ordered by physicians from the following organizations- if your present physician will not authorize the tests:

- o  The American Association of Naturopathic Physicians; naturopathic.org
- o  American Holistic Medical Association; holisticmedicine.org
- o  The Institute for Functional Medicine; functionalmedicine.org
- o  American Association of Integrative Medicine; aaimedicine.com
- o  On-line Home Diagnostic Testing can be performed without a physician referral from: Direct Labs and Canary Club

See chart on next page.

# Vibrant Aging Lab Tests

| |
|---|
| *Urine Organic Acid Testing (OAT): General Functional Medicine Screening. Helpful as a general metabolic; detoxification; oxidative stress; gut; and neurotransmitter functioning assessment. Also tests for bacteria, yeasts, parasites, fatty acids, and B vitamins. Additionally tests immunological factors and how well mitochondria make energy. |
| *Comprehensive Stool Analysis: Important for anyone with digestive problems. Tests for pathogenic bacteria; yeasts or parasites; colon inflammation; ulcerative colitis; Chrone's; IBS; pancreatic function; and carbohydrate, fat and protein digestion. |
| Essential Fatty Acid: Assesses essential fatty acid deficiencies as well as excesses. |
| Urinary Amino Acids and Plasma Amino Acids: Tests for amino acid levels and metabolism |
| Vitamin D; (25 OH) optimal range 50-80 ng/ml. See the website Grassrootshealth.com to view a chart showing dosages needed to reach optimal Vitamin D levels based on your lab tested vitamin D levels. |
| Lipid Peroxide Assays in Urine or Serum (or TBARS) Indicator of oxidative stress and oxidized fat from our cell membranes. |
| Antioxidant Enzyme Assays: Assesses the level of super oxide dismutase (SOD), glutathione peroxidase and catalase. |
| Chelation Challenge: Identifies the level of heavy metals in the system. One of the best heavy metal tests. |
| Homocysteine: Assesses homocysteine detoxification status. Ideal level: between 6-8 umol/l. Elevated homocysteine levels are linked to increased heart attack and stroke risk. |
| IGF-1: Measures the amount of the youth-enhancing Human Growth Hormone in the system. |
| ELISA/IgG Food Sensitivity. Identifies food sensitivities. (Metametrix Lab) |
| ELISA/RAST IgE (Mold and Environmental Allergy testing) Mold allergies can cause excessive inflammation and an irritated immune system. |
| Gluten Assessments: Cyrex Array 3; tTG-IgA; EMA; total serum IgA; Cyrex Array 4 (cross reactive foods) Gluten may cause inflammation, digestive issues and cognitive dysfunction. |
| Lipid Particle Size Via Nuclear Magnetic Resonance (NMR): Assesses whether cholesterol particles (LDL/HDL) are small (harmful) or large and fluffy. |
| Fasting Blood Sugar/Glucose Tolerance Test-1 and 2 hour Insulin and Glucose Levels after a 75gram Glucose Load: Assesses insulin resistance. |
| Triglycerides: Optimal under 100 (mg/dl) |
| HA1C. Measures blood sugar levels over the last 2-3 months. (diabetes/pre-diabetes test) |
| Adrenal Stress Index: Assesses whether the stress response is functioning well. |
| Melatonin: Measures the level of this antioxidant and sleep hormone. |
| Thyroid: TSH (ideal between 1 and 2), Free T4 (ideal 1-1.4 ng/dl), Free T3 (ideal 300-400 ng/dl), and Thyroid Antibodies (TPO) to test for Hashimoto's Thyroiditis (autoimmunity). Assesses total thyroid functioning. |
| Women's Hormone Blood Testing: FSH, LH, Estradiol, Progesterone, SHBG, Free testosterone, DHEA-S. Tests for hormone imbalances. |
| Men's Hormone Testing: Free testosterone, Total testosterone, DHEA-S and the PSA test |

| |
|---|
| <u>Methylation Testing</u>: (B6, B12, and Folate levels) Important for heart, mood, and brain health, and cancer prevention. (MCV should be 95 or below) |
| <u>Inflammation testing</u>: C-reactive Protein (CRP-hs): Optimal under 0.7<br>Fibrinogen: less than 300 is normal |
| <u>Nutrient Sufficiency</u>: Assesses vitamin, mineral, and CoQ10 status etc. |
| <u>Ferritin</u>: Tests for excess oxidizing iron. Should be in low to normal range. |
| <u>Ceruloplasmin and serum copper</u>: Tests for excess copper. An excess leads to the spread of cancer growth and anxiety. |
| <u>Gastrointestinal (GI) Function</u>: Tests for pathogenic microorganisms and beneficial gut bacteria; and digestive enzyme and gut inflammation status. |
| <u>Intestinal Permeability Assessment</u>: (Mannitol and lactulose test) Leaky Gut Assessment. |
| <u>Secretory IgA</u> (SIgA): Measures immune defenses in the gut. (Diminished by stress) Low SIgA increases gut permeability and anti-gliadin (gluten) antibodies in the bloodstream. |
| <u>Estrogen Metabolite Testing</u>: Measures the ratio of 2-hydroxyestrone (good estrogen) to 16a-hydroxyestrone (harmful estrogen.) Assesses risk for estrogen sensitive cancers. |
| <u>Iodine Loading Test</u>: Assesses whether there is a sufficient level of iodine in the body. Important for thyroid health and cancer prevention. Offered by Vitamin Research Products. |
| Telomere Lab Testing: Assesses telomere length. Spectra Cell Labs |
| Nitric Oxide Assays: Assesses vascular circulation functioning. Offered by Cell Biolabs, Inc. |
| Creatinine and Bun: Evaluates Kidney Function |

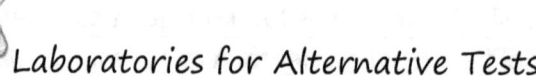 Laboratories for Alternative Tests

The above suggested lab tests can be performed at the following Labs:

- Diagnos-Techs, Inc.
- Genova Diagnostics
- Metametrix Clinical Laboratory
- Immuno Laboratories, Inc.
- Direct Labs (on-line testing)
- EnteroLab
- Metagenics
- Doctors Data
- Spectra Cell Labs
- Canary Club (on-line testing)

# Vibrant Aging Functional Self-Assessments

Many of us in midlife are accustomed to feeling less than ideal; consequently we come to ignore even major symptoms. However symptoms are the body's way of telling us that something is not functioning as well as it should. If we want to achieve high level health we need to understand our symptoms, and what they may signify. Additionally, most diseases have a 10-20 year antecedent; so assessing our health now can possibly head-off debilitating diseases in the future.

The following self-assessment lists symptoms that may occur when the body is imbalanced, or not functioning <u>optimally</u>. They are however not signs of disease. Most people by middle-age possess sub-optimal functioning in a number of these health areas. For that reason this questionnaire is not meant to cause any undue worry. The idea is to not become over-identified with any of these conditions; but to recognize and make note of the health areas that may be out of balance, or not functioning at their best; (health liabilities) and to also recognize your health assets. Taking preventative and corrective nutritional and lifestyle measures, as provided in this book, can often alleviate many symptoms, and improve overall functioning.

This quiz also asks you to note your nutrition and lifestyle habits. Responding to the following prompts will help you to take the vital first step in identifying areas in need of greater awareness, nutrition, and support. When you have finished checking each section, you can then refer to the corresponding chapters that outline some corrective, health enhancing nutrition and lifestyle protocols. After following the practices suggested in this guidebook, you will have made much progress in restoring natural balance and vitality, and in greatly cutting your risk of age-related diseases.

Directions: For each health topic you will be asked to check what is true for you currently, or if you experience the symptoms often. Starred statements are highly correlated with the particular condition. You will then total up and write down the number of check marks you have. This will be your score. Next, read the answer key for each health subject to determine your possible health status. There will be 33 different health areas to score; however not all chapters have a corresponding quiz. Subtests will be highlighted. It is suggested to complete each health topic assessment prior to reading the corresponding chapter. This will make the subject matter more relatable to you and therefore facilitate interest and comprehension.

In the interest of time and to avoid overload, begin with <u>addressing in your health plan only one to three</u> pressing health issues in need of the most support.

Note: This self-assessment is not meant to diagnose any disease states, nor is it a medical or scientific evaluation.

**CHAPTER 1: LONGEVITY (Health liabilities and assets):** Adapted from the *Longevity Prescription* by Robert Butler. Place a checkmark on all current positive nutrition/lifestyle habits and routines.

\_\_ I consume 5 to 10 servings of vegetables daily. (Leafy and crunchy) I consume 1-3 servings of fruit daily. (Especially berries) I eat <u>unprocessed</u> fiber-rich starches, such as whole grains, beans, and root/tuber vegetables daily.

\_\_ I drink at least 8 cups of purified water-based drinks. (Not coffee)

\_\_ I exercise at least 3 times a week (aerobic, weight bearing and/or range of motion). I don't sit for prolonged periods.

\_\_ I have good digestion. I don't experience gas, heartburn, constipation or diarrhea.

\_\_ I am not overweight.

\_\_ I avoid known toxic substances such as pesticide/chemical laden foods; personal care products; and household products as much as possible etc.

\_\_ I do not smoke.

\_\_ I drink alcohol in moderation. I don't drink more than one drink daily for a woman (1 1/2 oz.) or 2 drinks for a man. (3 oz.) One is better or none!

\_\_ I sleep 7-9 hours per night.

\_\_ I am in a marriage/partnership with someone I love, trust, and respect; and with whom I share physical intimacies.

\_\_ I am in regular and satisfying contact with children, siblings, and extended family.

\_\_ I maintain active loving friendships, and interact with a wide range of people.

\_\_ I have adequate emotional support.

\_\_ I am neither depressed, nor prone to prolonged anxiety.

\_\_ I don't obsessively relive unhappy times in the past. I have a hopeful attitude.

\_\_ I continue to challenge myself to learn new things.

\_\_ I regularly do something that stretches my mental muscles. (Crossword puzzles, Sudoku, cards, chess, games, trivia etc.)

\_\_ I find simple joys in my life that lift my spirit, and laugh a good deal.

\_\_ I have stress reduction strategies that I use to reduce anxiety or pressure such as gardening, baths, meditation, deep breathing, listening to calming music etc.

__ I do not harbor old grievances. I accept life's losses and look to new challenges.

__ I don't work more than 10 hours on a workday day on a consistent basis.

__ I spend time enjoying a creative hobby or art form.

____ Total checks. Answer Key: 15 or more checks indicate that you are living a longevity-promoting lifestyle.

*Research Study. The Medical Research Council at Cambridge University studied 20,000 healthy men and women between the ages 45 and 79 to determine mortality risk factors. The study concluded that If an individual was a combined smoker; heavy drinker; had a sedentary lifestyle; and did not eat at least 5 servings of fruits and vegetables daily; they would be almost four times more likely to die sometime in the next decade.

---

## CHAPTER 3: DIET EVALUATION- MALNUTRITION (Source of accelerated aging)

__ I eat packaged and/or processed foods often.

__ I eat out at fast food and chain restaurants often. (More than once a week)

__ I eat out at restaurants more than twice a week.

__ I drink regular sodas and/or diet sodas daily.

__ I consume products that contain MSG regularly. (Spice mixes, chips, packaged foods, Chinese food)

__ I use trans-fats or polyunsaturated margarine, or vegetable oils regularly. (Corn, soy, canola, sunflower, peanut, safflower oil)

__ I eat commercial (non-organic) meat, eggs and dairy products; and commercial fruits and vegetables often.

__ I eat refined carbohydrates regularly. (Sugar, white flour products, white rice, packaged cold cereals, and crackers)

__ I eat sweets daily or often (ice cream, cookies, cakes, muffins, pastries and candies)

__ I eat fried foods several times a week.

__ I eat pasta and breads several times a day. (Whole grain also)

__ I drink coffee more than once a day.

__ I don't eat 5 servings of vegetables on a daily basis

__ I don't eat 1-3 servings of fruit daily

__ I don't eat wild fish or seafood or take an omega-3 supplement.

__ I don't eat enough protein: .36 x (ideal weight in lbs.) = _____ grams of protein a day

__ I don't eat healthy fats very often (olive oil, olives, avocado, coconut oil, butter, nuts, seeds)

____ Total checks. Answer Key: 2 or more checks indicate that you may be in need of more corrective nutritional support.

**CHAPTER 4: IMPAIRED GUT HEALTH & BACTERIAL and FUNGAL IMBALANCE**

___ *I have excessive burping, bloating or gas immediately after meals

___ *I have excessive gas or bloating a few hours after meals

___ *I experience abdominal cramping a few hours after eating

___ *I have indigestion, heartburn, constipation, and/or diarrhea

___ I get an upset stomach easily after taking supplements

___ I have undigested food in my stool

___ I crave and eat sugar and refined carbohydrates often

___ I don't eat 25 grams or more of fiber-rich foods (beans, vegetables, fruits) per day

___ I have dark circles under my eyes

___ I Have iron deficiency anemia or low zinc levels

___ I experience or have experienced chronic stress

___ I have taken a round of antibiotics more than one time and/or birth control pills, NSAIDS, prednisone or cortisone

___ I have chronic fungal infections (on toes, athletes foot, jock itch etc.)

___ I have multiple food allergies, or sensitivities, and/or outdoor allergies or asthma

___ I have acne, eczema or other skin conditions

___ I frequently get colds or flu

___ I have a GI disease/condition? (Colitis, IBS, IBD, Chrone's disease, diverticulitis)

___ I have had urinary tract infections often?

_____ Total checks. Answer Key: Checking any of the first 4 statements or having 2 other checks indicate that you may be in need of digestive support and repair; and probiotics.

**CHAPTER 6 AND 22: SUGAR/PROTEIN GLYCATION (Source of accelerated aging)**

___ I eat foods sweetened with sugar, high fructose corn sweetener, maple syrup and/or honey almost daily

___ I eat fast foods and fried foods (French fries, fried fish etc.) more than twice a month

___ I BBQ and grill my foods more than twice a month

___ I eat highly processed and packaged foods daily

___ I eat junk foods (chips, pretzels, crackers etc.) daily

__ I have a high carb, grain heavy diet (Pastas, breads, baked goods, cereals etc. at almost every meal)

__ I smoke

__ I have premature wrinkles and age spots

__ I have rosacea

__ I have cataracts

__ I have osteoarthritis

__ I am obese

__ I have periodontal disease

__ I have asthma

__ I have a neurological impairment or poor memory

__ I have hypertension, high cholesterol, atherosclerosis, and/or cardiovascular disease

__ I am pre-diabetic or have Type 2 diabetes

_____Total checks. Answer Key: Checking 1 or more statements indicates glycation processes may possibly be occurring.

**CHAPTER 7: EMOTIONAL EATING, METABOLIC IMPAIRMENTS AND WEIGHT MANAGEMENT** The following quizzes identify emotional eating, and the 6 types of metabolic impairments (dysfunctional metabolism) that perpetuate poor health and weight problems. There are additional subtests in the hormone assessment. All quizzes relate to chapter 7.

### Chapter 7: Emotional Eating and Weight Gain

__ *I eat when I'm anxious, depressed, angry, shamed, hurt, or feel empty.

__ I eat when I'm lonely or bored

__ I always feel fat no matter what I weigh

__ I can't resist the urge to binge on my favorite foods

__ I constantly count calories

__ I can be secretive about my eating habits

__ I hide food to eat at a later time

__ I am a chronic dieter

__ I have one or more relatives with an eating disorder

_____Total checks. Answer Key: If you have checked the first statement or more than 2 other statements, emotional eating may be contributing to your weight gain.

## Chapter 7: Carbohydrate Sensitivity/Dysglycemia (I store rather than burn calories for energy)

___ I seldom eat more than two servings (combined) of fruits and vegetables daily

___ I consume 14 or more alcoholic drinks in a week.

___ I consume more than 20 oz. of soft drink daily

___ I seldom exercise 60 minutes or more in a week

___ I consume refined white carbohydrates and sugars at least several times daily

___ I frequently eat junk foods between meals

___ I consume foods such as hot dogs, hamburgers, pizza, fried chicken, fries or chips almost daily

___ I have a problem with stress eating or compulsive eating

___ I have a "pot belly" that has been growing bigger every year

_____ Total checks. Answer Key: If you have checked four or more statements, your lifestyle and genetics have probably joined to create carbohydrate sensitivity as a major factor in prolonging your weight problems, and keeping you from succeeding in a weight-loss program.

---

## Chapter 7: Metabolic Syndrome

___ My family history is positive for diabetes mellitus.

___ I have high triglycerides

___ I have borderline or confirmed high blood pressure

___ I have borderline blood sugar readings

___ I have a positive medical history for infertility, ovarian cysts, or unwanted facial hair

___ I gain weight in my upper body; especially in my belly and waist. (Apple shape)

___ I frequently crave sugar and/or carbohydrates

___ I experience erratic energy and/or mood swings

___ My ethnic roots are non-European

___ I have multiple tiny moles or skin tags on my upper body and neck

_____ Total checks. Answer Key: If you have checked five or more statements, your lifestyle and genetics have probably joined to create metabolic syndrome as a major factor in prolonging your weight problems, and keeping you from succeeding in a weight-loss program.

**Chapter 7: FOOD HYPERSENSITIVITY**

___*I eat wheat and other glutinous grains (rye, barley) and milk-based foods several times a day

___ *I have an emotional attachment to certain foods, and crave them

___ I suffer from brain fog

___ I have a tingling and/or a metallic taste in my mouth

___ I suffer from hives and other skin outbreaks/rashes

___ I suffer from asthma

___ I have chronic nasal congestion or sinus problems

___ I have taken NSAIDS or have a history of antibiotic use

___ I experience constipation and or diarrhea, indigestion, or bloating

___ I have a great deal of stress

___ I suffer from musculoskeletal aches and pains

___ I get excessive headaches

___ I have irritable bowel syndrome

_____ Total checks. Answer Key: If you have checked any of the first 2 statements, or more than 3 other statements, it is possible that food hypersensitivities are contributing to impaired health and weight problems.

**CHAPTER 7-HORMONAL IMBALANCES (thyroid, estrogen, leptin, cortisol subtests)**

**Sub-heading- hormone imbalances:**

1. **Chapter 7: Low Thyroid Function**

___ I frequently feel cold

___ I feel fatigued or exhausted more than usual (especially in the morning)

___ My hair appears to be unhealthy and dry and is falling out

___ My skin is rough, dry, scaly, thick and itchy

___ I have puffiness and swelling around my eyes, face or body

___ I have difficulty concentrating or remembering things

___ I have constipation

___ My nails are brittle

___ I have weight gain in my upper back or thighs and hips

_____ Total checks. Answer Key: If you have checked 3 or more statements, it is possible that low thyroid functioning is contributing to impaired health and weight problems.

2. **Chapter 7: Estrogen Dominance (for women)**

___ I eat sugars and refined foods on a regular basis

___ I experience food cravings and weight gain with PMS

___ My weight gain has been associated with perimenopause or menopause.

___ I take birth control pills or hormone replacement therapy

___ I have or have had chronic high stress

___ I have fibroids or fibrocystic breasts

___ I have borderline or low thyroid

___ I suffer from PMS and water retention

___ I use plastic containers and water bottles and/or commercial (nonorganic) meats, produce, and household and personal care products on a regular basis

_____ Total checks. Answer Key: If you have checked more than one statement, your lifestyle may have contributed to estrogen dominance and/or weight gain.

3. **Chapter 7: Leptin Resistance (the "I'm full" hormone)**

___ *I have an inability to feel full (best indicator)

___ I have difficulty losing weight

___ I have abdominal weight gain

___ I have fatigue

___ I have skin tags

___ I have skin discolorations/darkening around my neck, armpits, and folds that look like dirt

___ I have high blood pressure

_____ Total checks. Answer Key: If you have checked the first statement, and/or more than two other statements; your lifestyle may have contributed to leptin resistance.

4. **Chapter 7 And 18: Chronic Stress And Adrenal Dysfunction (cortisol dysregulation)**

___ *I feel stressed and run down

___ *I feel tired, but wired

___ *I have trouble sleeping or staying asleep

___ I am overwhelmed by life's daily demands

___ I am tired for no reason

___ I crave salty or sweet snacks

__ I am easily startled or have panic attacks

__ I have dark circles under my eyes

__ I need coffee, tea, energy drinks, or colas to keep me going

__ I have low blood pressure/and or get dizzy when I stand up

__ I have trouble bouncing back from stress or illness.

_____ Total checks. Answer key: If you have checked any of the first three statements or more than 2 other statements, your lifestyle may have contributed to adrenal dysregulation and weight gain.

---

**Chapter 7: TOXICITY AND WEIGHT GAIN (Toxins saturate the body and are stored in fat cells)**

__ *I frequently feel sick all over, like having the flu

__ *I am very sensitive to smoke, chemicals, perfumes, dyes, detergents, air fresheners, food additives, and/or fumes in the environment

__ *I used to tolerate caffeine and alcohol much better than I do now

__ *I am sensitive to medications

__ *I have chronic headaches: I also get headaches when I go into certain stores

__ *I have a negative reaction to MSG and sulfites (in wine, cheese, dried fruit etc.)

__ I am often itchy on my back

__ I frequently feel chronic fatigue

__ I have a stuffy nose/congestion, and or postnasal drip often

__ I have "foggy" thought processes

__ I have problem skin and or rosacea

__ I feel chronic achiness

__ I have a family history of fibromyalgia or chronic fatigue syndrome

__ I am or have in the past taken a lot of prednisone, Motrin, Advil, ibuprofen, antibiotics, antidepressants or other medications

__ I use commercial cosmetics, body products and/or perfumes, and use a variety of commercial household cleaning products. I cook with Teflon or aluminum cookware. I have numerous mercury amalgams.

__ I dry clean my clothes often

__ I drink water from plastic bottles often

_____ Total checks. Answer Key: If you have checked any of the first 6 statements or more than 2 other statements, your lifestyle may have contributed a high toxin level and /or impaired liver detoxification.

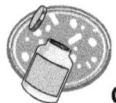

## Chapter 9: COMMON NUTRIENT INSUFFICIENCIES IN MIDLIFE

### Zinc

__ *I have paper thin/weak nails or white spots on my nails

__ *I have impaired taste or smell

__ *I have chronic anxiety/ repetitive negative thoughts

__ I have a poor mood or feel irritable

__ I have frequent colds or respiratory infections

__ I have acne

__ I have bad breath/fruity breath/body odor

__ My joints pop or crack or I have shoulder blade pain

__ I have cartilage problems

__ My wounds heal poorly

__ I get stretch marks easily

__ I have an enlarged or inflamed prostate gland, or erectile dysfunction

__ I am over age 65

_____ Total checks. Answer Key: If you have checked any of the first 3 statements or 2 or more other statements, this may signify a possible zinc insufficiency.

### Magnesium

__ *I have muscle or eye twitching; leg or hand cramps; or restless leg syndrome

__ *My heart flutters, skips beats, or I have heart palpitations

__ *I am sensitive to loud noises; I get irritated by things easily

__ I have constipation or IBS

__ I have PMS

__ I have depression or feel a "sense of doom"

__ I have excess stress and/or get headaches often

__ I suffer from mitral valve prolapse

__ I suffer from high blood pressure, heart disease, kidney stones or diabetes

_____ Total checks.  Answer Key: If you have checked any of the first 3 statements, and/or one or more other statements, it signifies a possible magnesium insufficiency

### Vitamin D

__ *I avoid the sun and wear sun block most of the time, and don't take Vitamin D supplements

__ I suffer from the winter blues (SAD)

__ I have had prostate cancer

__ I have tender bones (press on shin bone to see if it hurts)

__ I have broken more than two bones or have had a hip fracture

__ I have osteoarthritis, osteopenia, or osteoporosis,

__ I have frequent infections

__ I have dark skin

__ I have an autoimmune disease

__ I have poor memory and brain function

_____ Total checks.   Answer Key: If you have checked the first statement or more than one other statement, it signifies a possible vitamin D insufficiency

### B-Complex

__ I have fatigue (especially in the afternoon)

__ I have sores or cracks on my tongue or mouth

__ I have mood swings

__ I have chronic high stress

__ I have poor mental function and memory problems

__ I suffer from heart disease

__ I have prematurely gray hair

_____ Total checks.   Answer Key: One or more checks may signify a possible B-Complex insufficiency

### Vitamin B6

__ I have carpel tunnel syndrome

__ I have swollen, stiff fingers in the early morning (hard to bend fingers into palm)

__ I have a loss of balance or sensation in my feet

__ I have a poor mood/anxiety/depression

__ I suffer from motion sickness

__ I typically am not hungry for breakfast

__ I have poor dream recall

__ I suffer from PMS (headaches, cramps, poor mood)

__ I suffered from severe nausea when pregnant

__ I have or have had heart disease, stroke, cancer, M.S. or abnormal PAP test

_____ Total checks:   Answer Key: One or more checks may indicate a possible vitamin B6 insufficiency

### Chromium

__ I have blood sugar problems/imbalances (high or low) and/or pre-diabetes

__ I have sugar cravings

__ I have an afternoon energy slump

__ I have fatigue and shakiness

__ I have mood swings

_____ Total checks: Answer Key: One or more checks may signify a possible chromium mineral insufficiency

### Vitamin A

__ *I have poor night vision; a hard time seeing when walking into a darkened room from outside; or dry eyes

__ I have rough "chicken skin" on my upper arms or thighs

__ I have a history of Crohn's disease or ulcerative colitis or a peptic ulcer

__ I have a tendency toward recurrent infections (lung or urinary tract etc.)

__ I have frequent colds and flues

__ I have food allergies and/or diarrhea

__ I have acne

__ I have a hypothyroid condition

_____ Total checks:  Answer Key: If you checked the first statement, or 1 or more other statements, it may indicate a possible vitamin A insufficiency

### Vitamin C

__ I have puffy or bleeding gums

__ I have chronic soft tissue problems (tendonitis etc.)

__ I get ill easily (colds, flu)

__ I bruise easily

__ I have prematurely wrinkled skin

_____ Total checks.  Answer Key: One or more checks may signify a possible vitamin C insufficiency

**Calcium**

__ I have low bone density

__ I have had several fractures in adulthood

__ I have an irregular heartbeat

__ I am chronically nervous

__ I get muscle cramps

_____ Total checks. Answer Key: One or more checks may signify a calcium insufficiency

**Essential Fatty Acids**

__ I have a tendency towards constipation and hemorrhoids

__ I have rough "chicken skin" on my upper arms or thighs; or have eczema

__ I have soft, ridged cracking nails

__ I have dry brittle hair, or dandruff, or hair loss

__ I have cracks in my heals and/or cracks between my fingers and toes

__ I have dry itchy, scaling, or flaking skin

__ I have respiratory problems

__ I have joint or soft tissue problems (inflamed)

__ I have poor mood, depression, and/or memory loss

__ I have PMS

__ I have high blood pressure, and/or low HDL, and high triglycerides

__ I have fibrocystic breasts

__ I am of a North Atlantic genetic background: Irish, Scottish, Welsh, Scandinavian; or am Inuit or coastal Native American

_____ Total checks: Answer Key: Two or more checks may signify an essential fatty acid imbalance (GLA and/or Omega-3)

**CHAPTERS 10 AND 11: OXIDATIVE STRESS (A lack of antioxidants/Excessive free radical damage results in premature aging)**

__ I am chronically fatigued

__ I have chronic stress

__ I eat fewer than 5 deeply colored fruits and vegetables daily

__ I get less than 8 hours of sleep at night

__ I don't exercise regularly; or I exercise more than 15 hours a week

__ I drink more than 3 alcoholic beverages a week

__ I eat white flour and sugar more than 3 times a week

__ I take prescription, over-the-counter, and/or recreational drugs

__ I eat fried foods, margarine, and vegetable oils often (corn, sunflower, canola, soy, safflower, peanut)

__ I am exposed to a significant amount of environmental pollutants (home/work)

__ I am overweight

__ I am sensitive to perfume, smoke, or other chemicals or fumes

__ I smoke or am exposed to second hand smoke

__ I have chronic colds, infections, (cold sores, canker sores etc.)

__ I regularly experience deep muscle or joint pain

__ I have allergies and/or arthritis, diabetes or heart disease

__ I go to tanning booths or like to bake in the sun without sunscreen

_____ Total checks. Answer Key: Several checked statements may indicate some degree of oxidative stress. The more checks; the more oxidative stress may be occurring. Most everyone in middle age has some degree of oxidative stress and free-radical damage.

## CHAPTER 12: MITOCHONDRIAL DECAY (Our cellular batteries) Major contributor to accelerated aging.

__ I have high blood pressure, abnormal cholesterol, heart disease/stroke, and/or arrhythmias

__ I have pre-diabetes, and/or disordered glucose or insulin

__ I experience chronic fatigue and feel weak often.

__ I have chronic stress

__ I have trouble falling or staying a sleep; or I wake up too early; or I am not refreshed when I wake up

__ I am over-weight

__ I have muscle pain/or have fibromyalgia

__ I have some hearing loss

__ I am aging prematurely

__ I get migraine headaches

__ I have a poor tolerance for exercise, and I am incredibly tired afterward

__ My concentration and memory are poor and/or I have neurological problems and/or ADHD.

__ I eat processed/packaged foods and/or sugar daily

__ I am irritable and moody and/or suffer from depression, bipolar disorder or schizophrenia

__ I have Diabetes, Alzheimer's, Parkinson's, ALS disease, or Gulf War syndrome

__ I have been exposed to environmental chemicals

__ I have eye disorders

__ I get respiratory infections often, or have immune dysfunctions

__ I have kidney dysfunction

__ I don't exercise regularly

_____ Total checks. Answer Key: More than one checked statement may indicate an energy loss and decreased mitochondrial function.

**CHAPTER 13: TELOMERE LENGTH** "DNA time keepers:" Short telomeres increase aging.

__ I don't exercise regularly (3 times a week)

__ I am overweight by 20 pounds or more

__ I have chronic stress

__ I drink more than 7 alcoholic drinks a week and/or I smoke

__ I take unnecessary over the counter or prescription drugs

__ I have insomnia, or sleep less than 7 hours

__ I don't eat at least 3 servings of vegetables daily

__ I eat packaged and/ or processed foods often

__ I eat refined carbohydrates often (sugar, white flour products, packaged cereals)

__ I drink regular or diet sodas

__ I drink less than 8 glasses of water daily (dehydration)

__ I am pessimistic (I see the glass half empty) and/or worry about many things

__ I have hormone imbalances

__ I have a chronic condition such as rheumatoid arthritis, osteoarthritis, pre-diabetes or type 2 diabetes, or an immune dysfunction

__ I have high blood pressure, low HDL, and or high LDL

__ I have aged prematurely (premature wrinkles and gray hair)

_____ Total checks. Answer Key: If you have checked 3 or more statements, your lifestyle may have contributed to shortened telomeres.

## CHAPTER 14: ALKALINITY AND MINERAL RESERVES

__ I don't eat at least 5 vegetables daily (especially leafy greens)

__ I eat junk food often and/or drink soda daily

__ I have chronic stress

__ I have aching muscles

__ I have joint pain or arthritis

__ I am fatigued often

__ I suffer from stomach aches and nausea

__ I have prematurely aged skin/wrinkles

__ I suffer from osteoporosis or osteopenia

__ I have or have had kidney stones

__ I have had or have gout

__ I have diabetes

_____ Total checks. Answer Key: One or more checks may indicate an over-acid condition/mineral loss.

## CHAPTER 15: HIDDEN INFLAMMATION (Find out whether your immune system is optimized or dysfunctional)

__*I don't eat fish or take fish oil/cod liver oil at least 2-3 times a week

__*I have seasonal/environmental or food allergies or sensitivities or a stuffy nose

__ I eat sugar or high fructose corn sweetener almost daily

__ I eat processed and packaged foods almost daily

__ I eat junk food almost daily

__ I eat trans-fats and polyunsaturated vegetable oils (soy, safflower, corn, sunflower, canola, peanut) almost daily

__ I have a stressful life

__ I don't exercise at least 45 minutes- 3 times a week

__ I drink more than 7 alcoholic beverages a week

__ I am overweight

__ I don't sleep 7 hours or more nightly

__ I have aches/tender muscle points/swelling and stiffness or suffer from osteoarthritis

__ I am overweight

__ I suffer from skin rashes, dermatitis, eczema, or acne

__ I have breathing problems/asthma

__ I get frequent colds and infections

__ I have periodontal disease

__ I have IBS, colitis, or IBD

__ I have an autoimmune disease

__ I have had a heart attack or heart disease

_____ Total checks. Answer Key: If you have checked any of the first 2 statements and/or 2 other statements, your lifestyle may have contributed to an inflammatory state and poor immune health.

## CHAPTER 16: NITRIC OXIDE HEALTH (Optimal Blood/Oxygen Circulation)

__ *I have poor circulation

__ I have a poor memory/and poor brain function

__ I feel tired and worn out

__ I feel weak

__ I have hypertension

__ I have erectile dysfunction

__ I have heart disease

__ I have pre-diabetes/diabetes

__ I have asthma

__ I have arthritis

__ I have osteoporosis

_____ Total checks: Answer Key: If you have checked the first statement or more than one other statement, it may indicate a decreased production of nitric oxide and poor circulation of nutrients.

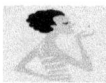 **CHAPTER 19: TOTAL LOAD AND TOXICITY**

__ I use commercial (chemical laden) cosmetics, perfumes and body products

__ I use commercial (not natural) household cleaning products

__ I dry clean my clothes often

__ I am exposed to pesticides and herbicides

__ I use Teflon or aluminum cookware

__ I drink water from plastic, crinkly bottles, and use plastic containers to store food

__ I use unfiltered tap water

__ I eat non organic animal products, fruits and vegetables

__ I eat shark, tuna, swordfish

__ I don't drink 8 glasses or more of filtered or mineral water daily.

__ I have a sweet tooth and indulge in sugary treats

__ I don't eat 5 plus servings of vegetables daily

__ I have more than a few amalgams

__ I am exposed to heavy metals through old peeling paint, aluminum cookware, commercial deodorants, vaccines etc.

_____ Total checks. Answer key: More than 2 checks may indicate a possible high "toxic load."

**CHAPTER 20: EMF's and ELECTRO SENSITIVITY**

__* I suffer from insomnia (most common symptom)

__ I have chronic headaches

__ I have chronic fatigue or fibromyalgia

__ I have had a miscarriage or infertility

__ I have excess sweating

__ I suffer from dizziness, ringing in the ears and earaches

__ I have balance problems and/or nausea

__ I have respiratory problems, asthma, coughing

__ I suffer from poor concentration, and/or memory loss, ADD, or cognitive problems

__ I have smarting eyes, tics, and deteriorating vision

___ I have fluctuating blood pressure

___ I suffer from mood problems such as depression, anxiety, anger, irritability and/or mood swings

___ I suffer from muscle and joint pain

___ I suffer from problems with my bladder

___ I have chemical, light, noise, and smell sensitivities

___ I suffer from upset stomachs and flatulence

_____ Total checks. Answer Key: If you suffer from insomnia and/or several of these symptoms; you may be suffering from a condition known as electro sensitivity.

## CHAPTER 22: FEMALE HORMONAL HEALTH (Perimenopause/menopause)

___ *I have excess chronic emotional or psychological stress, and don't manage it well (worst offender)

___ *I suffer from hot flashes and/or night sweats and/or sleep disturbances

___ I have heart palpitations

___ I have mood swings

___ I have a low sex drive

___ I suffer from a thyroid imbalance

___ I eat excess sweets

___ I drink more than 1 small alcoholic drink daily

___ I don't exercise regularly (3 times a week)

___ I make poor food choices almost daily

___ I use commercial body and home products

___ I drink unfiltered water on a daily basis

_____ Total checks: Answer Key: If you have checked the first 2 statements and/or more than one other checked item, it may indicate a need for corrective action to achieve symptom relief and hormonal balance.

## CHAPTER 23: MALE HORMONAL HEALTH

___ I am often fatigued and have reduced vitality

___ I consume processed/packaged foods, and/or eat out daily

___ My sex drive is reduced

___ I have muscle loss and feel weak

__ I have a pot belly

__ I have "man boobs"

__ I have erectile dysfunction

__ I have increased apathy and/or depression

__ I have low sperm counts

__ I have been exposed to a high amount of pesticides, toxins, and/or heavy metals

__ I have high blood pressure and/or cardiovascular disease

__ My insulin, triglyceride and blood sugar levels have increased

_____ Total checks:  Answer Key: One or more checks may indicate a need for corrective action

In order to achieve hormonal balance.

---

## Recording Your Score

Record your scores (number of checked statements) in the health goals chart on the next page. For the Longevity index, the greater the score, the more **health assets** you possess. Your goal is to try to increase your score throughout the next year to enjoy more health assets and benefits.

For the subsequent assessments, the more checks present, the more **health liabilities** you have; and your goal is to try to decrease your score over the next year. You will also mark the topic or condition's worst score or highest numbers (health liabilities) with a star by the corresponding topic/condition on the chart. These areas will be the first areas to address. However, it is advised to only address three issues or less at one time. Note: not all topics have the same amount of check-off statements. So a topic with the majority of statements checked should be the first area to address.

Mark your healthiest area of functioning (0-1 checks) with a smiley face. These will also be considered your health assets, and you can continue maintaining the health-enhancing routines that resulted in a low score.

After three months of following the advice in this book, take the test again; and see if your nutritional and lifestyle habits; and symptoms and conditions have improved. However, many conditions will take much longer to recover from. By following the recommendations outlined in this book, you will be able to chart the great results you will see and feel in your health.

## Vibrant Aging and Wellness Health Goals Worksheet

| Condition/Topic | Initial score Date: | 3 months later | 6 months later | 9 months later | 1 year later |
|---|---|---|---|---|---|
| Longevity: health assets | | | | | |
| Malnutrition | | | | | |
| Impaired Gut Health | | | | | |
| Glycation | | | | | |
| Emotional Eating | | | | | |
| Waist Circumference | | | | | |
| Carb Sensitivity | | | | | |
| Metabolic Syndrome | | | | | |
| Food Hypersensitivity | | | | | |
| Low Thyroid Function | | | | | |
| Estrogen Dominance | | | | | |
| Leptin Resistance | | | | | |
| Adrenal Dysfunction | | | | | |
| Toxicity | | | | | |
| Oxidative Stress | | | | | |
| Mitochondrial Dysfunction | | | | | |
| Telomere Length | | | | | |
| Alkalinity/Mineral Reserves | | | | | |
| Inflammation/Immunity | | | | | |
| Nitric Oxide/Circulation | | | | | |
| Total Load | | | | | |
| EMF'S/Electrosensitivity | | | | | |
| Female/Male Health | | | | | |

| Fitness | Initial amount Date: | 3 months later | 6 months later | 9 months later | 1 year later |
|---|---|---|---|---|---|
| Number of daily steps | | | | | |
| Amt. of time per week ex: 1hr.-3x/wk. | | | | | |
| Weight bearing exer. | | | | | |
| Yoga/other | | | | | |

## Health Goals Worksheet Continued

## Common Nutrient Insufficiencies in Midlife (from Quiz)

| Nutrient | Possible Insufficiency? Initial Score date: | 3 months later | 6 months later | 9 months later | 1 year later |
|---|---|---|---|---|---|
| Zinc | | | | | |
| Magnesium | | | | | |
| Vitamin D | | | | | |
| B-Complex | | | | | |
| Vitamin B6 | | | | | |
| Chromium | | | | | |
| Vitamin A | | | | | |
| Vitamin C | | | | | |
| Calcium | | | | | |
| Nutrients Pg. 136 | Date: | | | | |
| Essential Fatty Acid (EFA) | | | | | |
| NAC | | | | | |
| Vitamin K2 | | | | | |
| Iron | | | | | |
| Vitamin E | | | | | |
| Beneficial Bacteria | | | | | |
| Vitamin B12 | | | | | |
| Folate | | | | | |
| Iodine | | | | | |
| Vitamin B1/B2 | | | | | |

## Lab Tests/Results

| | | | |
|---|---|---|---|
| | | | |

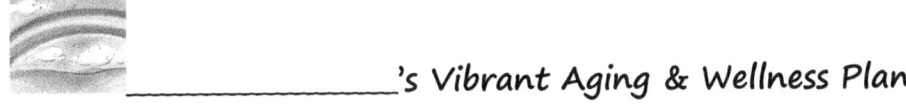     _____'s Vibrant Aging & Wellness Plan

Date:_____

Exer. 1: My personal motivators – Why I want to experience vibrant health & longevity.

1 _____

2 _____

3 _____

4 _____

5 _____

Exer. 2a: Five of my current "health assets" and strengths. I will "reframe" unconstructive thoughts about any health challenges by focusing on/affirming my health assets/strengths.

1. _____

2. _____

3. _____

4. _____

5. _____

Exer. 2b: Visualization Practice: My Health Vision. Short term health goals: (1-6 mo.)
_____

Long term goals: (1-3 years)_____

Exer. 2c: I set an intention every day to care for my physical, mental and spiritual wellbeing: 5 Affirmations that I can recite daily to encourage an upbeat attitude:

1. _____

2. _____

3._____

4._____

5._____

I will develop a life-affirming practice of _____ daily. (Gratitude, belly breathing, forgiveness, visualization, meditation, prayer, laughter and/or listening to calming music etc.)

<u>Exer. 3a</u>: Hydration: ½ my body weight in oz. of water based liquids: \_\_\_oz. or\_\_\_ cups/day

<u>Exer. 3b</u>: Beverage Substitution List/chart:_____

<u>Exer. 3c</u>: Food Substitution List/chart:_____

_____  _____  _____

_____  _____  _____

<u>Affirmation</u>: I treat my body as a temple. It is holy, clean and full of goodness.

<u>Exer. 3d</u>: Indulgent/Pleasure Food Frequency List: How often?

Fast Food/Chain restaurant Food: _____ Junk Food: chips, refined white foods:_____

Sweets-candies, pastries, cookies, cakes, ice cream: _____ Coffee/Decaf:_____

Alcohol:_____ Restaurant Food _____

<u>Exer. 4a</u>: My current optimal diet direction? Circle one: Building/Balancing/Cleansing (modify when needed) _____

<u>Exer. 4b</u>: Determine my protein needs: .36 x (ideal weight in lbs.) = _____ grams of protein a day/divide this amt. up-per meal. Check food labels and print out protein quantity gram chart. Possible protein excess or deficiency?
Yes/No_____

Exer. 4c: Healthy Protein Sources/Protein tips/cooking guidelines/glycation information:

_____    _____    _____
_____    _____    _____
_____    _____    _____
_____    _____    _____
_____    _____    _____
_____    _____    _____

Possible lactose intolerance? Yes/no _____ Possible casein sensitivity? Yes/no _____

Dairy options/substitutions/enzymes if needed: _____

_____    _____    _____
_____    _____    _____

Exer. 4d: Determine possible digestive status with baking soda test and symptom list: low/optimal/excessive HCL? _____ Pancreatic enzyme status? _____

Constipation? _____ GERD? _____ Foods/Supplements to support digestive fire and HCL production:_____

Other digestive support:_____

Exer. 5a: Fats: Possible oxidized cholesterol from symptom/lifestyle list? Yes/no _____
Nutrition/activities to reduce oxidized cholesterol:_____

_____

Unhealthy "bad" fats to eliminate:_____

_____    _____
_____    _____

*Exer. 5b*: Healthy fat sources:

Omega-3's:_____  Monounsaturated fats:_____
_____  _____
_____
                                    GLA fats (possible deficiency?)_____
Alpha Linolenic Acid: (ALA)_____  _____
_____
                                    Saturated fats:_____
Omega-6's:_____  _____

*Exer.5c*: ALA conversion problem? _____ Possible fat intolerance? _____ See symptom list. Fat digesting aids: _____

*Exer. 5d*: Fat needs/tips_____
_____

Cooking temps.: notes_____

*Exer. 6a:* Refined grains to reduce from diet:_____
_____

*Exer. 6b*: Possible gluten sensitivity/or celiac diseases? Yes/no_____ Get tested? Yes/no_____Lab: Cyrex Array 3   Eliminate gluten? Yes/no_____ Healthful gluten-free ingredients/print out wheat source chart:_____

*Exer. 6c* Print out the daily carb serving-sizes chart. Make note of some healthful carbohydrates gleaned from the chapter. _____

_____  _____
_____  _____
_____  _____
_____  _____
_____  _____

High-fiber carbohydrates. Try to get between 35-50 grams+ of fiber daily. Soak grains/beans/nuts/seeds in water with 1 tbsp. vinegar for every cup of grains etc. for 7-24 hours. (To dissolve mineral-binding phytates).   List high fiber foods:

Vegetables:_____

Fruits:_____

Grains:_____

Legumes/beans:_____

Nuts/seeds/etc.:_____

Exer. 6d: Useful glycemic control tips:_____
_____

Low glycemic load foods (or print out the chart) glycemic load value of 100 or less daily.

Vegetables:_____

Grain:_____

Nuts/Dairy:_____

Fruit:_____

Legumes:_____

Purchase *the Glycemic Load Counter* guidebook yes/no_____

Notes:_____

Exer. 6e: Input some blood sugar/glycation stabilizing meals/supplements: _____
_____
_____

Grain alternatives:_____

Sugar reduction strategies:_____

Tips & supplements to reduce sugar/carb cravings: _____
_____

Print-out carb food swap chart_____

Exer. 7a: Is emotional eating causing my weight gain? Yes/no. My emotional triggers are:
_____
_____

Healthful strategies to address triggers:._____
_____

Exer. 7b: Healthy Body Composition/My waist circumference: Goal is 35 in. or less for a women/40 in or less for a man. (To reverse insulin resistance) My waist size is:_____ inches

Exer. 7c: Possible carb sensitivity? _____ Possible insulin resistance?_____ Possible metabolic syndrome?_____ Possible food hypersensitivity?_____ Hormone imbalances with: Leptin?_____Adrenals?_____Thyroid?_____ Estrogen?_____Liver detoxification issues?_____ Is elimination diet needed?_____Get Lab work? ___Print out wheat sources chart. Record/remove xenoestrogens from my home:_____
_____

Follow nutritional support plan for dysfunctional metabolism issues from above.
Notes:_____
_____
_____

Exer. 7d: Print out and follow "Healthy Weight Loss Plan" and metabolism boosting meal plan. Refer to the carb food swap chart for healthy carb suggestions.
Notes:_____
_____

Exer. 8: Note several beneficial features of the four traditional diets. (Incorporate cultured/fermented foods into diet) See cookbook suggestions in the back of the book.

General traditional diet features: _____

_____

Mediterranean diet:_____

Okinawa diet:_____

Paleo diet:_____

Exer. 9a: Some of my likely nutritional deficiencies or excesses: Form/dosage suggestions?

_____     _____
_____     _____

Exer. 9b: Info on dietary supplements that I would like to remember including osteoporosis prevention: nutrients/supplements:_____

_____

Exer. 10a: Free radical offenders that I can limit or eliminate:_____

_____

_____

Exer. 10b: 5 or more antioxidant- ACESZ foods/supplements to quell oxidative stress:

vit.A (retinol)_____     vit. C:_____
_____         _____
_____         _____
                                         _____
vit.A (plant)_____
_____         vit E:_____
                                         _____

selenium:_____    zinc:_____
_____              _____

<u>Exer. 10c</u>: Several antioxidant/carotene rich foods and any supplements from each carotene group. Try to eat carotene sources 3 times a day or more.

Alpha/Beta carotenes_____    Lutein/zeaxanthin:_____
_____                _____
_____                _____

Lycopenes:_____      Astaxanthin:_____
_____                _____

<u>Exer. 10d:</u> several foods from each group of flavonoids and any supplements. Try to get one serving a day of most of these flavonoids.

Catechins:_____      Anthocyanins:_____
_____                _____
                                     _____
Hesperidin/Rutin:_____
_____                Glucosinolates:_____
                                     _____
Quercetin:_____
_____                Luteolin:_____
                                     _____
Resveratrol:_____
_____                Terpenes:_____
_____                _____

Ellagic Acid:_____      Pycnogenol:_____
_____                _____

<u>Exer. 10e:</u> High antioxidant "ORAC" foods. Try to get at least one from each group daily.

Spices/herbs:_____      Fruits:_____
_____                _____
_____                _____

Vegetables: _____  Nuts/seeds: _____

_____  _____

_____  Misc.: _____

Beans: _____  _____

_____  _____

**Exer. 11a**: Glutathione boosting foods (our own internal antioxidant) Try to get 3 in a day.

Vegetables: _____  Proteins: _____

_____  _____

Herbs: _____  Supplements: _____

_____  _____

Nuts/legumes/grains: _____  _____

_____  _____

**Exer. 11b**: Input SOD boosting foods (degenerative disease protectors) Try to get in 5 daily.

Veggies: _____  Nuts/seeds/beans: _____

_____  _____

_____  _____

_____  Other: _____

Fruits: _____  Catalase boosting foods: _____

_____  _____

**Exer. 12**: Include several mitochondrial boosting foods/activities (cellular power generators)

_____  _____  _____

_____  _____  _____

_____  _____  _____

_____  _____  _____

Supplements: _____

.

Mitochondrial multiplier (PQQ) foods: _____

_____

**Exer. 13a**: Telomere (timekeeper) shortening activities to eliminate:_____

_____

**Exer. 13b**: Input several telomere lengthening promoters: _____

Foods:_____   Activities:_____

_____   _____

_____   Supplements:_____

_____   _____

_____   _____

**Exer. 14**: Test pH/Possible acidosis? Yes/no _____ Alkalinizing-energy boosting foods/activities/supplements. _____

_____   _____   _____

_____   _____   _____

_____   _____   _____

**Exer. 15a**: Possible high inflammation? Yes/No_____ Substances/activities that trigger inflammation that I can eliminate/limit._____

_____

**Exer. 15b**: Anti-inflammatory foods/activities/supplements to reduce inflammation:

_____   _____   _____

_____   _____   _____

_____   _____   _____

_____   _____   _____

_____

_____

Exer.15c: Immune Boosting/Balancing foods & supplements etc.: _____
_____

Exer. 16: Possible low nitric oxide levels? Yes/no?_____ Foods/activities/ that can support my nitric oxide levels, and heart/brain health:_____

| _____ | _____ | _____ |
| _____ | _____ | _____ |
| _____ | _____ | _____ |
| _____ | _____ | _____ |

Supplements:_____

Exer. 17: Input exercise and HGH info, and any sports medicine info:_____
_____
_____

I set a fitness goal of _____ exercise daily/weekly

Exer. 18a: Am I suffering from a possible stress condition/adrenal dysfunction? ____ If so; what is the likely stage? _____

Exer. 18b: Stress Support. Input target foods, adaptogenic herbs, supplements, and stress-reduction activities to support chronic stress conditions, adrenal dysfunctions, and insomnia

_____
_____

| _____ | _____ | _____ |
| _____ | _____ | _____ |
| _____ | _____ | _____ |
| _____ | _____ | _____ |

Exer. 19a: "Total Load" Reduction. List my body's burdens/stressors that I can reduce to bolster my health: _____

_____     _____     _____
_____     _____     _____
_____     _____     _____
_____     _____     _____

Exer. 19a-con't: Health supportive diet/lifestyle substitutions (from chart) to lighten my "total load." _____

_____     _____     _____
_____     _____     _____
_____     _____     _____
_____     _____     _____

Exer. 19b: Daily detox support. Foods/lifestyle routines to boost liver detox

_____.    _____     _____
_____     _____     _____
_____     _____     _____
_____     _____     _____

Exer. 19c: Targeted nutrients to boost phase I and/or phase II liver detox:_____

_____     _____     _____
_____     _____     _____

Exer. 19d: Plan/schedule a seasonal cleanse: Print out seasonal cleanse information/ vegetable mineral broth recipe. Attempt a cleanse (level 1, 2, or 3) one to three times a year._____

_____

_Exer. 20_: Possible electro sensitivity? _____ EMF combating foods/herbs/supp's/devices:

_____   _____   _____
_____   _____   _____
_____   _____   _____

_Exer. 21_: Earthing. I will walk barefoot or sit/lay on the ground or on a moist cement floor in basement/garage (daily/weekly) _____ and/or purchase grounding devices to promote high level health and electron sufficiency.   Grounding info:
_____
_____

_Exer. 22/23_: Male/Female Health. Useful gender specific information, nutrients, supplements and lifestyle measures to enhance my hormonal and general health:_____

_____   _____   _____
_____   _____   _____
_____   _____   _____
_____   _____   _____
_____   _____   _____
_____

_Exer. 24_: Graceful Aging: Print-out/input any useful charts or information to help delay the visible signs of aging: _____

_____   _____   _____
_____   _____   _____
_____   _____   _____
_____   _____   _____
_____   _____   _____
_____

♥ If I criticize my looks, I will immediately find one aspect of myself that I like.

Exer. 25: Putting it all together: Print out any useful "vibrant aging" information; the meal plan, recipes, and the shopping list. Transfer the food lists from the wellness plan onto your shopping list.

Lab work/health test strips or supplies that may be useful for me:_____

_____   _____   _____
_____   _____   _____
_____   _____   _____
_____   _____   _____

Resources/Cookbooks: _____

_____

_____

Notes:

# References

Abel, R. 1999. *The Eye Care Revolution*. New York: Kensington Publications.

Abramson, J.L., and V. Vaccarino. 2002."Relationships between physical activity and Inflammation among apparently healthy middle-aged and older US adults." *Archives of Internal Medicine* 162 (11): 1286-92.

Aguilar, CA, G. Talavera, JM Ordovas et al. 1999. "The apolipoprotein E4 allele is not associated with an abnormal lipid profile in a Native American population following its traditional lifestyle." *Atherosclerosis*. 1999 Feb;142(2):409-14.

Aikata, H., H.Takaishi, K. Kawakami, S.Takahashi, M.Kitamoto, T.Nakanishi, ... and T. Ide. 2000. *"Telomere reduction in human liver tissue with age and chronic inflammation*. Exp. Cell Res., 256, 578–582.

Akan, Z, B. Aksu, A. Tulunay, S. Bilsel, and A. Inhan-Garip. 2010. "Extremely low-frequency electromagnetic fields affect the immune response of monocyte-derived macrophages to pathogens." *Bioelectromagnetics*. 31(8):603-612, 2010.

Allred, C. D., K. F. Allred, Y.H. Ju, T. s. Goeppinger, D. R. Doerge, and W. C. Helferich.2004. "Soy Processing Influences Growth of Estrogen-Dependent Breast Cancer Tumors." *Carcinogenesis* 25 (9): 1649-57. doi:10.1093/carcin/bgh178.

Alschuler, L.N. and K. Gazella. 2011. *Five to Thrive. The Definitive Guide to Thriving After Cancer: A Five-Step Integrative Plan to Reduce the Risk of Recurrence and Build Lifelong Health*. New York: Ten Speed Press.

Amen, D. 2005. *Making a Good Brain Great.* New York: Harmony Books

Ames, B. N. 2006. "Low Micronutrient Intake May Accelerate the Degenerative Diseases of Aging through Allocation of Scarce Micronutrients by Triage." *Proceedings of the National Academy of Sciences* 103 (47):17589-94.

Arasaki, S. 1983. *Vegetables from the Sea*, Tokyo: Japan Publishing.

Arem, R. 1999. *The Thyroid Solution: A Mind-Body Program for Beating Depression and Regaining Your Emotional and Physical Health*. New York: Ballantine Publishing Group.

Auld-Louis, M. Traditional Diets Promote Optimal Health. *www.optimumchoices.com/Traditional_Diets.htm* (accessed 4/19/14)

Avena, N.M., P. Rada, and B.G. Hoebel. 2008. "Evidence for sugar addiction behavioral and neurolochemical effects of intermittent, excessive sugar intake." *Neuroscience and Biobehavioral Reviews* 32 1): 20-39.

Bauman, E. and H. Waldman. 2012. *The Whole-Food Guide for Breast Cancer Survivors*. Oakland: New Harbinger Publications, Inc.

Bauman, E., and J. Friedlander. 2011. *Foundations of Nutrition*. Penngrove, CA: Bauman College.

Bauman, E., and J. Friedlander. 2011. *Therapeutic Nutrition Part One*. Penngrove, CA: Bauman College.

Bauman, E., and J. Friedlander. 2011. *Therapeutic Nutrition Part Two*. Penngrove, CA: Bauman College.

Beckwith M. B. 2008. Spiritual Liberation: Fulfilling Your Soul's Potential. New York: Simon & Schuster Inc.

Benbrook, C., X. Zhao, J.Yanez, N. Davies, and P. Andrews. 2008. "New Evidence confirms the nutritional superiority of plant-based organic foods." *State of Science Review*: Critical Issue Report, March, 1-50.

Benetos, A., K. Okuda, M. Lajemi, M. Kimura, F. Thomas, J. Skurnick,... and A. Aviv. 2001. "*Telomere lengths as an indicator of biological aging: the gender effect and relation with pulse pressure and pulse wave velocity.*" Hypertension, 37, 381–385.

Berger C, et. al. 2012. "Temporal trends and determinants of longitudinal change in 25-hydroxyvitamin D and parathyroid hormone levels." *J Bone Miner Res.* 2012;27(6):1381-9.

Berkson, D. L. 2000. *Hormone Deception: How Everyday Foods and Products Are Disrupting Your Hormones-and How to Protect Yourself and Your Family*. Chicago: Contemporary Books.

Berkson, L. 2000. *Healthy Digestion the Natural Way: Preventing Heartburn, Constipation, Gas, and Inflammatory Bowel*. New York: John Wiley and Sons, Inc.

Bland, J., L. Costarella, D. Liska. 2004. *Clinical Nutrition a Functional Approach.* Gig Harbor, Washington: Institute for Functional Medicine.

Body Ecology. 2008. "The 6 Benefits of Monounsaturated Fats (mufas)". http://bodyecology.com/articles/6_benefits_monosaturated_fats.php#.VHZ9T7l 0zs0.

Bowden. J., and S. Sinatra. 2012. *The Great Cholesterol Myth: Why Lowering Your Cholesterol Won't Prevent Heart Disease and the Statin-Free Plan That Will.* Beverly, MA: Four Winds Press.

Breus, M. 2006. *Good Night: the Sleep Doctor's 4-Week Program to Better Sleep and Better Health.* New York: Penguin Group.

Brimeyer, K. 2013. *The Leaky Gut Cure Stop Your Chronic Symptoms: Naturally and Permanently Stop Your Chronic Symptoms at the Source.* Copy write by K Brimeyer.

Brownstein, D. 2010. *Salt Your Way to Health. $2^{nd}$ed.* West Bloomfield MI: Medical Alternative Press.

Bryan, N.S., J. Zand, and B. Gottlieb. 2010. *The Nitric Oxide (NO) Solution: How to Boost the Body's Miracle Molecule to Prevent and Reverse Chronic Disease.* Austin: Neogenis.

Calzavara-Pinton,P, C. Zane, E. Facchinetti, R. Capezzera, and A. Pedretti "Topical Boswellic acids for treatment of photoaged skin." *Pub Med Publication*: 2010 Jan-Feb;23 Suppl 1:S28-32. doi: 10.1111/j.1529-8019.2009.01284.x.

CNN Report "Obesity may overtake tobacco as leading preventable cause of cancer": *ASCO* Posted 9:54 AM, October 1, 2014, by CNN, Updated at 10:11am, October 1, 2014

Center for Food Safety. 2011. "Genetically Engineered Crops." Washington D. C: Center for Food Safety.http.centerforfoodsafety.org/campaign/genetically-engineered-food/crops. (Accessed March 5, 2014).

Cooper, R.K., and L. L. Cooper. 2007. *Flip the Switch Lose the Weight: Proven Strategies to Fuel Your Metabolism & Burn Fat 24 Hours A Day.* New York: Rodale.

Corriher, S. 1997. *Cookwise: the Hows and Whys of Successful Cooking.* New York: Harper Collins Publisher's Inc.

Crinnion, W.J. 2000. "Environmental medicine, part 4: pesticides-biologically persistent and ubiquitous toxins." *Alternative Medicine Review* 5 (5): 432-437.

Dailyword: 2014. Unity Village, MO: Unity Publication

Dr. Robert Gould. 2012. "The 12 Types of Emotional Eaters" http://www.diet.com/dietblogs/read_blog.php?title=The+12+Types+Of+Emotional+Eaters&blid=15478. (Accessed January 2014)

Estruch, R, et al. 2013. "Primary Prevention of Cardiovascular Disease with a Mediterranean Diet." The New England Journal of Medicine, 368, 1279-1290. URL:http://www.nejm.org/doi/full/10.1056/NEJMoa1200303?query=featured_home&.

Fallon, S., and M.G. Enig.1999. *Nourishing Traditions: The Cookbook That Challenges Politically Correct Nutrition and the Diet Dictocrats.* Washington, D.C.: New Trends Publishing.

Farrer, K.T. H. 1987. *A Guide to Food Additives and Contaminants.* Nashville, TN: Parthenon Publishing Group.

Farrow, L. 2013. *The Iodine Crisis: What You Don't Know About Iodine Can Wreck Your Life.* Berkeley: Devon Press

Farshchi, H., M. Taylor, and I. Macdonald. 2005 "Deleterious effects of omitting breakfast on insulin sensitivity and fasting lipid profiles in healthy lean women 1,2,3 *American Society for Clinical Nutrition.*

Garavaglia, J. 2008. *How Not to Die.* New York: Crown Publishing

Garcia, O. 2008. *Redesigning 50: The No Plastic Surgery Guide to $21^{st}$ Century Age Defiance.* New York: Harper Collins.

Garza, L, Y Liu, Z. Yang, B. Alagesan, J. Lawson, and S. Norberg…G. Cotsarelis. 2012. "Prostaglandin $D_2$ Inhibits Hair Growth and Is Elevated in Bald Scalp of Men with Androgenetic Alopecia." Mar. 2012. 4 (126): 126ra34. *Sci. Transl. Med.*

Gates, D. 2010. *The Body Ecology Diet: Recovering Your Health and Building Your Immunity.* Atlanta: B.E.D. Publications.

Gates, D. 2011. *The Baby Boomer's Diet: Body Ecology's Guide to Growing Younger.* New York: Hay House Inc.

Gittleman, A. L. 2010. *Zapped: Why Your Cell Phone Shouldn't Be Your Alarm Clock and 1268 Ways to Outsmart the Hazards of Electronic Pollution.* New York: Harper Collins.

Gittleman, A.L. 1996. *Get the Sugar Out-501 Simple Ways to cut the Sugar out of Any Diet.* New York: Three Rivers Press.

Gittleman, A.L. 2001. *Guess What Came to Dinner: Parasites and Your Health.* New York: Avery.

Gittleman, A.L. 2010. *Fat Flush for Life.* Cambridge: Da Capo Press.

Gittleman. A.L. 2008. *The Gut Flush Plan.* New York: The Penguin Group.

Glassman, G. 2010. *The O2 Diet: the Cutting Edge Antioxidant-Based Program that Will Make You Healthy, Thin and Beautiful.* New York: Rodale.

Gould, R., M.D. 2007. *Shrink Yourself,* NY:Wiley and Sons

Gottfried, S. 2013. *The Hormone Cure: Reclaim Balance, Sleep, Sex Drive, and Vitality Naturally with the Gottfried Protocol.* New York: Scribner.

Green, R. A. and L. Feldon, 2005. *Perfect Balance: Dr. Robert Greene's Breakthrough Program for Finding the Lifelong Hormonal Health You Deserve.* New York: Clarkson Potter/Publishers.

Guarnet, F. and J.R. Malagelada. 2003. "Gut Flora in Health and Disease." *Lancet* 361361 (9356):512-19.

Harley,C.B. 1997. "Human ageing and telomeres." Ciba Found. Symp., 211, 129–139.

Hay, L. 2005. *You Can Heal Your Life Affirmations Kit Book Supplement.* Carlsbad, CA: Hay House.

Henderson, S.T. 2004. "High carbohydrate diets and Alzheimer's disease." *Med Hypotheses.* 2004;62(5):689-700.

Holt, S. 2014. "Telomeres and Telomerase as Natural Therapeutic Targets" http://www.naturalclinician.com/telomeresastherapeutics.cfm (accessed May 2014).

Hu, F.B., J. Manson, and W. Willett. 2001."Types of dietary fat and risk of coronary heart disease: a critical review. *J Am Coll Nutr*. 2001 Feb;20(1):5-19.

Huang TL, PP.Zandi, KL.Tucker et al. 2005. "Benefits of fatty fish on dementia risk are stronger for those without APOE epsilon4. *Neurology*." 2005 Nov 8;65(9):1409-14.

Hyman, M. 2009. *The Ultramind Solution: Fix Your Broken Brain by Healing Your Body First*. New York: Scribner.

Hyman, M. 2012. *The Blood Sugar Solution: The Ultra Healthy Program for Losing Weight, Preventing Disease, and Feeling Great Now*. New York: Little, Brown and Company.

Hyman, M. 2014. "Eggs Don't Cause Heart Attacks- Sugar Does." http://drhyman.com/blog/2014/02/07/eggs-dont-cause-heart-attacks-sugar/(accessed Feb. 13, 2014)

International working group of scientists, researchers, and public health policy professionals. 2012. *BioInnitiative 2012: A Rationale for Biologically-based Exposure Standards for Low-Intensity Electromagnetic Radiation*. Bioinnitiative .org

Janowiak, J.J. 2004. "A Practitioner's Guide to Hair Loss Part 2- Diet, Supplements, Vitamins, Minerals." Alternative and Complimentary Therapies. Aug. 2004: 10 (4) 200-205.

Kalish, D. 2012. *The Kalish Method: Healing the Body Mapping the Mind*. Richard Kalish Publishing.

Knoff, L. 2010. *The Whole food Guide to Overcoming Irritable Bowel Syndrome*. Oakland: New Harbinger Publications, Inc.

Kuljeet, K, R. Gupta, S. Saraf, and S.K. Saraf. 2014. "Zinc: The Metal of Life." *Comprehensive Reviews in Food Science and Food Safety*, 2014; 13 (4): 358 DOI: 10.1111/1541-4337.12067.

Lam, M. and D. Lam. 2012. *Adrenal Fatigue Syndrome: Reclaim Your Energy and Vitality with Clinically Proven Natural Programs*. Loma Linda, Ca: Adrenal Institute Press.

Leidy, H., L. Ortinau, S. Douglas, H. Hoertel. 2013. "Beneficial effects of a higher-protein breakfast on the appetitive, hormonal, and neural signals controlling energy intake regulation in overweight/obese, "breakfast-skipping," late-adolescent girls., Am J Clin Nutr. 2013 Apr;97(4):677-88. doi: 10.3945/ajcn.112.053116. Epub 2013 Feb 27.

Lesser, M. and C. Kapklein. 2002. *The Brain Chemistry Diet: The Personalized Prescription for Balancing Mood, Relieving Stress, and Conquering Depression Based on Your Personality Profile.* New York: G. P. Putman's Sons.

Leung, C.W., B.Laraia, B.Needham, D.Rehkopf, N. Adler, J. Lin, E. Blackburn, and E. Epel. "Soda and Cell Aging: Associations between Sugar-Sweetened Beverage Consumption and Leukocyte Telomere Length in Healthy Adults from the National Health and Nutrition Examination Surveys. *American Journal of Public Health*: December 2014, Vol. 104, No. 12, pp. 2425-2431. doi: 10.2105/AJPH.2014.302151

Li, Z., X. Dong, H. Liu, X. Chen, H. Shi, Y. Fan, D. Hou, and X.Zhang. 2013. "Astaxanthin protects ARPE-19 cells from oxidative stress via upregulation of Nrf2-regulated phase II enzymes through activation of PI3K/Akt." *Mol Vis*. 2013;19:1656-66.

Life Extension Media. 2003. *Disease Prevention and Treatment.* $4^{th}$ed. Hollywood, FL: Life Extension.

Lindberg, F. A. 2009. *The GI Mediterranean Diet: the Glycemic Index-Based Life-Saving Diet of the Greeks.* New York: Rodale.

"Link Between Vitamin D Deficiency and Dementia Confirmed." 2014. http://articles.mercola.com/sites/articles/archive/2014/11/06/vitamin-d-deficiency-dementia.aspx. (accessed Nov.6, 2014).

Lipski, E. 2012. *Digestive Wellness.* $4^{th}$ed. New York: McGraw-Hill.

Lipton, B.H. 2009. *The Biology of Belief: Unleashing the Power of Consciousness, Matter & Miracles.* New York: Hay House.

Littlejohns, T., W. Henley, I. Lang, et al. 2014. "Vitamin D and the risk of dementia and Alzheimer disease." *Neurology* August 6, 2014. Epub ahead of print.

Love, S. 2003. *Dr. Susan Love's Menopause & Hormone Book-Making Informed Choices.* New York: Three Rivers Press.

Lulli, M, E. Witort, L. Papucci, E. Torre, N. Schiavone, M. Dal Monte, and S. Capaccioli. "Coenzyme Q10 protects retinal cells from apoptosis induced by radiation in vitro and in vivo." *J Radiat Res*. 2012;53(5):695-703.

Magalie L., S.H. Ahmed L. Cantin, and F. Serre. 2007. "Intense Sweetness Surpasses Cocaine Reward" Published: August 01, 2007 DOI: 10.1371/journal.pone.0000698

McLean, L. 2011. *The Force: Living Safely in a World of Electromagnetic Pollution.* Victoria, Australia: Scribe Publisher's.

Mimers, Brunn. 2004. *Black on White: Voices and Witnesses about Electro-Hypersensitivity. The Swedish Experience.* Sweden: GranLund.

Mindell, E., and H. Mundis. 2004. *Earl Mindell's New Vitamin Bible.* New York: Warner Books.

Murray, M. 2003. *How To Prevent and Treat Diabetes with Natural Medicine.* New York: Riverhead Books.

Murray, M., J. Pizzorno, and L. Pizzorno. 2005. *The Encyclopedia of Healing Foods.* New York: Atria Books.

Northrup, C. 2012. *The Wisdom of Menopause-Creating Physical and Emotional Health during the Change.* New York: Bantam Books.

Ober, C., S.T. Sinatra, and M. Zucker. 2010. *Earthing: the Most Important Discovery Ever?* Laguna Beach, CA: Basic Health Publications.

Parvanch, K. et al., 2014. "Effect of probiotics supplementation on bone mineral content and bone mass density." *The Scientific World Journal*, Vol. 0214 (2014), Article ID 595962.

Perlmutter, D. 2013. "*Grain Brain: the Surprising Truth about Wheat, Carbs, and Sugar-Your Brains Silent Killers.*" New York: Little, Brown and Company.

Pick, M. 2011. *Are You Tired and Wired: Your Proven 30-Day Program for Overcoming Adrenal Fatigue and Feeling Fantastic Again.* New York: Hay House, Inc.

Pitchford, P. 2002. *Healing with Whole Foods: Asian Traditions and Modern Nutrition.* Berkeley: North Atlantic Books.

Pizzorno, J., M. Murray, and H. Joiner-Bey. 2008. *The Clinicians Handbook of Natural Medicine.* $2^{nd}$ ed. St. Louis: Churchill Livingstone Elsevier.

Pollan, M. 2009. *Omnivore's Dilemma: The Secret Behind What You Eat.* New York: Dial Books.

Price, W. A. 1945. *Nutrition and Physical Degeneration*. La Mesa CA: Price Pottenger Nutrition Foundation.

Q. Yang, Z. Zhang, E. Gregg, D.Flanders, R. Merritt, F. Hu. 2014. "Added Sugar Intake and Cardiovascular Diseases Mortality Among U.S. Adults." *JAMA Intern Med.* 2014;174(4):516-524. doi:10.1001/jamainternmed.2013.13563.

Qu, J, Y.Kaufman, and I.Washington "Coenzyme Q10 in the human retina." *Invest Ophthalmol Vis Sci.* 2009;50(4):1814-8.

Quinn, N. and J. Glaspey. 2012. *The Complete Idiot's Guide to Eating Paleo*. New York: Penguin Group.

Rector-Page, Linda. 1990. *Healthy Healing: An Alternative Healing Reference. 8th ed*. CA: Linda Rector Page.

Rigden, S. 2009. *The Ultimate Metabolism Diet: Eat Right for Your Metabolic Type*. Alameda, CA: Hunter House Inc., Publishers.

Rudolph, D. 2010. "PQQ - An Essential Micronutrient That Helps You Thrive". http://www.vegsource.com/pahy/pqq---an-essential-micronutrient-that-helps-you-thrive.html.(Accessed April 2014)

Santillo, Humbart. 1987. *Natural Healing with Herbs*. Prescott Valley, AZ: Hohm Press

Schmid, R. F. 1997. *Traditional Foods Are Your Best Medicine: Improving Health and Longevity with Native Nutrition*. Rochester, VT: Healing Arts Press.

Scholtz-Ahrens, K et al., 2007. "Prebiotics, probiotics and synbiotics affect mineral absorption, bone mineral content and bone structure". *J Nutr.* Vol 137, no 3 838S-846S, March 2007.

Scott, T. 2011. *The Anti-Anxiety Food Solution*. Oakland: New Harbinger Press.

Sears, A. 2010. *7 Pillars of Anti-Aging*. Royal Palm Beach: Wellness Research & Consulting

Sears, A. 2012. *12 Natural Ways to Stimulate Your Cells to Grow Younger*. Royal Palm Beach: Wellness Research & Consulting.

Sears, A. "Cell Secrets to Keep Doing What You Love-Telemere/Citruline." 2014. http://www.alsearsmd.com/2014/03/cell-secret-to-keep-doing-what-you-love/Telomerase-

Selye, H. 1956. *The Stress of Life*. New York: McGraw-Hill.

Shames, R., and K. Shames. 2002. *Thyroid Power: 10 Steps to Total Health*. New York: Harper Collins Publishers Inc.

Shoman, M. *2009. The Menopause Thyroid Solution: Overcome Menopause by Solving Your Hidden Thyroid Problems.* New York: Harper Collins Publishers Inc.

Shoman, M.J. 2006. *The Thyroid Hormone Breakthrough*. New York: HarperCollins Publishers, Inc.

Simopoulos, A. P. 2002. "The importance of the ratio of omega-6/omega-3 essential fatty acids." *Biomedicine and Pharmacotherapy* 56 (8):365-79.

Sinatra, S. 2014. "Saturated Fats Can Be Part of Heart-Healthy Diet." http://www.drsinatra.com/new-research-confirms-saturated-fats-are-not-the-villain. (Accessed 4/08/2014).

Stanway, P. 2010. *The Miracle of Apple Cider: Practical Tips for Health, Home, and Beauty*. London: Watkins Publishing.

Sundaram, H. 2003. *Face Value: the Truth about Beauty-and a Guilt-free Guide to Finding it*. New York: Rodale.

Tannis, A. 2009. *Feed Your Skin Starve Your Wrinkles*. Beverly, MA: Fair Winds Press.

Tsivgoulis, G, et al. 2013. "Adherence to a Mediterranean diet and risk of incident cognitive impairment." Neurology, 80(18), 1684-1692. URL: http://www.neurology.org/content/80/18/1684.abstract.

University of Delaware. April 4, 2012. "Soy and Menopause: Large-scale study finds soy may alleviate hot flashes in menopause." http://www.udel.edu/udaily/2012/apr/melby-soy-menopause-040412.html

Wahlqvist, M.L. *et al.* 1994. *Food Habits in Later Life: A Cross Cultural Study*. Tokyo: United Nations University Press.

Watson, B. 2008. *The Detox Strategy: Vibrant Health in 5 Easy Steps*. New York: Free Press.

Weed, S.S. 2002, *New Menopausal Years* the *Wise Woman Way.* Woodstock, N.Y.: Ash Tree Publishing

Wei. J. and S. Levkoff. 2000. *Aging Well: The Complete Guide to Physical and Emotional Health.* New York: John Wiley & Sons, Inc.

Weil, A. 2002. *Self-Healing Strategies- Simple Measures for Protecting Your Health, Staying Well and Living Longer.* Boulder: Sounds True Publishing.

Wilcox B. J., D. C. Wilcox and M. Suzuki 2001. *The Okinawa Program: How the World's Longest Lived People Achieve Everlasting Health and How You Can Too.* New York: Clarkson Potter Publishers.

Wilcox, B. and C. Wilcox, 2004. *The Okinowa Diet Plan. Get Leaner, Live Longer, and Never Feel Hungry.* New York: Clarkson N. Potter.

Wilcox, D.C., B. Wilcox, H.Todoriki, M. Suzki. 2009. "The Okinawan Diet: Health Implications of a Low-Calorie, Nutrient-Dense, Antioxidant-Rich *Dietary Pattern, Low in Gycemic Load.*" *Journal of the American College of Nutrition.* 28 (4) 500-516.

Williams, R. 2004. *Psych K: The Missing Piece (Peace) in Your Life.* $2^{nd}$ ed. Crestone CO: Myrddin Publication.

Williams, R.J. 1956. *Biochemical Individuality.* New Canaan, CT: Keats Publishing.

Wolfe, D. 2009. *SuperFoods: The Food and Medicine of the Future.* Berkeley: North Atlantic Books.

Wood, J.M., H. Decker, H. Hartmann, B. Chavan, H. Rokos, J.D. Spencer... and K. Schallreuter. June 2009. *"Senile hair graying: $H_2O_2$-mediated oxidative stress affects human hair color by blunting methionine sulfoxide repair."* The FASEB Journal 23 (7): 2065-2075.

Woodland Publishing Editors. 2009. *20 Essential Supplements. Revised and Updated.* Salt Lake City: Woodland Publishing.

Wright, H. 2013. *The Pre-diabetes Plan.* Berkeley: Ten Speed Press.

Wurtman, J. and N. Frusztajer. 2006. *The Serotonin Power Diet: Boost Serotonin to Switch off Your Appetite and Turn on a Good Mood.* New York: Rodale Books.

www.diet.com/dietblogs/print_blog.php?blid=15478

www.optimumchoices.com/Traditional_Diets.html

## About The Author

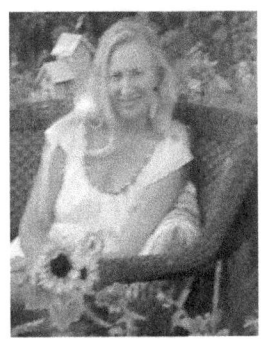 From her earliest memories, Linda has always had an interest in health. At the young age of 7 years old, Linda could be seen sprinkling wheat germ on her breakfast cereal every morning because the T.V. commercials stated that it was good for you! Throughout her life, Linda has enjoyed great energy and robust health, and attributes it to lifelong healthful eating, and a healthy lifestyle. In 2004, at the ripe old age of 44, Linda was able to effortlessly conceive and give birth to a healthy baby boy. At 51 years old, still experiencing youthfulness and vigor, Linda made a decision to use her extensive health knowledge and experience to obtain a nutrition consultant certificate from Bauman College in Berkeley, California. After graduating with honors in 2012, she then began a private practice in holistic nutrition consulting. She is also registered as a professional member of the *National Association of Nutrition Professionals*. Linda is passionate about inspiring and helping individuals to maintain or restore their vitality and wellbeing at any age.

Linda can be contacted concerning any questions or personal health issues related to the book. She offers half-hour and one hour consultations by phone for this purpose.

She also is available for ongoing nutrition consultations. Please refer to her website: vibranthealthconsulting.com for more information.

www.ingramcontent.com/pod-product-compliance
Lightning Source LLC
Chambersburg PA
CBHW081439070526
44586CB00019B/2177